PUBLIC HEALTH IN SUB-SAHARAN AFRICA

This fascinating collection shines a social epidemiological spotlight on the key public health issues affecting sub-Saharan Africa today.

Beginning with the legacy of colonial rule, this book outlines the complex interplay between population health and a range of social, economic, and cultural factors. It shows how social epidemiological methods can offer a deeper understanding of population health and features chapters on a range of infectious diseases that continue to have a devastating impact on the region, including Sickle Cell Disease, HIV/AIDS, Leprosy, and Ebola. The final section of this book includes a series of case studies in which social epidemiological methods have been used to explore specific public health issues.

Providing a timely overview of the relationship between social systems and human biology in the region, this important book will interest students and researchers across Public Health, Medicine, and African Studies.

John Fulton is Emeritus Professor of Social Inclusion at the University of Sunderland, which reflects his interest in social inequalities and their reproduction in education and health. He has been involved in a number of social epidemiology studies in Sub-Saharan Africa.

Philip Emeka Anyanwu is a reader in Public Health at Warwick Medical School (WMS), University of Warwick. He is an epidemiologist with research and teaching interests in infectious disease epidemiology, social epidemiology, global health, and digital health.

Catherine Hayes is Professor of Health Professions Pedagogy and Scholarship at the University of Sunderland, UK. She is Programme Leader for the

Professional Doctorate at Sunderland Campus and works predominantly with doctoral candidates undertaking PhDs, DBA, EdD, and DProf as well as those seeking to claim accreditation for doctorates by Existing Published Works and Higher Doctorates within postgraduate study.

Jonathan Ling is a former professor of Public Health at the University of Sunderland. He has a background in psychology and was the associate director for FUSE – The Centre for Translational Research in Public Health.

PUBLIC HEALTH IN SUB-SAHARAN AFRICA

Social Epidemiological Perspectives

Edited by John Fulton, Philip Emeka Anyanwu, Catherine Hayes and Jonathan Ling

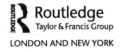

Routledge
Taylor & Francis Group

LONDON AND NEW YORK

Cover image credit line – Getty images, 1257717129

First published 2025
by Routledge
4 Park Square, Milton Park, Abingdon, Oxon OX14 4RN

and by Routledge
605 Third Avenue, New York, NY 10158

Routledge is an imprint of the Taylor & Francis Group, an informa business

© 2025 selection and editorial matter, John Fulton, Philip Emeka Anwanyu,
Jonathan Ling and Catherine Hayes individual chapters, the contributors

The right of John Fulton, Philip Emeka Anwanyu, Jonathan Ling and Catherine Hayes
to be identified as the authors of the editorial material, and of the authors for their
individual chapters, has been asserted in accordance with sections 77 and 78 of the
Copyright, Designs and Patents Act 1988.

All rights reserved. No part of this book may be reprinted or reproduced or utilised
in any form or by any electronic, mechanical, or other means, now known or
hereafter invented, including photocopying and recording, or in any information
storage or retrieval system, without permission in writing from the publishers.

Trademark notice: Product or corporate names may be trademarks or registered
trademarks, and are used only for identification and explanation without intent
to infringe.

British Library Cataloguing-in-Publication Data
A catalogue record for this book is available from the British Library

Library of Congress Cataloging-in-Publication Data
Names: Fulton, John, 1953– editor.
Title: Public health in sub-Saharan Africa : social epidemiological
perspectives / edited by John Fulton, Philip Anyanwu, Catherine Hayes,
and Jonathan L. Ling.
Description: Abingdon, Oxon ; New York, NY : Routledge, 2025. |
Includes bibliographical references and index.
Identifiers: LCCN 2024030577 (print) | LCCN 2024030578 (ebook) |
ISBN 9781032741109 (hardback) | ISBN 9781032171135 (paperback) |
ISBN 9781003467601 (ebook)
Subjects: LCSH: Epidemiology—Social aspects—Africa, Sub-Saharan. |
Public health—Social aspects—Africa, Sub-Saharan.
Classification: LCC RA650.8.A357 P83 2025 (print) | LCC
RA650.8.A357 (ebook) | DDC 362.10967—dc23/eng/20240711
LC record available at https://lccn.loc.gov/2024030577
LC ebook record available at https://lccn.loc.gov/2024030578

ISBN: 978-1-032-74110-9 (hbk)
ISBN: 978-1-032-17113-5 (pbk)
ISBN: 978-1-003-46760-1 (ebk)

DOI: 10.4324/9781003467601

Typeset in Times New Roman
by codeMantra

We dedicate this book to the students from Africa we have had the heartfelt privilege of working with and alongside over the last three decades.

We hope it can contribute to the ongoing agenda of the Africanisation of research, which acknowledges the shift in mindset needed in the recognition of new indigenous knowledge and the critical reflection on the past injustice of encroaching into this fundamentally unique research space, by the Western world.

We are hopeful that it is representative of our collaborative knowledge creation, which reflects the deep mutual respect of the contemporary cultures, praxes, and human relationships we share and value.

John Fulton
Philip Emeka Anwanyu
Jonathan Ling
Catherine Hayes
May 2024

CONTENTS

EDITORS

Professor John Fulton is Emeritus Professor of Social Inclusion at the University of Sunderland, which reflects his interest in social inequalities and their reproduction in education and health. He carried out a study on amateur and professional boxing and the ways in which boxing interacted with other aspects of the boxer's lives. He has been involved in a number of social epidemiology studies in Sub-Saharan Africa. John's background is in mental health and nurse education; before taking up his present position, he was Programme Leader for MSc Public Health. He is a principal fellow of the HEA. John is also interested in the development of practice and the approaches to researching practice and practice development. Since its inception, he has been involved with the University's Professional Doctorate Scheme in both teaching and supervision of this programme. A particular interest is in the ways in which appropriate methodologies can be developed to support and illuminate practice.

Dr Philip Emeka Anyanwu is a reader in Public Health at Warwick Medical School (WMS), University of Warwick. He is an epidemiologist with research and teaching interests in infectious disease epidemiology, social epidemiology, global health, and digital health. His research involves using population-level healthcare and routinely collected big data. He has experience leading and delivering research projects evaluating the mechanisms of the impact of policies/ interventions on antimicrobial stewardship, smoking in adults and children, COVID-19, and the inequalities therein. His scholarship activities include knowledge exchange on evidence-based pedagogic practices in higher education in low- and middle-income countries. He is a senior fellow of the Advanced Higher Education UK. He has previously held academic posts at the Universities of Sunderland, Suffolk, and Glasgow, Imperial College London, and Cardiff University.

Professor Catherine Hayes is Professor of Health Professions Pedagogy and Scholarship at the University of Sunderland, UK. She is Programme Leader for the Professional Doctorate at Sunderland Campus and works predominantly with doctoral candidates undertaking PhDs, DBA, EdD, and DProf as well as those seeking to claim accreditation for doctorates by Existing Published Works and Higher Doctorates within postgraduate study. Professor Hayes originally qualified in Podiatric Medicine in 1992, later becoming a founding fellow of the Faculty of Podiatric Medicine at the Royal College of Physicians and Surgeons (Glasgow) in 2012 after being awarded a fellowship in Podiatric Medicine in 2010 by the Royal Society of Chiropodists and Podiatrists (London). Having worked within Higher Education as an academic for over 25 years and with almost 400 peer-reviewed publications, Professor Hayes has also gained national recognition as a UK National teaching fellow and principal of the HE Advance (formerly the UK Higher Education Academy).

Dr Jonathan Ling is a former professor of Public Health at the University of Sunderland. He has a background in psychology and was the associate director for FUSE – The Centre for Translational Research in Public Health. He is interested in applying mixed methods to the study of a range of Public Health Issues, including alcohol use and the effects of ageing on health. Jonathan is now an independent researcher.

CONTRIBUTORS

Professor Ayo Adebowale is Faculty of Public Health, College of Medicine, University of Ibadan, Nigeria

Professor Vincent Adzahlie-Mensah is a professor of social justice and security education at the University of Education in Winneba, Ghana. He is a development researcher and strategy consultant. He is currently the principal of SDA, College of Education, Asokore-Koforidua, Ghana.

Dr Erhauyi Meshach Aiwerioghene is a senior lecturer in Health Care Management in the School of Health and Social Care, Swansea University, UK.

Benjamin Maduabuchi Aniugbo is a registered nurse, currently working as a clinical nurse manager 2, with the Health Service Executive's Department of Public Health, Dublin and Midlands Region, Ireland.

Dr Adilson José de Pina is Head of Malaria Elimination, CCS-SIDA/Ministry of Health, Cabo Verde.

Dr Judith Eberhardt is Associate Professor of Psychology at Teesside University, a chartered psychologist, and an associate fellow of the British Psychological Society.

Dr Adeniyi Francis Fagbamigbe is a senior lecturer in the Faculty of Public Health, College of Medicine, University of Ibadan, Nigeria.

Dr Ahmed Ali Hassan has been working as a medical doctor and researcher in Sudan and the UAE since 2004. He has managed several research projects. Currently, Dr. Ahmed is an independent researcher.

Dr Chinyere Ihejieto is a nursing lecturer at Leeds Beckett University, School of Health, City Campus, Leeds.

Dr Candidus Nwakasi is an assistant professor, Human Development and Family Sciences, and Affiliate Faculty, Africana Studies Institute, University of Connecticut, USA.

Dr Ade Ojelabi is a researcher and director of the Industrial Training Coordinating Centre, University of Ibadan, Ibadan Nigeria.

Dr Cynthia Okpokiri is a social work lecturer at the University of East Anglia. She provides independent, research-informed expertise in social work with people of the Global South and child welfare and protection to local authorities' social services and non-statutory organisations in UK and African countries.

David Olawade is Senior Research and Innovation Project Facilitator (Medway NHS Foundation Trust) and Public Health Lecturer (University of East London).

Florence Oseji is an optometrist working in Logos, Nigeria.

Dr Vivian Osuchukwu is a senior lecturer in the School of Health and Social Care, Swansea University, UK.

Dr Joseph Sunday is a senior lecturer in Public Health, University of South Wales.

Kareem Olusegun Thompson is a PhD student at the University of Sunderland.

Dr Jennifer Tyndall is an associate professor, Department of Public Health, American University of Nigeria.

PART 1

Exploring the Intersections of Health, History, and Methodology

Perspectives on Social Epidemiology in Africa

1

EXPLORING THE CURRENT TRENDS IN SOCIAL EPIDEMIOLOGY IN SUB-SAHARAN AFRICA

David B. Olawade

Introduction

Social epidemiology is a multidisciplinary field that has emerged at the intersection of epidemiology and the social sciences. A branch of public health and a sub-field of epidemiology, it examines the impacts of social, economic, and environmental determinants on health outcomes and disease prevalence within populations (PAHO, 2002; Honjo, 2004) to understand how social organization affects the distribution of health and diseases (Krieger, 2001). With the ever-evolving dynamics of societies and the increasing recognition of social determinants of health, social epidemiology has become key to understanding and addressing health disparities (Roux, 2022). Social epidemiology is distinguished from other fields by its insistence on focusing on the relationships between social determinants of health, such as socioeconomic status, education, employment, social support, and health outcomes (Krieger, 2001; Kawachi, 2002). Social epidemiology serves as a vital link between public health research and the formation of public policy (Roux, 2022). It informs activities and policies intended to advance health equity by providing insights into the structural and social factors that contribute to health disparities and recognizing that health disparities are not solely due to individual behaviors or genetic factors but are strongly influenced by the social context in which individuals live (Braveman and Gottlieb, 2014).

The origins of social epidemiology can be traced back to the mid-20th century, with an increasing acknowledgement that health inequalities could not be fully accounted for by individual behaviors or genetic determinants (Krieger, 2001; Honjo, 2004). Thomas McKeown, a Scottish physician who analyzed

DOI: 10.4324/9781003467601-2

mortality data for England and Wales from the mid-19th century, was one of the first to challenge the dominant notion that the drop in infectious diseases and mortality was primarily attributed to medical interventions and improvements in healthcare systems (McKeown, Record and Turner, 1975). According to McKeown, sociological changes, including improved nutrition, housing, and living conditions (such as sanitation and clean water), have a greater influence on health improvements than medical interventions (McKeown, Record and Turner, 1975).

During the 1960s and 1970s, other notable scholars such as Geoffery Rose and Sir Richard Doll in the United Kingdom, together with Richard Wilkinson in the United States, made significant contributions to the advancement of knowledge regarding the social determinants of health (Rose, 2001; Marmot and Wilkinson, 2005). Rose's concept of the "prevention paradox" argued that prioritizing the prevention of a substantial number of illnesses could yield more effectiveness than focusing solely on treating a few people at high risk (Rose, 2001). This notion underscores the significance of acknowledging and addressing the socioeconomic determinants that impact the population. Social determinants of health, as defined by the World Health Organization (WHO), are "non-medical factors that influence health outcomes; they are conditions in which people are born, grow, live, and age" (CSDH, 2008).

Moreover, health disparities take into account the relationship between social inequalities resulting from sociodemographic characteristics as well as the relationship between health and these inequalities (Bharmal et al., 2015). By identifying the root causes of health disparities and analyzing their intricate interactions, social epidemiology plays a pivotal role in public health efforts to improve overall health and well-being while addressing disparities within populations (Braveman and Gottlieb, 2014; Bradley et al., 2016; WHO, 2018). Social epidemiology is changing and broadening its scope to address new issues in our increasingly complex and interconnected society, including the impacts of urbanization, globalization, and digital technology on health (Huynen, Martens and Hilderink, 2005; Labonté and Schrecker, 2007; Eckmanns, Füller and Roberts, 2019).

At the global level, environmental degradation poses significant health risks, with poorer countries bearing the brunt of environmental pollution (Birn, Pillay and Holtz, 2009). The political landscape in many countries can also have detrimental effects on population health, particularly in regions torn by civil conflict or war with neighboring countries, impacting both military personnel and civilians (Birn, Pillay and Holtz, 2009). The post-colonial legacy continues to shape the health outcomes of many African countries, characterized by insufficient infrastructure and ongoing economic exploitation even after the departure of colonizers. While some nations, such as Botswana, have managed to develop robust health infrastructures despite these challenges (Azevedo, 2017), many others struggle due to limited capital and resources.

Cultural factors, including religious beliefs, play a significant role in shaping health outcomes, although it is essential to avoid oversimplification and recognize the broader socio-political context (Said, 1978). The education of women emerges as a crucial determinant of both economic growth and child health outcomes (Oztunc, 2015; Rodriguez, 2015), highlighting the interconnectedness of social and health factors. Post-colonial legacies have often marginalized indigenous medical practices, which encompass not only physical but also social and spiritual dimensions (Moïsi, Madhi and Rees, 2019). Additionally, Harris (2023) discusses the discounting of treatments from the Global South in the so-called developed world, despite their effectiveness and affordability, reflecting broader issues of inequity and power dynamics in global health discourse.

Addressing the multifaceted determinants of health in Sub-Saharan Africa requires a comprehensive understanding of environmental, political, socio-economic, and cultural factors. Efforts to improve health outcomes must be contextually sensitive, acknowledging historical legacies and power imbalances while promoting equity, inclusivity, and collaboration on a global scale. By adjusting to these emerging trends, social epidemiology continues to be an important topic in the global effort to improve health outcomes and lessen health disparities. This chapter aims to explore the current trends in social epidemiology and emphasize the urgent need for concerted efforts in this field, particularly in Sub-Saharan Africa.

Current Trends in Social Epidemiology

Current trends in social epidemiology in Sub-Saharan Africa are characterized by a growing recognition of the complex interplay between social determinants and health outcomes in the region. Researchers are increasingly exploring the intersectionality of social factors, acknowledging the unique challenges faced by various population subgroups based on factors such as gender, ethnicity, socio-economic status, and geographic location. Additionally, there is a heightened focus on understanding the impact of structural factors such as poverty, inequality, and discrimination on health disparities within the region. The role of social networks and community dynamics in shaping health outcomes is also receiving attention, with efforts aimed at leveraging social capital to improve health outcomes and promote community resilience. Furthermore, there is an emerging emphasis on the importance of addressing mental health disparities and integrating mental health services into broader public health initiatives. These trends, as discussed below, reflect a growing commitment to advancing social epidemiology research in Sub-Saharan Africa to inform evidence-based interventions and policies aimed at reducing health inequities and improving population health outcomes.

Intersectionality

Intersectionality in social epidemiology in Sub-Saharan Africa represents a critical lens through which researchers examine the compounding effects of multiple social disadvantages on health outcomes within the region. Recent trends in social epidemiology underscore the importance of recognizing that individuals in Sub-Saharan Africa can experience intersecting forms of disadvantage simultaneously, shaping their lived experiences and health trajectories (Harari and Lee, 2021). Originating from the work of Kimberlé Crenshaw in 1989, intersectionality has since become a fundamental framework for understanding the complexities of social identities and inequalities (Crenshaw, 1989). It acknowledges that factors such as gender, race, ethnicity, class, and other social constructs are intertwined and intersect to create unique experiences of privilege or discrimination (McCall, 2005; Bauer, 2014). At the individual level, intersectionality highlights how these intersecting identities influence access to resources, opportunities, and healthcare services, ultimately shaping health outcomes. Moreover, at the structural level, intersectionality elucidates the intricate interactions of various systems of power, privilege, and oppression that contribute to health disparities. This framework recognizes that the intersection of multiple social disadvantages can exacerbate health inequities, with marginalized populations facing heightened vulnerabilities and barriers to accessing quality healthcare and achieving optimal health outcomes.

In Sub-Saharan Africa, where a diverse range of social, cultural, and economic factors intersect, understanding intersectionality is paramount for developing effective interventions that address the unique challenges faced by different population subgroups. For example, research has shown that women in rural areas may experience intersecting forms of disadvantage related to gender, socioeconomic status, and geographic location, leading to disparities in maternal and child health outcomes (Bharmal et al., 2015). Similarly, ethnic minorities may face intersecting barriers related to discrimination, language barriers, and limited access to healthcare services, exacerbating health disparities within these communities. By adopting an intersectional approach, researchers can uncover the complex interplay of social determinants and identify the root causes of health inequities, informing targeted interventions and policies that address the specific needs of diverse population subgroups.

Furthermore, intersectionality in social epidemiology emphasizes the importance of considering the intersecting effects of social disadvantages on health outcomes. Factors such as race, gender, ethnicity, and class intersect to shape health trajectories, with individuals experiencing compounded disadvantages that contribute to disparities in health outcomes (Roux, 2022). For example, research has shown that individuals from marginalized racial and ethnic groups may face higher rates of chronic diseases such as diabetes, hypertension, and cardiovascular disease due to intersecting factors such as limited access to healthcare, socioeconomic disadvantage, and environmental exposures. By understanding these intersections, researchers can develop interventions that address the underlying structural determinants of health inequities and promote health equity within Sub-Saharan Africa.

In summary, intersectionality in social epidemiology provides a comprehensive framework for understanding the intersecting forms of disadvantage that shape health outcomes in Sub-Saharan Africa. By acknowledging the complex interplay of social factors such as race, gender, ethnicity, and class, researchers can develop targeted interventions that address the unique challenges faced by different population subgroups, ultimately advancing efforts to reduce health inequities and promote health equity within the region.

Social Networks and Health

Social networks play a vital role in shaping health outcomes across Sub-Saharan Africa, with recent studies highlighting their multifaceted impact on individual well-being and community resilience (Martire and Franks, 2014; Zhang and Centola, 2019). In this region, characterized by diverse cultural contexts and socio-economic disparities, social networks serve as crucial conduits of social support, social capital, and social cohesion, all of which are fundamental for maintaining and improving health. Social cohesion, for instance, reflects the quality of interpersonal relationships within communities, encompassing aspects such as trust, solidarity, and a sense of belonging (Kawachi and Berkman, 2014). Such cohesive social structures foster a supportive environment where individuals can access resources and support from their peers, thus enhancing their ability to cope with stressors and navigate health challenges effectively (Okafor and Rihan, 2023).

Central to the concept of social cohesion is the notion of social capital, which refers to the collective resources embedded within social networks that individuals can access for mutual benefit (Kawachi and Berkman, 2014). These resources may include tangible forms of assistance, such as financial support or access to healthcare, as well as intangible benefits like emotional support and guidance (Berkman and Glass, 2000). In Sub-Saharan Africa, where formal support systems may be limited, social networks serve as critical sources of social capital, particularly in rural and underserved communities. Individuals rely on these networks not only for material aid but also for emotional sustenance and a sense of community belonging, which are essential for maintaining mental and emotional well-being (Christian et al., 2020).

Moreover, research indicates that robust social networks can act as protective factors against various diseases, particularly non-communicable diseases (NCDs; Christian et al., 2020). Individuals with strong social ties are more likely to engage in health-promoting behaviors, seek timely medical care, and adhere to treatment regimens, thereby reducing their risk of chronic conditions such as hypertension, diabetes, and cardiovascular disease. Conversely, social isolation and a lack of social connections have been linked to adverse health outcomes, including increased mortality rates and poorer mental health (Holt-Lunstad, 2021). In Sub-Saharan Africa, where social bonds are deeply ingrained in cultural norms and traditions, efforts to strengthen social networks and foster community resilience have the potential to yield significant improvements in population health.

Exploring the dynamics of social networks in Sub-Saharan Africa can inform targeted interventions aimed at bolstering social support systems and enhancing community well-being. Strategies may include the promotion of community-based support groups, the facilitation of social gatherings and community events, and the implementation of peer support programs for vulnerable populations. By harnessing the power of social networks, public health initiatives can leverage existing resources and social capital to address health disparities, improve health outcomes, and promote equitable access to healthcare services across Sub-Saharan Africa.

Structural Racism and Discrimination

The impact of structural racism and discrimination on health outcomes has garnered significant attention within the field of social epidemiology, particularly in the context of Sub-Saharan Africa. Structural racism refers to the normalization and justification of a variety of dynamics, encompassing historical, cultural, institutional, and interpersonal dimensions (Churchwell et al., 2020). This recognition underscores the multifaceted nature of racism and its pervasive influence across different socio-ecological levels, including individual, community, and societal levels (Gee and Ford, 2011).

In Sub-Saharan Africa, structural racism manifests in various forms, perpetuating health disparities and inequities. Historical legacies of colonialism and imperialism have left enduring impacts on social, economic, and political structures, shaping contemporary patterns of discrimination and inequality. Moreover, the legacy of slavery and the transatlantic slave trade has left lasting scars on the collective psyche of African societies, contributing to entrenched systems of racial hierarchy and marginalization.

Subtle and overt forms of discrimination further exacerbate health disparities within the region. Racial profiling, unequal access to healthcare services, and disparities in educational and employment opportunities are just a few examples of systemic injustices faced by marginalized communities in Sub-Saharan Africa (Williams and Mohammed, 2009). Discriminatory practices within healthcare systems, such as differential treatment based on race or ethnicity, can result in delayed diagnoses, inadequate treatment, and poorer health outcomes for racial and ethnic minorities.

Moreover, structural racism intersects with other forms of social disadvantage, such as poverty, gender inequality, and geographic marginalization, creating intersecting systems of oppression that compound health inequities. For example, women from marginalized racial or ethnic groups may face intersecting forms of discrimination based on both race and gender, resulting in unique health challenges and barriers to accessing healthcare services.

Recognizing and addressing structural racism are essential steps toward achieving health equity in Sub-Saharan Africa. Efforts to dismantle systemic barriers and promote social justice must encompass policy reforms, institutional changes, and community empowerment initiatives. Interventions aimed at reducing health disparities should adopt an intersectional approach, taking into account the intersecting forms of disadvantage faced by marginalized populations.

Furthermore, fostering anti-racist attitudes and promoting cultural competence within healthcare systems are crucial for ensuring equitable access to healthcare services and improving health outcomes for all individuals. By confronting the root causes of structural racism and discrimination, Sub-Saharan Africa can move closer toward realizing the goal of health equity and creating a more just and inclusive society for future generations.

Neighborhood and Built Environment

The characteristics of neighborhoods and built environments wield significant influence over health outcomes within Sub-Saharan Africa, underscoring the pivotal role of environmental factors in shaping population health. Access to essential resources such as healthy food, green spaces, safe housing, and reliable transportation infrastructure profoundly impacts the well-being of individuals and communities alike (Duncan, Kawachi and Diez Roux, 2018). However, disparities in access to these resources are often stark, with marginalized populations facing greater challenges in accessing the elements necessary for a healthy lifestyle. For instance, urban areas may be characterized by food deserts, where access to affordable, nutritious food is limited, exacerbating malnutrition and diet-related illnesses among vulnerable populations. Similarly, inadequate housing conditions, such as overcrowding and a lack of sanitation facilities, contribute to the spread of infectious diseases and undermine overall health outcomes.

Moreover, geographically specific environmental factors may reinforce existing socioeconomic and racial or ethnic disparities, further exacerbating health inequalities within Sub-Saharan Africa (Woolf and Aron, 2013). Neighborhoods with limited access to healthcare facilities and educational opportunities may perpetuate cycles of poverty and ill health, particularly among marginalized communities. Additionally, environmental hazards such as pollution, inadequate sanitation, and unsafe drinking water pose significant health risks, disproportionately affecting residents in low-income and informal settlements.

Understanding the intricate relationship between neighborhoods and health is crucial for guiding urban planning, policy development, and interventions aimed at creating healthy environments in Sub-Saharan Africa. Efforts to improve access to essential resources, enhance housing conditions, and promote sustainable transportation infrastructure can have profound implications for population health and well-being. For example, initiatives to increase the availability of affordable fresh produce through farmers' markets or community gardens can address food insecurity and promote healthy eating habits. Similarly, investments in green spaces and recreational facilities can provide opportunities for physical activity and social interaction, thereby mitigating the risk of chronic diseases and improving mental health outcomes.

Furthermore, addressing the underlying social determinants of health, such as poverty, inequality, and social exclusion, is essential for creating equitable and healthy neighborhoods in Sub-Saharan Africa. By prioritizing investments in infrastructure, education, and social services, policymakers can create environments that support health and foster community resilience. Collaborative approaches that engage local communities, stakeholders, and policymakers are integral to developing sustainable solutions that address the complex challenges facing neighborhoods in Sub-Saharan Africa. Ultimately, building healthy environments requires a multi-sectoral approach that integrates urban planning, public health, and social development efforts to create vibrant, inclusive, and equitable communities for all residents.

The Urgent Need for Action in Sub-Saharan Africa

The urgency for action in Sub-Saharan Africa is paramount as the region grapples with multifaceted challenges that threaten the health and well-being of its populations. Persistent health disparities, exacerbated by factors such as poverty, inadequate healthcare infrastructure, and environmental hazards, continue to plague communities across the region. Addressing these disparities requires concerted efforts from governments, policymakers, healthcare providers, and community stakeholders to implement evidence-based interventions that prioritize health equity and social justice. Urgent action is needed to strengthen healthcare systems, improve access to essential services, and address the root causes of health inequities, including structural racism, discrimination, and socio-economic disparities. Moreover, as the region confronts emerging health threats such as infectious diseases, climate change, and NCDs, proactive measures must be taken to build resilience and enhance preparedness at all levels of society. Collaborative approaches that engage local communities and leverage existing resources are essential for achieving sustainable progress and fostering a healthier future for all in Sub-Saharan Africa. The following points below highlight the urgent need to prioritize social epidemiology in the region.

Health Inequities

Health inequalities represent an urgent and pervasive challenge in Sub-Saharan Africa, where the region grapples with some of the most significant disparities in health outcomes worldwide. Socioeconomic disparities, limited access to education and healthcare, and gender-based inequalities contribute to a disproportionate burden of disease, exacerbating existing health inequities (Deaton and Tortora, 2015). The pervasive presence of poverty, weak health systems, poor governance, and the historical legacy of colonization have all played significant roles in perpetuating health disparities and contributing to poor population health outcomes (Wamai and Shirley, 2022). At the proximal level, high maternal mortality rates serve as a stark reminder of the dire consequences of inadequate access to quality healthcare services for women, highlighting the urgent need for comprehensive maternal health interventions (Wamai and Shirley, 2022). Additionally, mental health illnesses, substance abuse, anxiety, and hopelessness are prevalent in communities characterized by unequal wealth distribution, underscoring the complex interplay between socioeconomic factors and mental health outcomes (Wilkinson and Pickett, 2009).

Addressing health inequalities in Sub-Saharan Africa requires a multifaceted approach that encompasses both structural and proximal determinants of health. By understanding the social determinants of health, interventions can be designed to target the root causes of health inequities effectively. This entails implementing policies and programs that aim to reduce poverty, improve access to education and healthcare, and promote gender equality. Furthermore, tackling health inequalities will necessitate significant reforms in health policies, both at the local and international levels. Unfortunately, progress in policy reforms has been slow, hindering efforts to address health disparities and promote health equity in the region (Wilkinson and Pickett, 2009).

Addressing health inequalities in Sub-Saharan Africa is an urgent imperative that requires comprehensive, coordinated, and sustained action from governments, policymakers, healthcare providers, and civil society organizations. By prioritizing investments in health system strengthening, poverty alleviation, education, and gender equality, the region can work toward achieving equitable health outcomes for all its inhabitants. Moreover, fostering partnerships and collaboration among stakeholders at the local, national, and international levels is essential for driving meaningful change and realizing the vision of a healthier, more equitable future for Sub-Saharan Africa.

Communicable and Non-Communicable Diseases

In Sub-Saharan Africa, the urgent need for action against the dual burden of communicable and NCDs is paramount, given the region's complex socio-economic and health challenges. Social factors such as poverty, limited access to healthcare, and inadequate infrastructure contribute significantly to the spread and impact of both types of diseases (Wamai and Shirley, 2022). Alarmingly, studies have projected substantial increases in both communicable and NCDs by 2030, underscoring the urgent need for proactive intervention efforts (Osetinsky et al., 2019; Wamai and Shirley, 2022).

The region's vulnerability to the spread of infectious diseases is compounded by factors such as poor outbreak response, inadequate risk assessment, and low financial resources (Paintsil, 2020). In fact, infectious diseases account for a staggering 50% of deaths in Africa, highlighting the devastating toll of these diseases on public health (Fenollar and Mediannikov, 2018). The epidemiology of tuberculosis in Sub-Saharan Africa exemplifies the intersection of social determinants and disease burden, with rapid population growth, poor housing conditions, environmental factors, and financial barriers contributing to the high prevalence and difficulty in accessing appropriate healthcare facilities (Hargreaves et al., 2011).

Meanwhile, the rising prevalence of NCDs in the region is closely associated with poor living standards, illiteracy, and unhealthy behaviors (Yaya et al., 2018). Sedentary lifestyles, alcohol abuse, and unhealthy diets are behavioral factors that contribute significantly to the increasing incidence of cardiovascular diseases and premature mortality (Riley et al., 2017). These trends underscore the urgent need for comprehensive interventions aimed at addressing the social determinants and behavioral risk factors driving the burden of NCDs in Sub-Saharan Africa.

Social epidemiology offers a valuable framework for understanding the social drivers of disease transmission and identifying strategies to prevent and manage both communicable and NCDs in Sub-Saharan Africa. By examining the complex interplay of social, economic, and environmental factors, social epidemiology can inform targeted interventions that address the root causes of health disparities and promote equitable access to healthcare services. Moreover, by integrating social epidemiological approaches into public health policies and programs, policymakers can develop evidence-based strategies that effectively address the dual burden of disease and improve health outcomes for all populations in the region.

Community Engagement and Empowerment

In Sub-Saharan Africa, community engagement and empowerment emerge as urgent imperatives in the realm of public health, underpinned by the recognition within social epidemiology of their pivotal roles in health promotion and disease prevention (Wallerstein, Yen and Syme, 2011). Acknowledging the diverse cultural landscapes, social structures, and contextual nuances across the region, community-based interventions tailored to local contexts hold immense potential for yielding substantial improvements in health outcomes. Community engagement entails active participation and collaboration between community members, stakeholders, and healthcare providers in identifying health priorities, designing interventions, and implementing sustainable solutions. By involving community members in decision-making processes and leveraging local knowledge and resources, interventions can be better aligned with the needs and preferences of the target populations, thereby enhancing their effectiveness and relevance.

Moreover, community empowerment serves as a catalyst for fostering self-determination, resilience, and collective action within communities, thereby enabling them to address health challenges proactively. Empowerment initiatives empower individuals and communities to advocate for their rights, access healthcare services, and implement health-promoting behaviors. By building capacity, enhancing leadership skills, and fostering social cohesion, empowerment initiatives lay the foundation for sustainable improvements in health and well-being.

Furthermore, community engagement and empowerment are essential for overcoming barriers to healthcare access and utilization, particularly in marginalized and underserved communities. By fostering trust, fostering dialogue, and addressing cultural and linguistic barriers, community engagement initiatives can enhance healthcare-seeking behaviors and promote equitable access to services. Additionally, empowering communities to take ownership of their health enables them to address underlying social determinants of health, such as poverty, education, and housing, thereby addressing the root causes of health inequities.

In the context of Sub-Saharan Africa, where healthcare infrastructure may be limited and access to services may be constrained by geographical, economic, and cultural factors, community engagement and empowerment emerge as indispensable strategies for achieving meaningful improvements in health outcomes. By fostering partnerships between communities, governments, civil society organizations, and healthcare providers, stakeholders can leverage collective expertise and resources to address the complex challenges facing the region's health systems. Ultimately, community-driven approaches that prioritize local ownership, cultural relevance, and sustainability are essential for realizing the vision of health equity and social justice in Sub-Saharan Africa.

Policy and Resource Allocation

In Sub-Saharan Africa, urgent action is needed to prioritize policy development and resource allocation strategies informed by evidence from social epidemiology.

By generating robust evidence on the social determinants of health, social epidemiology plays a crucial role in identifying areas where investments are most needed to address health inequities (Whitman et al., 2022). This evidence can inform policy decisions and resource allocation strategies aimed at addressing the root causes of poor health outcomes in the region. For instance, investments in education can empower individuals to make informed health choices, promote healthier lifestyles, and enhance overall well-being. Similarly, poverty reduction initiatives can alleviate economic disparities, improve access to healthcare services, and mitigate the impact of social determinants on health. Moreover, strengthening healthcare infrastructure and social support systems can enhance the resilience of communities and improve health outcomes, particularly among vulnerable populations.

Evidence-based policies grounded in social epidemiology have the potential to contribute to more equitable resource distribution and foster positive health outcomes across Sub-Saharan Africa. By aligning policy priorities with the social determinants of health, policymakers can ensure that limited resources are allocated efficiently and effectively to address the most pressing health needs. Moreover, adopting a holistic approach that integrates health considerations into broader development agendas can yield synergistic benefits and promote sustainable improvements in population health. For example, initiatives that address both health and education simultaneously can yield significant returns on investment by breaking the cycle of poverty and ill health.

However, translating evidence into policy action requires political will, multisectoral collaboration, and sustained advocacy efforts. Policymakers must prioritize investments in data collection, research, and capacity-building to strengthen the evidence base and inform decision-making processes effectively. Furthermore, engaging stakeholders across sectors, including government agencies, civil society organizations, academia, and the private sector, is essential for fostering buy-in and ensuring the successful implementation of evidence-based policies. Overall, policy development and resource allocation informed by evidence from social epidemiology are urgently needed to address health inequities and improve population health in Sub-Saharan Africa.

Strengthening Health Systems

In Sub-Saharan Africa, the urgent need to strengthen health systems underscores the critical role that social epidemiology can play in informing evidence-based interventions aimed at addressing barriers to healthcare access and utilization. By identifying and understanding the social determinants of health-seeking behaviors, social epidemiology can provide valuable insights into the factors that impede individuals' ability to access healthcare services (Wallerstein, Yen and Syme, 2011). Common barriers include financial constraints, geographical distance, cultural beliefs, and a lack of awareness about available services. By addressing these barriers, interventions can be designed to improve health service utilization and promote equitable access to care for all populations.

One key aspect of strengthening health systems in Sub-Saharan Africa involves improving healthcare infrastructure and service delivery mechanisms to ensure that essential services are available and accessible to all (Duncan, Kawachi and Diez Roux, 2018). This may involve expanding the reach of healthcare facilities, particularly in rural and underserved areas, through the construction of new facilities or the implementation of mobile clinics and outreach programs. Additionally, investments in medical equipment, supplies, and trained healthcare personnel are essential for enhancing the quality and efficiency of healthcare delivery.

Moreover, addressing financial barriers to healthcare access is crucial for ensuring equitable access to services. Social epidemiology can help identify populations most at risk of facing financial hardship when seeking care and inform policies aimed at reducing or eliminating user fees, expanding health insurance coverage, and implementing targeted subsidy programs for vulnerable groups. By making healthcare services more affordable and accessible, health systems can better meet the needs of the population and reduce disparities in health outcomes.

Cultural factors also play a significant role in shaping health-seeking behaviors and healthcare utilization patterns. Social epidemiology can help identify cultural beliefs, practices, and norms that influence individuals' attitudes toward healthcare and inform culturally sensitive interventions designed to promote health-seeking behaviors. Engaging community leaders, traditional healers, and local stakeholders in healthcare planning and delivery can help bridge the gap between traditional and modern healthcare systems and improve health service utilization among diverse populations.

Furthermore, strengthening health systems requires a comprehensive approach that addresses not only healthcare delivery but also health workforce capacity, health information systems, finance mechanisms, and governance structures. Social epidemiology can provide valuable insights into the broader social, economic, and political factors that influence health system performance and inform strategies for building resilient and responsive health systems that can effectively address the diverse health needs of populations in Sub-Saharan Africa.

Strengthening health systems in Sub-Saharan Africa is an urgent and imperative need that requires a multidimensional approach informed by social epidemiology. By identifying and addressing social barriers to healthcare access, improving healthcare infrastructure, addressing financial barriers, and promoting culturally sensitive interventions, health systems can be better equipped to meet the needs of diverse populations and promote equitable access to quality healthcare services for all. Collaborative efforts involving governments, policy-makers, healthcare providers, civil society organizations, and local communities are essential for achieving meaningful improvements in health system performance and advancing health equity in the region.

Building Research Capacity

In Sub-Saharan Africa, building research capacity in social epidemiology emerges as an urgent imperative to address the region's unique health challenges and contribute to global knowledge on population health (Petteway et al., 2019). Enhancing research capacity is essential for generating context-specific evidence, fostering local expertise, and informing evidence-based interventions that are tailored to the region's diverse social, economic, and cultural contexts. Investments in research infrastructure are critical for building research capacity in Sub-Saharan Africa (Roux, 2022). This includes establishing and strengthening research institutions, laboratories, and data repositories to support high-quality research initiatives. Additionally, expanding access to research funding and resources can enable researchers to conduct comprehensive studies that address priority health issues and contribute to evidence-based decision-making.

Training programs play a crucial role in developing a skilled workforce capable of conducting rigorous research in social epidemiology. Capacity-building initiatives, such as graduate programs, workshops, and mentorship opportunities, can help cultivate a new generation of researchers equipped with the necessary knowledge and skills to address complex health challenges. Furthermore, fostering interdisciplinary collaborations and partnerships with international institutions can provide valuable opportunities for knowledge exchange, skill transfer, and collaborative research endeavors.

By investing in research capacity-building efforts, Sub-Saharan Africa can strengthen its contribution to global knowledge on social epidemiology while addressing the specific challenges faced by its population. Research findings generated through local studies can inform the development and implementation of targeted interventions that are contextually appropriate and culturally sensitive. Moreover, building research capacity can empower local researchers to take ownership of the research agenda, advocate for evidence-based policies, and drive positive change within their communities. Furthermore, strengthening research capacity in social epidemiology can enhance the region's resilience to health threats, such as infectious diseases, NCDs, and emerging health challenges. By building a robust evidence base and fostering local expertise, Sub-Saharan Africa can better anticipate, monitor, and respond to health crises, ultimately improving population health outcomes and promoting health equity.

Overall, building research capacity in social epidemiology is an urgent need in Sub-Saharan Africa, requiring concerted efforts from governments, policymakers, research institutions, and international partners. Investments in research infrastructure, training programs, and interdisciplinary collaborations are essential for developing a skilled workforce, generating context-specific evidence, and addressing the region's unique health challenges. By strengthening research capacity, Sub-Saharan Africa can harness the power of research to drive positive health outcomes, promote equity, and advance the well-being of its population.

Conclusion

Social epidemiology emerges as a critical framework for understanding and addressing health disparities in Sub-Saharan Africa. By focusing on the social determinants of health, social epidemiology provides valuable insights into the underlying root causes of inequities and guides interventions aimed at promoting health and well-being across diverse populations. The current trends in social epidemiology underscore the importance of adopting a comprehensive approach for tackling health disparities, including addressing intersectionality, understanding social networks, confronting structural racism, and addressing neighborhood factors. As highlighted by the International Monetary Fund, there is an urgent need for governments to prioritize healthcare and education, as these sectors play a crucial role in improving population health outcomes over the long term. Moreover, robust campaigns against diseases that pose significant threats to Sub-Saharan Africa, coupled with efforts to reinforce social safety nets in communities, are imperative for protecting vulnerable populations and fostering resilience. Urgent action is required to prioritize social epidemiology in Sub-Saharan Africa, with investments in research, policy development, and resource allocation strategies that effectively address the social determinants of health. By adopting a holistic and evidence-based approach, Sub-Saharan Africa can make meaningful strides toward achieving health equity and improving the well-being of its population for generations to come.

References

Azevedo, M.J. (2017). The State of Health System(s) in Africa: Challenges and Opportunities. *Historical Perspectives on the State of Health and Health Systems in Africa*, 1–73. https://doi.org/10.1007/978-3-319-32564-4_1.

Bauer, G.R. (2014). Incorporating Intersectionality Theory into Population Health Research Methodology: Challenges and the Potential to Advance Health Equity. *Social Science & Medicine*, 110, pp. 10–17. https://doi.org/10.1016/j.socscimed.2014.03.022.

Berkman, L.F. and Glass, T. (2000). Social Integration, Social Networks, Social Supports and Health. In: L.F. Berkman and I. Kawachi, eds., *Social Epidemiology*. New York: Oxford University Press, pp. 137–173.

Bharmal, N., Derose, K.P., Felician, M.F. and Weden, M.M. (2015). *Understanding the Upstream Social Determinants of Health* [online]. *Rand.org*. Santa Monica, CA: RAND Corporation. Available at: https://www.rand.org/pubs/working_papers/WR1096.html [Accessed 18 August 2023].

Birn, A.-E., Pillay, Y. and Holtz, T.H. (2009). *Textbook of International Health*. New York and Oxford: Oxford University Press.

Bradley, E.H., Canavan, M., Rogan, E., Talbert-Slagle, K., Ndumele, C., Taylor, L. and Curry, L.A. (2016). Variation in Health Outcomes: The Role of Spending on Social Services, Public Health, and Health Care, 2000–09. *Health Affairs*, 35(5), pp. 760–768. https://doi.org/10.1377/hlthaff.2015.0814.

Braveman, P. and Gottlieb, L. (2014). The Social Determinants of Health: It's Time to Consider the Causes of the Causes. *Public Health Reports*, 129(Suppl 2), pp. 19–31. https://doi.org/10.1177/00333549141291s206.

Christian, A.K., Sanuade, O.A., Okyere, M.A. and Adjaye-Gbewonyo, K. (2020). Social Capital Is Associated with Improved Subjective Well-being of Older Adults with Chronic Non-communicable Disease in Six Low- and Middle-Income Countries. *Globalization and Health*, 16(1). https://doi.org/10.1186/s12992-019-0538-y.

Churchwell, K., Elkind, M.S.V., Benjamin, R.M., Carson, A.P., Chang, E.K., Lawrence, W., Mills, A., Odom, T.M., Rodriguez, C.J., Rodriguez, F., Sanchez, E., Sharrief, A.Z., Sims, M. and Williams, O. (2020). Call to Action: Structural Racism as a Fundamental Driver of Health Disparities: A Presidential Advisory from the American Heart Association. *Circulation*, 142(24), pp. e454–e468. https://doi.org/10.1161/cir.0000000000000936.

Crenshaw, K. (1989). Demarginalizing the Intersection of Race and Sex: A Black Feminist Critique of Antidiscrimination Doctrine, Feminist Theory and Antiracist Politics. *University of Chicago Legal Forum* [online], 8, pp. 139–167. Available at: https://chicagounbound.uchicago.edu/uclf/vol1989/iss1/8/ [Accessed 19 August 2023].

CSDH (2008). *Closing the Gap in a Generation: Health Equity through Action on the Social Determinants of Health. Final Report of the Commission on Social Determinants of Health*. Geneva: World Health Organization.

Deaton, A.S. and Tortora, R. (2015). People in Sub-Saharan Africa Rate their Health and Health Care among the Lowest in the World. *Health Affairs*, 34(3), pp. 519–527. https://doi.org/10.1377/hlthaff.2014.0798.

Duncan, D.T., Kawachi, I. and Diez Roux, A.V. eds. (2018). *Neighbourhoods and Health*. 2nd ed. New York: Oxford University Press.

Eckmanns, T., Füller, H. and Roberts, S.L. (2019). Digital Epidemiology and Global Health Security; An Interdisciplinary Conversation. *Life Sciences, Society and Policy*, 15(2), pp. 1–13. https://doi.org/10.1186/s40504-019-0091-8.

Fenollar, F. and Mediannikov, O. (2018). Emerging Infectious Diseases in Africa in the 21st Century. *New Microbes and New Infections*, 26, pp. S10–S18.

Gee, G.C. and Ford, C.L. (2011). Structural Racism and Health Inequities. *Du Bois Review: Social Science Research on Race*, 8(1), pp. 115–132. https://doi.org/10.1017/s1742058x11000130.

Harari, L. and Lee, C. (2021). Intersectionality in Quantitative Health Disparities Research: A Systematic Review of Challenges and Limitations in Empirical Studies. *Social Science & Medicine*, 277, p. 113876. https://doi.org/10.1016/j.socscimed.2021.113876.

Hargreaves, J.R., Boccia, D., Evans, C.A., Adato, M., Petticrew, M. and Porter, J.D. (2011). The Social Determinants of Tuberculosis: From Evidence to Action. *American Journal of Public Health*, 101(4), pp. 654–662.

Harris, M. (2023). *Decolonizing Healthcare Innovation: Low-Cost Solutions from Low-Income Countries.* Taylor & Francis, Oxford, United Kingdom.

Holt-Lunstad, J. (2021). Loneliness and Social Isolation as Risk Factors: The Power of Social Connection in Prevention. *American Journal of Lifestyle Medicine*, 15(5), pp. 567–573. https://doi.org/10.1177/15598276211009454.

Honjo, K. (2004). Social Epidemiology: Definition, History, and Research Examples. *Environmental Health and Preventive Medicine*, 9(5), pp. 193–199. https://doi.org/10.1007/bf02898100.

Huynen, M.M., Martens, P. and Hilderink, H.B. (2005). The Health Impacts of Globalisation: A Conceptual Framework. *Globalization and Health*, 1(1), p. 14. https://doi.org/10.1186/1744-8603-1-14.

Kawachi, I. (2002). Social Epidemiology. *Social Science & Medicine*, 54(12), pp. 1739–1741. https://doi.org/10.1016/s0277-9536(01)00144-7.

Kawachi, I. and Berkman, L.F. (2014). Social Capital, Social Cohesion, and Health. In: *Social Epidemiology.* New York: Oxford University Press, pp. 290–319. https://doi.org/10.1093/med/9780195377903.003.0008.

Krieger, N. (2001). A Glossary for Social Epidemiology. *Journal of Epidemiology & Community Health*, 55(10), pp. 693–700. https://doi.org/10.1136/jech.55.10.693.

Labonté, R. and Schrecker, T. (2007). Globalization and Social Determinants of Health: Introduction and Methodological Background (part 1 of 3). *Globalization and Health*, 3, p. 5. https://doi.org/10.1186/1744-8603-3-5.

Marmot, M. and Wilkinson, R. (2005). *Social Determinants of Health.* 2nd ed. Oxford: Oxford University Press.

Martire, L.M. and Franks, M.M. (2014). The Role of Social Networks in Adult Health: Introduction to the Special Issue. *Health Psychology*, 33(6), pp. 501–504. https://doi.org/10.1037/hea0000103.

McCall, L. (2005). The Complexity of Intersectionality. *Signs*, 30(3), pp. 1771–1800. https://doi.org/10.1086/426800.

McKeown, T., Record, R.G. and Turner, R.D. (1975). An Interpretation of the Decline of Mortality in England and Wales during the Twentieth Century. *Population Studies*, 29(3), pp. 391–422. https://doi.org/10.2307/2173935.

Moïsi, J., Madhi, S.A. and Rees, H. (2019). Vaccinology in Sub-Saharan Africa. *BMJ Global Health*, 4(5), e001363.

Okafor, A.E. and Rihan, J.I. (2023). Influence of Social Capital on the Health of Individuals. *Open Journal of Social Sciences*, 11(4), pp. 107–118. https://doi.org/10.4236/jss.2023.114009.

Osetinsky, B., Hontelez, J.A.C., Lurie, M.N., McGarvey, S.T., Bloomfield, G.S., Pastakia, S.D., Wamai, R., Bärnighausen, T., de Vlas, S.J. and Galárraga, O. (2019). Epidemiological and Health Systems Implications of Evolving HIV and Hypertension in South Africa and Kenya. *Health Affairs*, 38(7), pp. 1173–1181. https://doi.org/10.1377/hlthaff.2018.05287.

Oztunc, H., Oo, Z.C. and Serin, Z.V. (2015). Effects of Female Education on Economic Growth: A Cross Country Empirical. *Educational Sciences: Theory and Practice*, 15(2), pp. 349–357.

Paintsil, E. (2020). COVID-19 Threatens Health Systems in Sub-Saharan Africa: The Eye of the Crocodile. *The Journal of Clinical Investigation*, 130(6), pp. 2741–2744.

Pan American Health Organization (2002). *Introduction to Social Epidemiology.* [online] Paho.org. Available at: https://www3.paho.org/english/sha/be_v23n1-socialepi.htm [Accessed 25 November 2023].

Petteway, R., Mujahid, M., Allen, A. and Morello-Frosch, R. (2019). Towards a People's Social Epidemiology: Envisioning a More Inclusive and Equitable Future for Social Epi Research and Practice in the 21st Century. *International Journal of Environmental Research and Public Health*, 16(20), p. 3983. https://doi.org/10.3390/ijerph16203983.

Riley, L., Gouda, H., Cowan, M. and World Health Organization. Noncommunicable Diseases Progress Monitor, 2017. Available at: http://apps.who.int/iris/bitstream/10665/258940/1/9789241513029-eng.pdf (Accessed 5 April 2024).

Rodríguez, D. C., Shearer, J., Mariano, A. R., Juma, P. A., Dalglish, S. L., & Bennett, S. (2015). Evidence-informed policymaking in practice: country-level examples of use of evidence for iCCM policy. *Health Policy and Planning*, 30(suppl_2), ii36–ii45.

Rose, G. (2001). Sick Individuals and Sick Populations. *International Journal of Epidemiology*, 30(3), pp. 427–432. https://doi.org/10.1093/ije/30.3.427.

Roux, A.V.D. (2022). Social Epidemiology: Past, Present, and Future. *Annual Review of Public Health*, 43, pp. 79–98. https://doi.org/10.1146/annurev-publhealth-060220-042648.

Said, E. (1978). *Orientalism: Western Concepts of the Orient*. New York: Pantheon.

Wallerstein, N.B., Yen, I.H. and Syme, S.L. (2011). Integration of Social Epidemiology and Community-engaged Interventions to Improve Health Equity. *American Journal of Public Health*, 101(5), pp. 822–830. https://doi.org/10.2105/ajph.2008.140988.

Wamai, R.G. and Shirley, H.C. (2022). The Future of Health in Sub-Saharan Africa: Is There a Path to Longer and Healthier Lives for All? In: *African Futures*. Leiden, Netherlands: Brill, pp. 67–98. https://doi.org/10.1163/9789004471641_008.

Whitman, A., De Lew, N., Chappel, A., Aysola, V., Zuckerman, R. and Sommers, B. (2022). *Addressing Social Determinants of Health: Examples of Successful Evidence-based Strategies and Current Federal Efforts*. [online]. Available at: https://aspe.hhs.gov/sites/default/files/documents/e2b650cd64cf84aae8ff0fae7474af82/SDOH-Evidence-Review.pdf [Accessed 20 August 2023].

Wilkinson, R.G. and Pickett, K.E. (2009). Income Inequality and Social Dysfunction. *Annual Review of Sociology*, 35, pp. 493–511.

Williams, D.R. and Mohammed, S.A. (2009). Discrimination and Racial Disparities in Health: Evidence and Needed Research. *Journal of Behavioral Medicine*, 32(1), pp. 20–47. https://doi.org/10.1007/s10865-008-9185-0.

Woolf, S.H. and Aron, L. (2013). *Physical and Social Environmental Factors*. [online] National Library of Medicine. Available at: https://www.ncbi.nlm.nih.gov/books/NBK154491/ [Accessed 20 August 2023].

World Health Organisation (2018). *Health Inequities and their Causes* [online]. World Health Organization. Available at: https://www.who.int/news-room/facts-in-pictures/detail/health-inequities-and-their-causes [Accessed 18 August 2023].

Yaya, S., Uthman, O.A., Ekholuenetale, M. and Bishwajit, G. (2018). Socioeconomic Inequalities in the Risk Factors of Noncommunicable Diseases among Women of Reproductive Age in Sub-saharan Africa: A Multi-Country Analysis of Survey Data. *Frontiers in Public Health*, 6, p. 412663.

Zhang, J. and Centola, D. (2019). Social Networks and Health: New Developments in Diffusion, Online and Offline. *Annual Review of Sociology*, 45, pp. 91–109. https://doi.org/10.1146/annurev-soc-073117-041421.

2

HEALTH LEGACY OF COLONIALITY IN AFRICA

John Fulton and Philip Emeka Anyanwu

Introduction

This chapter will examine colonisation and the legacy of colonisation. There are two broad themes to the chapter: the ways in which the colonisation process constructed an identity for the colonised and the implications that this could have for health and the health status of the individual. Both indirectly through the creation of structures and the ways in which the former colonised countries were set up to allow a particular focus and approach. The second part will focus on economic structures and how the economic position of the former colonies continues economic exploitation and perpetuates the existence of economic disadvantage. This, in turn, has an effect on the health status of individuals, perpetuating health issues and health problems.

Colonisation

Colonisation is the process of establishing a territory in another country that is inhabited by indigenous people and, in doing so, establishing control over the area. While colonisation is as old as civilisation, modern colonisation began with the discovery of the Americas by Christopher Columbus in 1492 and was followed quickly by the colonisation of Central and South America by Spain and Portugal. Since the 16th century, Europeans have been actively engaged in the process of colonising other countries. The practice of colonisation meant exploitation for many of the indigenous peoples. Specifically, their economic resources were exploited to create wealth for the colonising countries (Andrews,

2021). To further develop this point, the colonisation of America was associated with widespread genocide:

> when they arrived, they found millions of people living in complex societies who needed to erased in order to clean the slate necessary for Western progress. The genocide in the Americas is without precedent- wiping up to 99% of the natives off the face of the earth.
>
> *(Andrews, 2021: 17)*

Northern European countries engaged in colonialism. First, Spain and Portugal rapidly colonised Mexico and the South American countries, followed by Britain, which became a strong colonising force in Southeast Asia, particularly in India.

The colonisation of Africa came later, climaxing with the Berlin Conference (1884–1885), where Africa was carved up among the European superpowers (Pakenham, 2015). By the 20th century, most of Africa was colonised by European powers, mainly France, Belgium, Britain, Italy and Germany. "By the 1930s, 84% of the globe was colonised" (Hoffman, 2015). Colonisation is claimed to be altruistic and civilising, but the raison d'etre of colonisation is economic dominance, resulting in exploitation, domination and repression (Omanga with Ndlovu-Gatsheni, 2020). The presence of the colonisers persisted well into the 20th century, and it was only after World War Two that many of the former colonies gained their independence from their sovereigns. The colonisers took over the country and imposed their laws and regulations on it. Through the imposition of laws and regulations and the control of the economy, a dependency on the dominant country was created. In addition to this economic dominance came the imposition of the dominant country's customs, culture and religion on the conquered country (Butt, 2013) and the suppression of local customs and traditions.

De-Colonisation

Following the Second World War and peaking in the 1960s, the colonisers left the dependent countries, and the withdrawal of the colonisers left a vacuum in many of the countries. On leaving, the coloniser often set up artificial boundaries, which were, to say, the least problematic. There are numerous examples of this; one example that stands out is the country of Nigeria. There are, in Nigeria, several tribal groups, the dominant ones being the Yoruba, the Igbo and the Hausa. When Nigeria achieved its independence in 1960, the country was divided into three groups: the Yoruba in the Southwest, the Hausa-Fulani in the North and the Igbo in the Southeast. The Nigerian Civil War, better known as the Biafran War, was the result of the Igbo being dissatisfied with the central government, and they set up their own independent country. Arguably, this war was the result of Britain's colonisation (Falola and Ezekwem, 2016).

Decolonisation means the process of withdrawal of the former colony gaining independence; this was far from a straightforward process. Colonialism had a massive impact on African societies not only in a material sense but also in a metaphysical sense (Woldegiorgis, 2021). To develop this point, Ndlovu-Gatsheni (2021) discusses what he terms the three empires and three trajectories of decolonisation. The physical empire, the commercial or non-territorial empire and the metaphysical empire were all part of the colonisation process, and it logically follows that the process of decolonisation is political, economic and epistemic (Gebremariam, 2021). It is important to unpick the terminology used to describe the process, as all of it has important implications for health.

Ndlovu_Gatsheni (2015) uses the term coloniality to explain and encapsulate the continuation of colonialism in the contemporary world. Coloniality is more about colonisation and emphasises the hold the coloniser has over the indigenous people in terms of control over the economy, control over authority, gender, sexuality, knowledge and subjectivities, and as such, it imposes an invisible power structure.

Coloniality is different from colonialism. Colonialism denotes a political and economic relation in which the sovereignty of a nation or a people rests on the power of another nation, which makes such a nation an empire. Coloniality, instead, refers to long-standing patterns of power that emerged as a result of colonialism but that define culture, labour, intersubjectivity relations, and knowledge production well beyond the strict limits of colonial administrations. Thus, coloniality survives colonialism. It is maintained alive in books, in the criteria for academic performance, in cultural patterns, in common sense, in the self-image of people, in aspirations of self and in so many other aspects of our modern experience. In a way, as modern subjects, we breathe coloniality all the time and every day (Maldonado-Torres, 2007: 243 as cited by Ndlovu-Gatsheni, 2015).

Physical Withdrawal

Once the physical presence of the coloniser has been withdrawn, the influences of the previous regime could strongly remain within the colonised country (Ndlovu-Gatsheni, 2013). The former president of Ghana Kwane Nkrumah, writing in 1965, discussed what he referred to as neo-colonialism: many countries remained dependent on their former masters, who continued to influence and direct. This was tied in with economics and economic dependence. Colonialism was very much about imposing their laws on the country being colonised, thus creating a dependency that could remain. The countries were, in terms of governance, immature, and this led to, in many countries, civil war, bad government and corrupt systems, which were an obvious hindrance to development (Collier, 2008).

Economic Decolonisation

Physical decolonisation was relatively straightforward in comparison to economic withdrawal, and there still could be economic dependency, the result being that "foreign capital is used for exploitation rather than development" (Nkrumah, 1965). Nkrumah was writing in 1965, and this still holds true today. Financial institutions investing in Africa exert an influence on policy in every African country (Gebremariam, 2021).

The argument put forward for the lack of economic development in many countries is encapsulated in modernisation theory, such as Rostow's Model of Development (Rostow, 2013). This theory demonstrates a hierarchy of countries at the bottom of the ladder, which are the traditional countries, followed by pre-conditions where the global West helps with aid and industrial development. Followed by continuing economic growth and development, which pushes towards maturity and continued economic development and the age of mass consumption. The lack of significant development is due to a focus on traditional values of ascription, particularism and collectivism.

The World Bank and free-market reforms attempt to invest in countries and promote modernism. Western investment in factories and education is all driven by the promotion of modernism and the encouragement of economic growth and development. It aims to develop the entrepreneurial middle class and a high urban population. These theories ignore coloniality and the associated inequalities between the West and developing countries. It benefits small elites and thereby adds to the gulf between the rich and the poor.

A more convincing alternative to modernisation theories is dependency theory (Frank and Gills, 1996), which views the world as consisting of a metropolis and peripheral nations. The peripheral nations are in a state of dependency due to their background of slavery and colonialism and, in the post-colonial world, dependency on their formal colonial masters. Foreign investment is concerned with extractive industries, and as a result, many nations are in a state of underdevelopment.

Wallerstein (2000) developed the "World Systems Theory" by examining why many countries fail to develop. He classifies countries into core, semi-periphery and periphery. Core countries are in a developed state because they exploited the resources of the countries they colonised. The countries on the periphery remain underdeveloped because of the inequalities. Foreign investment is to exploit these countries, not to build and develop them. Global capitalism perpetuates these inequalities; developing nations cannot compete against the highly technologically developed West. The main product is agriculture, and this does not allow competition.

Decolonising Healthcare Systems

Colonialism and its legacies have had a significant impact on the healthcare system and practices in Africa. Most societies in Africa experienced the displacement of traditional indigenous medicine by Western medical practices led by European powers during the colonial era. Colonialism imposed the Western medical systems, stigmatising African indigenous medical practice as primitive and backward, undermining its legitimacy and efficacy and disrupting the psychological, social and cultural dimensions of indigenous medicine and its role in the African tribes.

One of the profound differences between Western medicine and indigenous medicine in Africa is the latter's rich psychosocial connotation. Indigenous medical practice in Africa is deeply intertwined with cultural practices and spirituality, a unique aspect that sets it apart from Western medicine. For instance, in the Igbo tribe rooted in West Africa, mostly Nigeria, the "Dibia" is a healer, diviner, and mediator between the human world and the spirit world, among other roles. The word "Dibia" is also the Igbo translation of the English word doctor, underscoring the cultural significance of indigenous medicine.

Despite the challenges posed by colonialism, indigenous medicine in Africa has demonstrated remarkable resilience and adaptability. The importance of indigenous medicine to healthcare systems in Africa is seen more in rural and remote areas where such practices are more common and augment the lack or poor access to Western healthcare facilities and services.

The legacy of colonialism on contemporary healthcare systems and attitudes towards indigenous medicine is a barrier to maximising the potential of indigenous medicine in Africa. Colonial ideologies continue to shape healthcare policies and practices in post-colonial Africa. Therefore, understanding colonial legacies is essential for decolonising healthcare systems in Africa, addressing the ongoing challenges faced by indigenous medicine and promoting culturally sensitive healthcare practices.

Metaphysical (epistemic)

The final category is the most pervasive, and that is the metaphysical category, and this is the most enduring of all Ndlovu-Gatsheni's categories. Colonisation, which was not just the physical taking over of territories but was all pervasive as such, led to a radical change in African society. Woldegiorgis (2021) discusses Chinua Achebe's *"Things Fall Apart"* and the ways in which the organised and functioning society was changed. The tribal system was a fluid and flexible system, yet this was reinvented by the coloniser to be a tighter, more organised entity than it was in reality (Hobsbawm and Ranger, 1983). There was a system of learning and a world view that were destroyed by the colonised under the guise of being a civilising force. The languages of education were French and English, representing the dominant colonising countries in Africa, and local languages were negated, and much of the indigenous knowledge and traditions were lost.

Ndlovu-Gatsheni (2015) uses the term coloniality to explain and encapsulate the continuation of colonialism in the contemporary world. Coloniality is more about colonisation and emphasises the hold the coloniser has over the indigenous people in terms of control over the economy, control over authority, gender, sexuality, knowledge and subjectivities, and as such, it imposes an invisible power structure.

Post Colonialism

Perhaps the commonest term is post-colonialism, which can differentiate the divide between the period of colonisation and its aftermath and the subsequent exploration of the former colonies by the developed world. It is used in a second way to encapsulate the experience of the colonised individual, that is, those who have both directly experienced colonisation and its remnants. It is not a single theory but a set of ideas or ways of examining the experience and position of the formally colonised. As such, it defies grand narrative and cannot provide a universal encapsulation of experience and position (Abrahamsen, 2003). As such, it can be described as a post-modern theory that can illuminate and explain.

Abrahamsen (2003) discussed this in some detail and argued that while obvious control is now over, the situation for many is still that of subordination and subservience to the dominant and so-called first-world countries. This has a profound effect on those in the subordinate position; the psychiatrist Franz Fanon developed this thinking that colonisation had a destructive effect on the individual (Fanon, 2016). Spivak, another post-colonial writer, coined the term, Subaltern, to emphasise the way in which the colonised are excluded, and by this, she means totally excluded from society and not involved in the current discourses (Spivak, 1996).

Postmodernism, and particularly the work of Foucault, has been used to explain the post-colonial condition. Post-colonialism is not synonymous with Foucauldian theory. However, many scholars working in this tradition have drawn on these theories to illuminate and explain orientation and practice. Foucault did not present a unified theory, but his work has been explained as a toolkit that can be used to illuminate and explain (Allen, 2012). Discourses and power are useful explanatory concepts in both colonial and post-colonial situations.

Discourse, in the context, is used as a noun and, as such, is used to illustrate the way in which language not only reflects our perceptions and actions but also can illuminate and influence our perceptions and actions. The concept of discourse is, for Foucault, very much tied to power. Foucault saw power as initially being repressive and centrally administered in a controlling and authoritative way. With enlightenment, there came a shift in power, which was diverse and operated throughout society through institutions like medicine, the judicial system and education. Stemming from his examination of the prison system based on the panopticon, which ensured continuous surveillance. Modern medicine, which emerged in late 18th-century Europe, further developed surveillance of the population. Populations were measured, objectified and classified. Power in the Foucauldian sense is no longer a central controlling factor but is rather diffuse and pervasive, running through society, and is present in every aspect of society. Through surveillance, people were treated as objects or objectified; from this objectification, they became subjects who actively participated in the surveillance; as Foucault described it, they became "docile bodies" (Foucault, 1975).

The scholar Edward Said, a Christian Palestinian, in 1978, published "Orientalism," which examined the oriental position and the ways in which a binary was created between East and West. While not explicitly writing in the tradition of Foucault, Said drew from insights from Foucault's writing, particularly the idea of discourses. The Eastern position is seen in opposition to the rational West, and the East is perceived as the other (Said, 1978). The other is an important concept, and in his analysis, he argues that the Western world sees the East as strange and different in opposition to the rational West and, importantly, as inferior to the West. Relations with the East are conducted from this standpoint. While Said's analysis was explicit about the East, that is, the Muslim world, many of his insights can be applied to Africa and the ways in which people can be seen as the other.

This can be applied to the African situation, the representation of Africa and Africans and, through the rejection of what Africa is perceived to be, "Africa still constitutes one of the metaphors through which the west represents origins of its own norms develops a self-image and integrates this image into a set of signifiers asserting what is supposed to be an identity" (Mbembe, 2001).

The construction and re-construction of society is another important feature of colonialism. The colonisers came into a country or region and re-constructed that society according to the norms and ideals of the conquering country. Vaughan (1991) rightly makes the point that the experience of colonisation could vary depending on the colonising country, and this is particularly a British consideration. The colonisers justified their interventions as bringing order and civilisation to a deficient country. Part of this justification lay in seeing the indigenous people as the other and being intrinsically different.

What Does this Mean in Terms of Social Epidemiology?

The main aim of this book is to discuss the many factors that can influence health, ranging from global issues such as environmental pollution to bacteria or viruses infiltrating the body. It is a mixture of these factors that can cause ill health and an illness trajectory. The social construction of health and illness is an important factor in social epidemiology; that is not to say that there is no biological basis for illness, but how illnesses are perceived by society and how groups of people are constructed is an important part of the social epidemiological landscape. Scientific rationalism and social construction are what make medicine different (Comeroff), and they are also what make it so interesting.

Modern medicine relies as its basis on scientific rationalism and is based on empirical research and scientific rationalism in the past 50 years, and certainly, in the past 30 years, the evidence-based discourse has been at the forefront of modern health care. Medical intervention should be based on sound scientific evidence. Similarly, public health interventions are based on epidemiological evidence, and much effort lies in translational research, which translates the findings from epidemiological studies into public health interventions.

Social constructionism also plays a part in health care, the discourse of eugenics. While few would hold the principles of the 19th and early 20th centuries, there are various ways in which these differences are perceived. Eugenics developed at the very time that colonialism was at its peak. Colonialism, while exploiting the indigenous people, was justified in an altruistic way, and it was seen as a civilising force for the poor natives. The ideas were in vogue at the time of many of the developments in medicine.

Vaughan (1991) applied Foucauldian theory to colonial Africa to explain the construction and operation of medicine in colonial Africa. Vaughan discussed the ways in which power was created and maintained within the African context and argues that clearly, in colonial Africa, there was a repressive and restrictive power that was between the ruling class (the coloniser) and the African people (the colonised), who were in a subordinate position. Africans were regarded as strange and inferior to white Europeans; in the 1920s and 1930s, this was replaced by a focus on cultural differences and the African being seen as maladaptive; medicine played an important part in this construction (Vaughan, 1991).

Vaughan (1991) gives many examples of the ways in which Africa and Africans were constructed through medicine and the assumption that Africans are prone to particular diseases. The example of mental health is important in that the African was not seen as an individual but as part of a group, with mental illness being viewed as deviance from the norm. In particular, mental illness could be explained by exposure to European culture, which could challenge the so-called traditional values. Foucault viewed asylum as a place for others, that is, those outside of society who, in turn, because of their otherness, defined society. The Africans were already the other, and the culture was seen as "sick." Boundaries in the colonial regime were seen as important, both in the geographical sense and in the sense of people and behaviour, and the Africans could be defined as deferent and alien because their behaviour did not fit with that which was deemed appropriate in European society.

Eugenics

A justification for colonialism was that the indigenous people were savages, and the colonisers served as a civilising force; it was no coincidence that the eugenics movement was strong in the late 19th and early 20th centuries. Dominant in many of the Victorian explorations of race are attempts to identify different physiological attributes. In the 20th century, these physiological theories have been replaced by an exploration of cultural differences. Importantly, this did not mean that there was a sudden paradigm shift and all notions of physiological differences were abandoned, but cultural differences were used to justify the otherness, and in many discourses, there were (and still are) elements of the African being seen as being physically different.

To start with the physiological differences, in the 18th century, there was an interest in eugenics, which is the superiority of one group of people over another. Eugenics lost credibility after the atrocities of Nazi Germany (Rutherford, 2021, 2022), and most of the ideas are refuted, although there are still elements in current discourse, as we will see in later discussions. It was a very powerful movement in the 18th and early parts of the 20th centuries and influential both implicitly and explicitly in much of the thinking of the time.

The term eugenics was coined by Francis Galton, and his work was based on Darwin's evolutionary theories, particularly those of natural selection (Rutherford, 2021). He founded the Eugenics Records office at University College London (Rutherford, 2021), which continued well into the 20th century. It was subsequently headed by the notable statisticians Karl Pearson and Ronald Fisher. Groups of people within Britain were seen as inferior, that is, sectors of the working class, and this very easily took on racial overtones.

Foucault, in discussing surveillance (REF), was highly prophetic, and in the 20th and early 21st centuries, the collection of information about people has greatly increased. People continue to be categorised, and the ways in which this categorisation takes place are very socially constructed. For example, the way in which race is categorised can vary from survey to survey. People can find themselves in a group to which they have no affinity, and the term mixed race can apply to a number of "mixes," which often has no particular relevance. Of course, surveys, etc., are useful in highlighting and demonstrating areas of disadvantage, but they are still socially constructed and reflective of particular discourses.

Not only in medicine but in other areas of activity. To give an example, which is cited by Rutherford (2021), The notion of an underclass was posited by Charles Murray in the 1960s, and the underclass were groups of people who were excluded from society and functioned outside of society, existing mainly on benefits (and the fruits of crime). It had racial overtones, and the underclass were largely African Americans, while their disadvantaged position in society can explain much. This was not an argument put forward by supporters of the underclass, who saw them as morally inferior to those in mainstream society and as less intelligent than white Americans. The reason why Americans are less successful than their white counterparts is because they are less inherently intelligent (Herrnstein and Murray, 1994).

While these ideas no longer hold any credibility, they were very influential, and, as Sowemino (2023) argues, colonial ideologies were influential in the development of modern medicine. In her book, she gives examples of the ways in which medicine was influenced by the premises of eugenics, much of which is still in evidence today. To focus on one of her healthcare examples, that of pain and pain control in health care. The concept of different groups or, more accurately, different races experiencing pain in a different way is an idea prevalent in health care; it is not based on any empirical evidence but nonetheless is a commonly held assumption.

Sowemino (2023) gives the example of a textbook on nursing practice in which the authors had to retract their representation of different racial groups' experiences of pain. Pain is a highly individual experience, but the authors of this textbook were reflecting (unfortunately) a commonly held assumption that different groups have different pain thresholds. She argues that the authors of the book took a series of racial stereotypes and made a general statement as to how different, arbitrary classifications of so-called races behaved. The example Sowemino gives is that the authors present "black people" as having a fatalistic attitude towards pain, with no evidence for this statement, and by using the collective term black people, this reflects the discourses around the racial groups rather than an observation based on empirical evidence. She also makes the point that there was no category for white people who presumably behave in an appropriate and socially acceptable way when experiencing pain. This example, perhaps rather obviously, shows the ways in which discourses can infiltrate and thereby influence modern health care. It is also interesting that the publishers issued an apology for this particular section of the book, and it raises the question of how often these assumptions are not challenged or, more importantly, how often are they not made explicitly but serve as the basis for a discussion or intervention?

Vaughan (1991) analysed psychiatry in colonial Africa and the way in which it played its part in the construction of the African. There is a legacy of this which is played out in contemporary life; an example of this is the perception of young black males in both the UK and the US. Black men, in particular those from Afro-Caribbean backgrounds, are more likely to be diagnosed as suffering from psychosis than their white counterparts (mind). Similarly, young men from Afro-Caribbean backgrounds are more likely to be diagnosed as suffering from psychosis than their white counterparts (mind). There is no evidence that they have a stronger genetic disposition to psychosis. There are a number of factors that can affect the development of severe mental illness, and one is stress and the position of the individual in society. While it can be argued that there can be a variety of factors associated with this, one factor is how the individual is perceived and how this perception can affect the individual. This construction of Black men as being aggressive is arguably similar, in the sense that it is a social construction, to the construction of colonial Africans as outlined by Vaughan.

Economics

Government health expenditure, a significant component of public finance, plays a key role in shaping a nation's healthcare sector development and the well-being of its population. As a measure of economic growth based on the value of goods and services produced during a given period, a country's gross domestic product (GDP) is an important determinant of its health spending power. It is not surprising that countries or regions with high GDP per capita allocate more resources to healthcare for improved access, advanced treatment, and better health outcomes. The economic position of many African countries means they have less income than the countries of the West and, consequentially, less money to spend on health care. Africa faces significant constraints in funding its healthcare systems, which can exacerbate the burden of diseases. Limited healthcare expenditure may lead to inadequate infrastructure, shortages of medical supplies and insufficient healthcare personnel, all of which contribute to poorer health outcomes and a higher burden of disease, especially the persistent prevalence of communicable diseases and the double burden of communicable and non-communicable disease in this setting compared to high-income countries.

Conclusion

In this chapter, we have explored the colonial legacy and its influences on health care in particular, both in terms of economic inequalities that are still being perpetuated. This crudely means that in the so-called developing countries, there is insufficient income to spend on health care and to develop healthcare infrastructure. An additional feature is in the colonisation process indigenous people were categorised, and through this process, they were looked on as inferior to their (white) European counterpart, as evidenced in the eugenics movement. These attitudes, while perhaps not as explicit, are nonetheless evident in today's world. In social epidemiological terms, it focuses on how the wider issues, in this case colonialism and decolonisation, can have a profound effect on the healthcare experiences of individuals, particularly those in the global south.

References

Abrahamsen, R., 2003. African Studies and the Postcolonial Challenge. *African Affairs*, *102*(407), pp. 189–210.

Allen, A., 2012. Using Foucault in Educational Research. *British Educational Research Association, 13*(7), p. 2012. https://www.bera.ac.uk/publication/using-foucault-in-education-research

Andrews, K., 2021. *The New Age of Empire: How Racism and Colonialism Still Rule the World.* Penguin UK.

Butt, D. (2013). Colonialism and Postcolonialism. In *The International Encyclopedia of Ethics.* Wiley-Blackwell.

Collier, P., 2008. *The Bottom Billion: Why the Poorest Countries Are Failing and What Can Be Done about It.* Oxford University Press.

Falola, T. and Ezekwem, O. eds., 2016. *Writing the Nigeria-Biafra War.* Boydell & Brewer.

Fanon, F., 2016. Black Skin, White Masks. In Longhofer, W., & Winchester, D. (Eds). *Social theory re-wired: New connections to classical and contemporary perspectives* (pp. 394–401). Routledge.

Frank, A.G. and Gills, B.K. eds., 1996. *The World System: Five Hundred Years or Five Thousand?.* Psychology Press.

Foucault, M., 1975. *Discipline and Punish.* A. Sheridan, Tr. Gallimard.

Gebremariam, E.B., 2021. Reflections from Teaching African Development Using Decolonial Perspectives at LSE. https://blogs.lse.ac.uk/internationaldevelopment/2021/05/25/reflections-from-teaching-african-development-using-decolonial-perspectives-at-lse/

Herrnstein, R. J., & Murray, C. (1994). The bell curve. *Library Quarterly, 66*(1), 89–91.

Hobsbawm, E. and Ranger, T., 1983. *The Invention of Tradition.* Cambridge University Press.

Hoffman, P.T., 2015. How Europe Conquered the World. Foreign Affairs. https://www.foreignaffairs.com/articles/europe/2015-10-07/how-europe-conquered-world

Maldonado-Torres, N., 2007. On the Coloniality of Being: Contributions to the Development of a Concept. *Cultural Studies, 21*(2–3), pp. 240–270.

Mbembe, A., 2001. *On the Postcolony* (Vol. 41). University of California Press.

Ndlovu-Gatsheni, S.J., 2015. Decoloniality as the Future of Africa. *History Compass, 13*(10), pp. 485–496.

Nkrumah, K., 1965. Neo-colonialism, the Last Stage of Imperialism. https://www.marxists.org/subject/africa/nkrumah/neo-colonialism/introduction.htm

Omanga, D., 2020. Decolonisation, Decoloniality and the Future of African Studies. A Conversation with Dr Sabelo

Ndlovu-Gatsheni, S. J. (2015). Decoloniality as the future of Africa. *History Compass, 13*(10), 485-496.

Pakenham, T., 2015. *The Scramble for Africa.* Hachette UK.

Rostow, W.W., 2013. The Stages of Economic Growth. In Sanderson, S. K. (ed.). *Sociological worlds: comparative and historical readings on society* (pp. 130–134). Routledge.

Rutherford, A., 2021. A Cautionary Tale of Eugenics. *Science, 373*(6562), p. 1419.

Rutherford, A., 2022. *Control, the Dark and Troubling History of Eugenics.* W.W. North and co.

Said, E., 1978. *Orientalism: Western Concepts of the Orient.* Pantheon.

Sowemimo, A. (2023). *Divided: Racism, medicine and why we need to decolonise healthcare.* Profile Books.

Spivak, G.C., 1996. *The Spivak Reader: Selected Works of Gayatri Chakravorty Spivak.* Psychology Press.

Vaughan, M., 1991. *Curing their Ills: Colonial Power and African Illness.* Stanford University Press.

Wallerstein, I., 2000. Globalization or the Age of Transition? A Long-term View of the Trajectory of the World-System. *International Sociology, 15*(2), pp. 249–265.

Woldegiorgis, E.T., 2021. Decolonising a Higher Education System Which Has Never been Colonised. *Educational Philosophy and Theory, 53*(9), pp. 894–906.

3

BIOSTATISTICAL METHODS IN SOCIAL EPIDEMIOLOGY

Philip Emeka Anyanwu, Adeniyi Francis Fagbamigbe and Ayo Adebowale

Introduction

> Epidemiology without statistics is like a bicycle without wheels.
>
> *– Mervyn Susser*

As the evidence of the link between social factors and health outcomes becomes increasingly apparent, the need for precise, robust, and innovative statistical tools in the domain of social epidemiology has never been greater. Statistical methods have proven useful in identifying and quantifying causal pathways between social factors such as socioeconomics, housing and neighbourhood, and disease and health. Biostatistics, as a subdiscipline in statistics, focuses on the application of statistical methods in the collection, analysis, interpretation, and presentation of data in health-related research. Biostatistical tools and techniques are necessary to analyse and interpret complex data, allowing researchers to uncover patterns, relationships, and insights that can inform evidence-based decision-making. These tools and techniques have become increasingly important to public health with advancements in digital health and big data.

This chapter is designed to expose readers to the applications of biostatistical methods in social epidemiology. It is aimed at showcasing how statistics can be harnessed to investigate the social determinants of health.

Biostatistics in Social Epidemiology

The application of biostatistical methods is crucial in understanding the link between social factors and health within and between populations. Such methods

DOI: 10.4324/9781003467601-4

enable the quantification of associations and the establishment of causality between social determinants (such as education, employment, housing, income, and gender) and health outcomes, informing public health interventions. The abilities of biostatistical methods to identify priority areas for intervention and evaluate the effectiveness of social and health policies and programmes make them critical to evidence-based decision-making in public health.

Given the intersectionality between social factors in determining health and health outcomes, biostatistical methods play an important role in teasing out the individual and combined impacts of social factors and how they mediate or moderate the effects of other factors on health.

Establishing causality remains an important challenge in epidemiology, especially in social epidemiology. Contemporary biostatistical methods offer robust techniques that strengthen causal inference in epidemiology. Techniques such as propensity score matching and causal mediation analysis enable researchers to navigate the complexities of observational data towards causal inference on the impact of social factors on health outcomes.

The design of social epidemiological studies increasingly benefits from the contributions of biostatisticians, driving interdisciplinarity in social epidemiology. Biostatisticians' contributions in this area include, but are not limited to, study design, sample size calculation, sampling strategies, statistical analysis plan and execution, and integrating approaches to promote study validity and generalisability of findings.

Biostatistics also enables the use of big data in social epidemiology by offering techniques to manage and analyse complex multimodal big datasets commonly encountered in social epidemiology. Techniques like multivariate analysis, hierarchical modelling, and machine learning algorithms empower researchers to optimise insights from large and diverse datasets.

Sources of Data for Social Epidemiology Research

Social epidemiology relies on strong data to make a meaningful evaluation. The data are from diverse sources. In general, these sources can be categorised into routine and non-routine (ad hoc) sources. Routine sources are established systems for the continuous collection of health-related data. They are usually cheaper and readily available, but they often suffer from incompleteness, inaccuracy, and the unavailability of crucial characteristics of interest. Examples of routine data include censuses, vital registration systems, notification centres (e.g., infectious diseases, cancer registries, school health, hospitals, health centres, and veterinary clinics), electronic health data, accident records, police and prison records, and traffic records. Non-routine sources are well-designed with measurable objectives. Examples are interviews, surveys, experiments, planned studies (research), outbreak monitoring, special sample surveys, environmental health ad-hoc surveys, and monitoring of underserved or vulnerable populations. The non-routine sources are scheduled data collections occasioned by the inadequacy of statistics derived from routine data. They guarantee reliability, completeness, and accuracy, but they require enormous resources, planning, personnel, and logistics.

Based on methods of data collection, data sources can be categorised into primary and secondary data. For primary data, data are collected directly from participants for a particular purpose. This method is common in surveys and most public health studies. While secondary data are extracted from existing records such as hospital case files/notes and surveillance systems. Secondary data are not originally collected for a specific research purpose but can be used for different purposes. However, secondary data are not necessarily routinely collected.

Often, data could be linked to or pooled from different sources in social epidemiology. For example, primary data may be triangulated with secondary data or secondary data pooled across multiple settings (Fagbamigbe et al., 2021). However, African social epidemiologists face huge challenges as a result of poor funding and the poor or non-existent linkage of different data. Despite the limitations, they have sourced data using different strategies, such as the use of secondary data.

Measurement of the Frequency of Diseases

- Social epidemiologists are often interested in measuring the frequency of diseases in a society. Different statistical tools can be used for such measurements.
- Numbers/counts: These are the number of individuals who meet a specific description. Example: The number of pregnant women who attended a health talk.
- Ratios: These are the relative magnitudes of two quantities (usually expressed as a quotient) (A/B). An example is the ratio of pregnant women aged 15–24 years and those aged 25–49 years who attended a health talk.
- Proportions: This is the ratio that relates the part (the numerator) to the whole (the denominator)—the numerator is always part of the denominator (A/A+B). An example is the proportion of pregnant women aged 15–24 years who attended a health talk. This will be the number of pregnant women aged 15–24 years who attended a health talk divided by the total number of pregnant women aged 15–24 years. It usually ranges from 0 to 1.
- Percentages: This is similar to proportions, except that the proportions are multiplied by 100. It is the ratio that relates the part (the numerator) to the whole (the denominator) * 100. That is, the numerator is always part of the denominator (A/A+B*100).
- Rates: Rates are similar to proportions but multiplied by certain figures, such as 1,000 or 100,000, to ease the understanding and comparability of the estimates across time and domains. An example is the under-five mortality rate,

defined as the number of deaths before the 60th birthday divided by the number of live births * 1,000.

Descriptive Measures

Descriptive measures provide important information in understanding the patterns and characteristics of diseases and health-related events.

Morbidity

Morbidity statistics are essential to public health agencies for the control of disease and epidemics. They are used for the location, design, and administration of public health and medical care facilities and services, including rehabilitation programs. Morbidity data may originate either from a survey of the population or from some reporting system as part of administrative procedures.

Sources of morbidity data include the National Health Survey (NHS), single-visit surveys, periodic visit surveys, cohort studies, case-finding surveys, notifiable disease records, public accident records, case registers, hospital records, records of private physicians, school records, industry records, defence activity records, etc.

Measures of Morbidity

The measures of morbidity are indicators of the extent of illness in a population or community. Morbidity statistics are obtained or gathered to know the number of cases or persons unwell due to a particular health problem.

The following terms are used in measuring morbidity:

- *Prevalence Rate (PR)*
  This is the proportion of the population that has the health problem under study.

$$PR = \frac{Number\ of\ existing\ cases\ of\ the\ health\ problem\ at\ a\ specified\ point\ in\ time}{Total\ population\ in\ that\ period} \times 1,000$$

The denominator includes people diagnosed with the health problem and those who do not have the health problem.

- *Incidence Rate (IR)*
  This is the number of new cases of a health problem that occur in a population at risk within a specified period. When the rate is based on the assumption that the entire population at risk is followed up from the onset to the

end of the observation period, such a rate is referred to as the *cumulative incidence* rate.

$$IR = \frac{Number\ of\ new\ cases\ of\ disease\ during\ a\ specified\ period\ of\ time}{Total\ population\ at\ risk} \times 1,000$$

- *Incidence Density (ID)*
  This is the number of new cases of a health problem during a given period per 1,000 total person-times of observation during the period. It is otherwise known as the instantaneous rate at which disease develops in a population.

$$ID = \frac{Number\ of\ new\ cases\ of\ disease\ during\ a\ specified\ period\ of\ time}{Total\ person\ time\ of\ observation} \times 1,000$$

  where total person-time of observation is the total amount of time the individual contributed by all persons involved in the study. The total person-time of observation must reflect time, which could be in days, weeks, months, or years.

- Attack Rate (AR)
  This is the number of cases reported during an epidemic per 1,000 total populations at risk.

$$AR = \frac{Number\ of\ cases\ reported\ during\ an\ epidemic}{Total\ population\ at\ risk} \times 1,000$$

Mortality

Mortality (death) is the permanent disappearance of all evidence of life at any time after birth has taken place. It is the post-natal cessation of vital functions of the body cells without the capacity for resuscitation.

Sources of Mortality Data

Sources of mortality data are basically censuses and surveys, but these are subject to errors. Other sources are civil registers, statistics yearbooks, United Nations Demographic books, Annual World Health Statistics, etc.

Measuring Mortality

Mortality is measured by relating deaths in periods among different categories of individuals (classified by sex, age, religion, occupation, income, etc.) to the total numbers at risk in these groups. In mortality measurement, two significant rates can be identified. These are observed rates and adjusted rates. The adjusted rates are more complex than the observed rates in the sense that they are hypothetical representations of the level of mortality for a given population group. Adjusted rates required many assumptions for their estimates. The basic measures of mortality are:

- Crude Death Rate (CDR)
    This is defined as the number of deaths in a year per 1,000 mid-year population.

$$CDR = \frac{D}{P} \times 1,000$$

    where D is the total number of deaths in a year and P is the mid-year population.
    Factors affecting CDR are population distribution and composition, e.g., climatic conditions, occupational distribution, population structure, natural disasters, etc.

- Age-Specific Death Rate (ASDR or ASMR)
    This is defined as the number of deaths in a particular age group in a year per 1,000 mid-year population in that age group.

$$ASDR \text{ or } =_n M_x = \frac{_n D_x}{_n P_x} \times 1,000$$

    Where: $_n D_x$ is the number of deaths to persons aged x, $x+n$; $_n P_x$ is the mid-year population of persons aged x, $x+n$

- Cause-Specific Death Rates and Ratios

  - Cause-Specific Death Rates (CSDR)
      This is the number of deaths from a given cause or causes during a year per 100,000 mid-year population. It makes use of 100,000 since there are relatively few deaths from many of the causes.

$$CSDR = \frac{Number\ of\ deaths\ from\ a\ cause}{Total\ population} \times 100,000$$

  - Cause-Specific Death Ratio (CSDR)
      This measures the distribution of deaths by cause and can be computed for intercensal years. It represents the percentage of all deaths due to a particular cause.

$$CSDR(ratio) = \frac{Number\ of\ deaths\ from\ a\ cause}{Total\ population} \times 100,000$$

- Infant Mortality Rate (IMR)

    This is the number of deaths among children below 1 year of age per 1,000 live births during the year. It reflects a country's level of socio-economic development and quality of life. IMR is used for monitoring and evaluating population and health programmes and policies (Akinyemi et al., 2019).

$$IMR = \frac{Number\ of\ Infants\ deaths}{Number\ of\ livebirths} \times 1,000$$

- Neonatal Mortality Rate (NMR)

    This is the number of deaths of infants under 4 weeks (under 28 days) of age during a year per 1,000 live births during the year (Morakinyo & Fagbamigbe, 2017).

$$NMR = \frac{Number\ of\ Infants\ deaths\ under\ 28\ days}{Number\ of\ livebirths} \times 1,000$$

The NMR of a country is an indicator of the levels of attendance at antenatal and postnatal care, and it reflects the organisation of the health care system. For instance, the figure can raise a question about what percentage of deliveries takes place in an institution. NMR is a combination of early neonatal and late neonatal mortality rates.

- Early neonatal mortality rate (ENMR)

    This is the number of deaths among infants aged between 5 and 7 days divided by the number of live births.

$$ENMR = \frac{Number\ of\ Infants\ deaths\ under\ 7\ days}{Number\ of\ live\ births} \times 1,000$$

- Late Neonatal Mortality Rate (LNMR)

    This is the number of deaths among infants aged between 7 and 28 days divided by the number of live births

$$LNMR = \frac{Number\ of\ Infants\ deaths\ between\ 7\ and\ 28\ days}{Number\ of\ livebirths} \times 1,000$$

- Post-Neonatal Mortality Rate (PNMR)

    This is the number of deaths aged between 28 days and 1 year divided by the number of live births.

$$PNMR = \frac{Number\ of\ Infants\ deaths\ between\ 28\ days\ and\ 1\ year}{Number\ of\ livebirths} \times 1,000$$

- Perinatal Mortality Rate (PMR)

  Perinatal deaths are composed of pregnancy losses occurring after seven completed months of gestation (stillbirths) and death within the first seven days of life (early neonatal deaths). Perinatal mortality refers to the total number of stillbirths and deaths of children aged under 7 days per 1,000 total births (live + stillbirths).

  $$PMR = \frac{Number\ of\ still\ births + deaths\ aged\ under\ 7\ days}{Total\ number\ of\ births\left(live + still\ births\right)} \times 1,000$$

- Maternal Mortality Measure

  Maternal mortality has three different measures (Adebowale et al., 2010). These are:

  - *Maternal mortality ratio*

    This is defined as the number of maternal deaths from causes related to pregnancy and childbirth per 100,000 live births. It provides insight into women's health more broadly: their access to health care, the adequacy of the healthcare system in meeting their needs, and even their social status and economic standing.

    $$MM\ Ratio = \frac{Number\ of\ maternal\ deaths\ in\ a\ year}{Number\ of\ livebirths} \times 100,000$$

  - *Maternal Mortality Rate*

    This is defined as the number of maternal deaths in a year per 100,000 women of reproductive age in that year

    $$MM\ Rate = \frac{Number\ of\ maternal\ deaths\ in\ a\ year}{Number\ of\ women\ aged\ 15-49\ years} \times 100,000$$

Disability

Disability is a body or mind condition that makes it more difficult for an individual with the condition to do certain activities or interact with the world around him or her (Bovbjerg, 2019).

Measuring Disability

Disability is heterogeneous; therefore, its measurement is complex. The identification of people with disabilities is not static and can differ depending on why it is being conceptualised. Disability can be measured using three different approaches in line with the international classification of functioning, disability, and health.

- Direct Questioning on Disability: Direct questions can be asked of individuals to respond to how they perceive themselves in terms of disability (whether they view themselves as being disabled or having a disability). This approach will produce an underestimation of the prevalence of disability because many people may not consider themselves as being disabled.
- Self-reported Functioning: Disability can be measured through self-reported functioning in terms of whether they experience difficulties in the six different domains of functioning: seeing, hearing, walking, cognition, communicating, and self-care.
- Extended Self-reporting Questions: This measurement approach captures a more complete picture of disability, involves the use of about 35 sets of questions, and can be used in surveys depending on time availability.

Quality of Life

The World Health Organization defines quality of life as an individual's perception of their position in life in the context of the culture and value systems in which they live and about their goals, expectations, standards, and concerns. WHO, in an attempt to have a quality-of-life assessment that would be applicable cross-culturally, developed an assessment of quality of life tool (WHO-QOL) in collaboration with 15 international field centres. Adaptations have been developed for people with HIV (WHOQOL-HIV), and an additional 32-item instrument has been developed to assess aspects of spirituality, religiousness, and personal beliefs (WHOQOL-SRPB).

Life Tables

A life table is a tabular representation that displays the likelihood, for individuals of different ages, of not surviving to their next birthday. It is a table that contains the life history of a hypothetical group or cohort of people, as it is diminished gradually by death. The record begins at the birth of each member and continues until all have died. The cohort loses a pre-determined proportion at each age and thus represents a situation that is artificially conceived. It is a form of combining the mortality rates of a population at different ages into a single statistical model. Life tables can be constructed for both sexes together, but the differences between male and female mortality at most ages are sufficient to justify treating them separately.

Types of Life Tables

- Period life table: This is based on the experience after a short period, such as a year, 3 years, or an intercensal period, in which mortality has remained the same. This represents the combined mortality experienced by age of the population in a particularly short period. It does not represent an actual cohort but a hypothetical one and is subject to the prevailing ASDR.

- Generation life tables: This is otherwise known as a cohort life table. This life table describes the actual survival experience of a group, or cohort, of individuals born at about the same time. Theoretically, the mortality experience of the people in the cohort would be observed from their moment of birth through each consecutive age in successive calendar years until all the group members die. This life table is based on the mortality rates experienced by a particular birth cohort, e.g., those born in 2022.

Life Table Functions

Life table functions can be classified into two categories. These are;

1 Those that refer to intervals of age. They are rates, probabilities, deaths, and populations.
2 Those that refer to an exact age: They are people surviving to an exact age, population over a given age, and expectation of life at an exact age. These are useful for computing the exact age of x.

Definition and Notation of Life Table Functions

a *Age (x)*
This is used individually and is the exact number of completed years that have elapsed since birth. For instance, the exact age "30" in a life table means when a person has lived exactly 30 full years. Therefore, a person is said to have reached exact age x when he has reached his xth birthday.

b *Number of survivors at age x (l_x)*
This is the number of people alive at the exact age of x, out of the original number of births. It is the survivors of a cohort of babies born alive to the exact age x.

c *Probability of dying between age x and x+n ($_nq_x$)*
This is the probability that a person aged x dying within the interval x to $x+n$. It is the probability of dying between the exact ages x and $x+n$. This is represented mathematically as:

$$q_x = {}^n\frac{d_x}{l_x} = \frac{l_x - l_{x+n}}{l_x} = \frac{l_x}{l_x} - \frac{l_{x+n}}{l_x} = 1 - \frac{l_{x+n}}{l_x}$$

d *Number of deaths between ages x and x+n ($_nd_x$)*
This is the number of deaths between the exact ages x and $x+n$. It is the number of people in the population who attained age x but died before they reached age $x+n$. For instance, if $l_{30} = 350$, $l_{31} = 300$, and $l_{32} = 230$. This means

that at age 30, 50 people died before reaching age 31. Also, at age 30, 120 people died before they reached age 32.

e *Probability of surviving between age x and x+n* $\left(_n p_x\right)$

This is the probability of surviving from exact age x to exact age x+n.

$$_n P_x = \frac{l_{x+n}}{l_x}$$

f Number of person-years lived between age x and x+n $\left(_n L_x\right)$

This is the average number alive in the interval between exact ages x and x+n, i.e., the age distribution of the stationary population. It is also the number of person-years that would be lived within the indicated age interval (x to x+n) by the cohort of 100,000 (or any radix) births assumed. This is mathematically represented as: $_n L_x = \frac{1}{2} n \left(l_x + l_{x+n} \right)$. For the first few years of life, it is not reasonable to use the average of l_x and l_{x+1} as an approximation of L_x. This is because deaths are not evenly distributed throughout the year. Instead, they are concentrated in the earlier part of the year. Therefore, values of L_x for the first few years should be closer to l_{x+1} than to l_x.

Practically, we use:

$$L_0 = 0.3 l_0 + 0.7 l_1 \text{ for age } 1$$

$$L_1 = 0.4 l_1 + 0.6 l_2 \text{ for age } 2$$

$$^4_4 L_1 = 1.3 l_0 + 2.7 l_5 \text{ for age } (1-4)$$

For older ages, i.e., 5 or more:

$$L_x = \frac{1}{2} \left(l_x + l_{x+1} \right) \text{ for single-year ages}$$

$$_n L_x = \frac{n}{2} \left(l_x + l_{x+1} \right) \text{ for age group}$$

g *Total number of person-years lived after age x (T_x)*

This is the total population aged x and over. It represents the total number of person-years that would be lived after the beginning of the indicated age interval by the cohort of the chosen radix. This means the number of person-years lived after the exact age x. It is derived directly from the $_n L_x$ column by taking the summation of the $_n L_x$ column. The summation starts with the beginning of the stationary population and is a cumulative frequency obtained from the $_n L_x$ column. $T_x = \sum_{y=x}^{r} L_y$, where r is the highest attainable age.

h *Life expectancy at age x* $(\overset{\circ}{e}_x)$

This is called life expectancy. It is the expectation of life at exact age x, i.e., the average number of years lived by a person from exact age x. It represents the average remaining lifetime (in years) for a person who survives to the beginning of the indicated age interval. It is often used as an index for summarising the mortality risk of a country. This is mathematically represented as: $\overset{\circ}{e}_x = \dfrac{T_x}{l_x}$

Analytical Study Designs in Social Epidemiology

Analytical studies investigate the association between variables/factors to understand their impact on specific health outcomes or events. It involves a systematic determination of disease risk associations with exposure or non-exposure. Such studies aim to test whether certain factors are "associated", whether the association is a statistical concept, or to compare estimates among different groups (Bovbjerg, 2019). Analytical studies include cross-sectional studies, case-control studies, cohort studies (longitudinal studies), controlled trials, etc.

Cross-Sectional Studies

A one-time study or survey to assess the presence or absence of both exposure and disease is assessed at the same single point in time to provide a "snapshot" of health experience. Its major disadvantage is that it provides only a temporal relationship between exposure and disease that is not always distinguishable. Its estimates do not imply causality.

Case-Control Studies

Case-control studies start after an "outbreak" or occurrence of certain health conditions of interest. The study helps to compare exposure to a specified risk among individuals who had the disease (case) and those who did not (control). The studies start with the identification of cases and determine exposures. If the observed exposures are higher than expected, then identify the comparison group (controls) needed to find out what is expected. The main statistical tool is the odds ratio (OR).

	Cases	*Control*	*Total*
Exposed	a = 20	b = 5	25
Not Exposed	c = 5	d = 20	25
Total	25	25	50

$$Odds\ Ratio = \frac{odds\ in\ cases}{odds\ among\ control} = \frac{a/c}{b/d} = \frac{a \times d}{b \times c}$$

Example: The distribution of cases and controls according to bottled water consumption in a case-control study is tabulated above.

$$OR = \frac{20 \times 20}{5 \times 5} = 16$$

$$\text{The 95\% CI} = \exp\left(\ln\left(\widehat{OR}\right) \pm z\sqrt{\frac{1}{a} + \frac{1}{b} + \frac{1}{c} + \frac{1}{d}} \right)$$

$$= \exp\left(\ln\left(16\right) \pm 1.96\sqrt{\frac{1}{20} + \frac{1}{5} + \frac{1}{5} + \frac{1}{20}} \right) = \left(3.398, 81.172\right)$$

An OR > 1 suggests higher odds of exposure among the cases.
An OR < 1 suggests lower odds of exposure among the control.
A 95% CI that excludes 1 is considered statistically significant.

Cohort Studies

Cohort studies start with the identification of a group of people sharing the same experience and are followed for a specified period, either prospectively or retrospectively. Four methodological issues consisting of (i) age, cohort, and period effects; (ii) direction of causality; (iii) state dependence; and (iv) residual heterogeneity must be addressed before the study starts. A certain group of the cohort is exposed to certain conditions, while others are not. The main statistical tool is relative risk (RR).

	Diseased	Healthy	Total
Exposed	a = 30	b = 10	a+b = 40
Not Exposed	c = 5	d = 25	c+d = 30
Total	35	35	70

$$Relative\ Risk = \frac{Risk\ in\ exposed}{Risk\ in\ unexposed} = \frac{a/(a+b)}{c/(c+d)}$$

Example: The distribution of illness according to exposure in a cohort study is shown above.

$$Relative\ Risk\ (RR) = \frac{30\backslash(30+10)}{5\backslash(5+25)} = 4.5$$

$$\text{The 95\% CI} = \exp\left(\ln\left(\widehat{RR}\right) \pm z\sqrt{\frac{(1-p_1)}{x_1} + \frac{(1-p_2)}{x_2}}\right)$$

$$= \exp\left(\ln\left(4.5\right) \pm 1.96\sqrt{\frac{\left(1-\frac{30}{40}\right)}{30} + \frac{\left(1-\frac{5}{30}\right)}{5}}\right) = \left(1.982, 10.216\right)$$

A $RR > 1$ suggests an increased risk of that outcome in the exposed group.

A $RR < 1$ suggests a reduced risk in the exposed group.

A 95% CI that excludes 1 is considered statistically significant.

Other names for relative risk are risk ratio and relative rate.

Rate Ratio: This is the ratio of the incidence rate in an exposed group divided by the incidence rate in an unexposed (or less exposed) group.

$$Rate\ Ratio = \frac{Incidence\ rate\ in\ exposed}{Incidence\ rate\ in\ unexposed}$$

Relative risk from OR.

However, an approximate relative risk can be obtained from the OR and vice versa using

$$\widehat{RR} = \frac{Odds\ Ratio}{1 - risk\ in\ unexposed + \left(risk\ in\ unexposed\ group * odds\ ratio\right)}$$

- Controlled Trials: These are studies in which data are obtained or characteristics are measured of treatment and control populations after an intervention/exposure/event to measure differences between responses in the two groups. Sometimes participants are randomised into groups.

Natural Experiment

Some situations present a need to study the impact of exposure to events, policies, or interventions that researchers have no control over. These exposures could be social or public health policies, such as the smoke-free public places legislation, or events like the COVID-19 pandemic. The COVID-19 pandemic has been studied as a natural experiment for the impact of social restrictions on health, an intervention that would have been unethical in normal situations. Therefore, a natural experiment approach provides an alternative to randomised controlled trials (RCTs), especially in evaluating large-scale population-wide interventions/events that are not amenable to experimental manipulations (Craig et al., 2012, 2017). It provides researchers with an opportunity to study causal relationships by making the most of naturally occurring events or conditions, such as policy changes, disasters, or historical events, that mimic the random assignment of subjects to treatment groups, similar to controlled experiments.

Natural experiments are common in evaluating public health policies. Their adoption in policy/intervention evaluations is appropriate in specific circumstances, such as when exposed and unexposed groups have comparable and accurate data on exposure, outcomes, and confounders exist for a large sample size (Craig et al., 2017). Studies adopting this approach are observational and can assess the impact of policies and interventions with differences in implementation between nations, regions, or local areas. The exposure is usually a "naturally" occurring situation that researchers can take advantage of to study impacts, rather than one created by the researchers as in an RCT. The differences in policy/intervention/event implementation offer the opportunity to assign groups to treatment and control groups. This difference could be based on the time of implementation (for example, Province A banned smoking in cars carrying children in 2015, whereas the ban came into effect in Province B in 2016), how comprehensive the policy is (for example, smoke-free public places legislation was implemented in both Province A and B; however, the implementation in Provinces A is comprehensive (a complete ban on smoking in enclosed public places), while that of Province B is not (a smoking ban in bars and restaurants only), among others.

Natural experimentation draws on statistical methods such as difference-in-difference (DID), propensity score matching, instrumental variables, regression discontinuity, machine learning, and causal inferential methods. In the bullet points below, we have provided a brief description of these methods and examples of studies that have applied them in natural experiments.

Difference-in-Differences (DID) Analysis

DID is a widely used statistical method for evaluating the causal impact of a treatment or intervention in a natural experiment and involves comparing the change in outcomes over time between a treatment group (exposed to the intervention) and a control group (not exposed). The difference in these changes before and after the intervention represents the causal effect.

Laverty et al. (2020) *adopted a natural experiment approach in assessing the effects of the English ban on smoking in cars carrying children using logistic regression within a DIDs framework, adjusting for all time-invariant differences between the intervention (England) and comparison (Scotland) populations.*

Matching Methods

In observational studies, receiving the intervention/exposure is usually influenced by participant characteristics. These constitute confounding factors. Propensity score methods mimic an RCT experimental design to address confounding issues such that the treatment and control groups are similar with respect to covariates. It is used to reduce observational data's confounding bias and create comparable treatment and control groups in natural experiments. These techniques estimate the probability of an individual or unit being exposed to the treatment based on observed covariates. Matching methods pair each treated unit with one or more control units that have similar propensity scores. Thus, in a set of subjects all of whom have the same propensity score, the distribution of observed baseline covariates will be the same between the treated and untreated subjects.

In a natural experiment in Medellín, Colombia, Cerdá et al. (2012) examined the effects of exogenous change in the built environment on violence using a propensity score matching method.

Instrumental Variable Analysis

Instrumental variable analysis, originally used by economists, holds potential in epidemiological research, especially when there is endogeneity or self-selection bias in the treatment assignment (Angrist et al., 1996). An instrument variable is used to predict the treatment assignment, and it should satisfy certain conditions (e.g., relevance and exclusion restrictions). The analysis of instrumental variables estimates the causal effect by using the instrument to create exogenous variation in treatment assignment. Glymour (2006), in their book chapter, demonstrate in detail the use of natural experiments and instrumental variable analyses in social epidemiology.

Neve et al.'s (2015) natural experiment estimating the causal effects of length of secondary schooling on the risk of HIV infection in Botswana is a good example of the application of instrumental variables in social epidemiologic research.

Regression Discontinuity Design

Similar to instrumental variable analysis, the regression discontinuity design was long used by economists. In social epidemiology research, it is used in studies where assignment to a treatment/experimental group is determined by a cutoff point or threshold (such as age, school year group, test score, etc.), and units just above and below this threshold are compared. Regression discontinuity designs permit strong causal inference with relatively weak assumptions (Hilton Boon et al., 2021). The causal effect is estimated by examining the discontinuity in the outcome variable at the threshold. Both parametric and non-parametric regression models can be applied in an analysis of regression discontinuity.

Davies et al. (2018) *employed a regression discontinuity design in estimating the causal effect of education on health outcomes by exploiting the raising of the minimum school leaving age in the UK in September 1972 as a natural experiment.*

As with other research designs, natural experiments have some limitations. Given that researchers have no control over the exposure/event, establishing causation using natural experiments is a major challenge. The absence of randomisation and the possibility of selective exposure in natural experiments can result in differences in the exposed and unexposed groups, especially on factors associated with the outcomes (confounders). However, natural experiments are very useful in studying issues where manipulating exposure is impractical or unethical. Although it can be argued that a natural experiment has the features of an observational study, it requires weaker assumptions for observed effects to be interpreted as causal than in most observational epidemiological studies (Anyanwu et al., 2018). Another advantage of natural experiments is their cost-effectiveness in comparison to experimental studies.

Mediation Analysis

The evaluation of public health interventions and policies goes beyond understanding what works—that is, the effect of interventions/exposures on outcomes. The "why" and "how" questions are important in social epidemiology for understanding the interaction between factors that determine the impact of interventions and policies on health. Mediation analysis is one of the techniques employed in answering the "how" question, as it explores the underlying mechanisms through which intervention/policy X impacts on Y health outcome. It investigates the role of intermediate variable Z (referred to as mediator) in the causal pathway between interventions/exposures and outcome variables. When mediation occurs, the relationship between two variables X (intervention) and Y (outcome) can be explained by another variable Z (the mediator). As such, the mediator variable Z can be said to transmit the effects of X on Y as it lies between the causal pathways between both variables (see Figure 3.1).

Mediation analysis teases out the total ©ffect of an intervention/policy on an outcome into the direct and indirect effects through a mediator (Mittinty & Vansteelandt, 2020). In basic terms, the analysis involves:

- Calculating the direct effect (c'), i.e., the effect of intervention (X) on outcome (Y), while controlling for the mediator (Z).
- Calculating the mediating effect (a*b), i.e., the associat(ion between the intervention (X) and mediator (Z) and the association between mediator (Z) and the outcome (Y), and multiplying their coefficients (a*b) to compute the mediating effect.

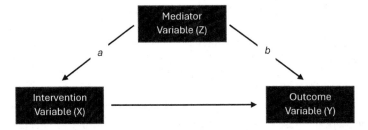

FIGURE 3.1 "Mediation analysis causal pathway", demonstrates three variables x-Intervention, y-Outcome , z-Mediator. Mediator interacts with both Intervention and the Outcome, whereas the intervention effects the Outcome.

- The total effect (c) is the sum of the direct and indirect effects of the intervention variable X.

The outcome of a mediation analysis suggests whether the effect of an intervention/exposure on the outcome changes with changes in the mediator variable. In other words, examining whether the mediator (Z) accounts for a significant portion of the total effect (c) from X to Y. As such, the proportion of the mediating effect can be full/complete, partial, or no mediation.

In a full/complete mediation, the effect of X on Y is 100% mediated by the mediator variable. That is, the mediation effect (a*b) is significant, but the direct effect (c') is not. A full/complete mediation effect is rare; the most common is partial mediation. In partial mediation, the mediator variable only mediates a proportion (part) of the effect of X on Y, so both the mediation effect (a*b) and the direct effect (c') are significant. In a no-mediating effect scenario, a*b is not significant, implying that X affects Y independently of Z.

Fitting a mediation analysis model requires prior consideration of key assumptions of causal ordering, no unobserved confounders, linearity in associations, and sequential ignorability (Forastiere et al., 2018), among others. Violations of these assumptions can lead to biased estimates. An important limitation of making causal inferences in observational studies using mediation analysis is the potential for uncontrolled biases. A detailed description of statistical methods to assess mediation analysis and contemporary comprehensive approaches is described in the articles by MacKinnon et al. (2007) and Lange et al. (2012).

Control and Analysis of Confounders and Effect Modifications

The notions of confounders, interactions, and effect modifications are issued in social epidemiology to gain a better understanding and identification of variables or factors that may not directly influence the relationship between dependent and independent variables, the combinations of such factors, and how the factors are related to the dependent and independent variables. They indicate different concepts but sometimes have interdependent notions in multivariate analysis (Bovbjerg, 2019).

Confounders

Confounders are those factors that influence both the exposure and the outcome, thereby causing a suspicious or unreasonable association between them. Confounding belongs to the concept of causal factors. For example, it is not right to just conclude that eating red meat could cause heart disease; smoking could lead to heart disease if an individual smokes. Therefore, failure to include smoking status in the study may lead to the wrong conclusion. All confounders that may influence the exposure and the outcome should be identified and considered at the conceptual stage of research, and concerted efforts should be made to address them irrespective of the study design (Figure 3.2).

Effect Modifications

Confounders are used to separate the effects of an exposure. The motivation for the identification of effect modifiers is to identify whether the effect of a treatment (or exposure) differs across different categories of study members with different characteristics. Sometimes, the effects are the same. If they are the same, the effect of the exposure is homogeneous; otherwise, they are heterogeneous. Effect modification is useful in identifying a group (such as males or young people) that may not benefit from an intervention.

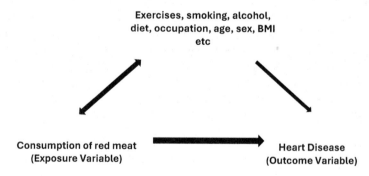

FIGURE 3.2 Diagram which demonstrates a pathway with a triangulation of three variables that have confounding effects: exercise, smoking, alcohol, diet, occupation, age, sex, BMI, etc.

Interactions

Interactions evaluate both individual and combined, often additive, effects of exposures. They are used to identify the joint effect of at least two exposures on a health outcome. If the joint effect is higher than the effect expected by the sum of the individual effects of the exposures, the interaction is referred to as synergistic; otherwise, it is antagonistic. Assessment of interaction helps determine if two or more different interventions can be combined to bring about a change in an outcome.

Conclusion

In this chapter, we explored the fundamental role of biostatistics in the field of social epidemiology. We introduced rigorous statistical approaches, including contemporary methods for causal inference in observational data, such as propensity score matching and mediation analysis. The methods covered in this chapter can be applied to investigating and quantifying the impact of social determinants such as income, education, race, and neighbourhood environment on health outcomes, as well as understanding the mechanisms and differential impacts of social and public health policies. As the field of social epidemiology further develops, contemporary biostatistical methods will remain important for advancing our understanding of the complex interaction between society and health.

References

Adebowale, S., Fagbamigbe, F., & Bamgboye, E. (2010). Rural-urban differential in maternal mortality estimate in Nigeria, sub-Saharan Africa. *Journal of Medical and Applied Biosciences*, *2*(1), 74–91.

Akinyemi, J. O., Odimegwu, C. O., Banjo, O. O., & Gbadebo, B. M. (2019). Clustering of infant deaths among Nigerian women: Investigation of temporal patterns using dynamic random effects model. *Genus*, *75*(1), 12. https://doi.org/10.1186/s41118-019-0058-x

Angrist, J. D., Imbens, G. W., & Rubin, D. B. (1996). Identification of causal effects using instrumental variables. *Journal of the American Statistical Association*, *91*(434), 444–455. https://doi.org/10.1080/01621459.1996.10476902

Anyanwu, P. E., Craig, P., Katikireddi, S. V., & Green, M. J. (2018). Impacts of smoke-free public places legislation on inequalities in youth smoking uptake: Study protocol for a secondary analysis of UK survey data. *BMJ Open*, *8*(3), e022490. https://doi.org/10.1136/bmjopen-2018-022490

Bovbjerg, M. L. (2019). *Foundations of epidemiology*. Oregon State University.

Cerdá, M., Morenoff, J. D., Hansen, B. B., Tessari Hicks, K. J., Duque, L. F., Restrepo, A., & Diez-Roux, A. V. (2012). Reducing violence by transforming neighborhoods: A natural experiment in Medellín, Colombia. *American Journal of Epidemiology*, *175*(10), 1045–1053. https://doi.org/10.1093/aje/kwr428

Craig, P., Cooper, C., Gunnell, D., Haw, S., Lawson, K., Macintyre, S., Ogilvie, D., Petticrew, M., Reeves, B., Sutton, M., & Thompson, S. (2012). Using natural experiments to evaluate population health interventions: New Medical Research Council guidance. *Journal of Epidemiology and Community Health, 66*(12), 1182–1186. https://doi.org/10.1136/jech-2011-200375

Craig, P., Katikireddi, S. V., Leyland, A., & Popham, F. (2017). Natural experiments: An overview of methods, approaches, and contributions to public health intervention research. *Annual Review of Public Health, 38,* 39–56. https://doi.org/10.1146/annurev-publhealth-031816-044327

Davies, N. M., Dickson, M., Davey Smith, G., van den Berg, G. J., & Windmeijer, F. (2018). The causal effects of education on health outcomes in the UK biobank. *Nature Human Behaviour, 2*(2), Article 2. https://doi.org/10.1038/s41562-017-0279-y

Fagbamigbe, A. F., Oyinlola, F. F., Morakinyo, O. M., Adebowale, A. S., Fagbamigbe, O. S., & Uthman, A. O. (2021). Mind the gap: What explains the rural-nonrural inequality in diarrhoea among under-five children in low and medium-income countries? A decomposition analysis. *BMC Public Health, 21*(1), 575. https://doi.org/10.1186/s12889-021-10615-0

Forastiere, L., Mattei, A., & Ding, P. (2018). Principal ignorability in mediation analysis: Through and beyond sequential ignorability. *Biometrika, 105*(4), pp. 979–986. https://doi.org/10.1093/biomet/asy053

Glymour, M. M. (2006). Using causal diagrams to understand common problems in social epidemiology. *Methods in social epidemiology*, 393–428.

Hilton Boon, M., Craig, P., Thomson, H., Campbell, M., & Moore, L. (2021). Regression discontinuity designs in health. *Epidemiology, 32*(1), 87–93. https://doi.org/10.1097/EDE.0000000000001274

Lange, T., Vansteelandt, S., & Bekaert, M. (2012). A simple unified approach for estimating natural direct and indirect effects. *American Journal of Epidemiology, 176*(3), 190–195. https://doi.org/10.1093/aje/kwr525

Laverty, A. A., Hone, T., Vamos, E. P., Anyanwu, P. E., Taylor-Robinson, D., de Vocht, F., Millett, C., & Hopkinson, N. S. (2020). Impact of banning smoking in cars with children on exposure to second-hand smoke: A natural experiment in England and Scotland. *Thorax, 75*(4), 345–347. https://doi.org/10.1136/thoraxjnl-2019-213998

MacKinnon, D. P., Fairchild, A. J., & Fritz, M. S. (2007). Mediation analysis. *Annual Review of Psychology, 58*(1), 593–614. https://doi.org/10.1146/annurev.psych.58.110405.085542

Mittinty, M. N., & Vansteelandt, S. (2020). Longitudinal mediation analysis using natural effect models. *American Journal of Epidemiology, 189*(11), 1427–1435. https://doi.org/10.1093/aje/kwaa092

Morakinyo, O. M., & Fagbamigbe, A. F. (2017). Neonatal, infant and under-five mortalities in Nigeria: An examination of trends and drivers (2003–2013). *PLOS ONE, 12*(8), e0182990. https://doi.org/10.1371/journal.pone.0182990

Neve, J.-W. D., Fink, G., Subramanian, S. V., Moyo, S., & Bor, J. (2015). Length of secondary schooling and risk of HIV infection in Botswana: Evidence from a natural experiment. *The Lancet Global Health, 3*(8), e470–e477. https://doi.org/10.1016/S2214-109X(15)00087-X

4

ADOPTING QUALITATIVE RESEARCH METHODS IN UNDERSTANDING HIV/ AIDS IN AFRICA

Joseph Sunday and John Fulton

Introduction

This chapter will explore the ways in which qualitative research is a valuable tool of social epidemiology. Public health is rightly founded on epidemiological principles and patterns, and trends can tell us much about the trajectories and transmission patterns of disease. To demonstrate this point, Autoimmune Deficiency Syndrome (AIDS) and HIV in the context of Africa will be used to illustrate how qualitative research can bring in the individual and group perspective.

To further illustrate the uses of qualitative research in social epidemiology, we are taking HIV/AIDS within African countries as an exemplar. AIDS is caused by the transmission of a virus, and while this is relatively straight forward, there are various factors that play a role in the distribution of HIV/AIDS, extending from economic interactions at the global level through political, social and cultural issues to the experiences of individuals within local and family groups. Social epidemiology provides a robust framework for a deeper insight into the distribution of these conditions among affected populations.

Epidemiology and social policy studies can tell us much about the wider factors and the relationships between them. To deeply unpack the societal dimensions associated with health conditions like HIV/AIDS, there is an increasing recognition that qualitative research is an important dimension in epidemiology (Bannister-Tyrrell and Meiqari, 2020).

This chapter will outline some of the principles of qualitative research and consider its application to social epidemiology. The latter part of the chapter will examine how qualitative research can aid our understanding of the wider determinants of HIV and AIDS.

DOI: 10.4324/9781003467601-5

Qualitative Research

Methodology is an overarching framework that gives direction and focus to the research process. In qualitative research, the main methodological approaches are ethnography, phenomenology and grounded theory. Phenomenology is concerned with the lived experiences of individuals and, thus, is an overarching approach that can help individuals with lived experiences thus being studied. Grounded theory aims to generate theory from the research process.

Ethnography is a qualitative approach where the researchers immerse themselves in the research setting, interact with participants in that setting and thereby become part of the setting they are studying. Ethnography as a research method is well established and was popular in the 19th century, with anthropologists studying other cultures. In the early 20th century, the approach became popular in the US, particularly in Chicago, with ethnographic studies such as William Foote Whyte's (2012) *Street Corner Society*. The aim is to illuminate the experiences of individuals and gain an understanding of why there are certain habits and practices. According to the American anthropologist Clifford Geertz, through a detailed description, one can gain an understanding of the rationale and meaning of certain actions. This allows us to understand and establish the meanings of certain practices; it also allows us to understand the position of the people involved (Geertz, 2008).

The work of the doctor and activist Paul Farmer is of note; he was both a doctor and an anthropologist, and while his main focus was not on Africa and his studies were in Haiti, he meticulously detailed the experiences of people in Haiti suffering from AIDS. At the time of his study, treatment was available but not accessible to those with lower incomes. He detailed their experiences and the social conditions that could impact their plight, based on this understanding of the ways in which social conditions could interact with treatment and at a time when they were considered.

Methods, as distinct from methodology, are the approaches that collect data about the phenomenon being studied. Traditionally, the main approaches in qualitative research are interviews and observation. Interviews can be unstructured, and the respondent is encouraged to talk freely, an approach used in narrative research where people are allowed and encouraged to tell their personal stories. Semi-structured interviews are also commonly used where the researcher has a series of questions that can be used as a guide, but the researcher can also follow up on issues that arise in the interview. Observation, particularly in ethnography, is also a common approach; there is participant and non-participant observation. In ethnography, the researcher participates in the area of study by becoming an active part of the situation and people being studied.

Another important distinction is that qualitative research tends to be inductive, that is, theory arises through the data analysis, and quantitative research tests theory and theoretical assumptions. However, the reality is that often quantitative research can be used to identify patterns and trends; for example, in epidemiology, studies establish trends, and patterns can arguably be thought to be inductive. Qualitative research is useful in giving us insights into people's experiences, for example, what it's like for people with AIDS to manage their symptoms and the different illness experiences of people from different social classes and the associated income differentials.

As a methodological approach, mixed methods is a common approach where more than one type of data are collected. It goes well beyond collecting both qualitative and quantitative data. In mixed methods research, the data should both complement and interact with each other, thereby facilitating an understanding of complex situations. The example from epidemiology where the researcher explores both broader trends and patterns and then explores individual experiences illustrates this very well.

There are various qualitative approaches used in research in addition to the ones considered. It is not within the scope of this chapter to discuss each of these approaches. There are important texts one can consult for deeper insight into the major types and intricacies of each relevant qualitative approach (Denzin and Lincoln, 2011; Creswell and Creswell, 2017; Creswell, 2018). However, other common approaches have included ethnography, case studies, action (and participatory action) research, narrative analysis, phenomenology and discourse analysis (Denzin and Lincoln, 2011; Safdar et al., 2016; Creswell, 2018). Of the major qualitative methodological approaches and their relevance in social epidemiology towards delineating the social factors or dimensions consistent with this branch of epidemiology, ethnography appears to be the most utilised and recommended qualitative research approach.

The Case for Qualitative Approaches in Social Epidemiology

As an area of study, social epidemiology can help identify the factors playing a role in the pattern of diseases and the distribution of health within society while at the same time providing valuable insight into the systems and infrastructures within which they operate (von dem Knesebeck, 2015).

> [s]ocial epidemiology…is a branch of epidemiology concerned with the way that social structures, institutions, and relationships influence health. Social epidemiologists are concerned with the ways that societies are organized [sic] to produce or impede the development and maintenance of good health.
> *(Berkman et al., 2014, p. 1).*

Bannister-Tyrrell and Meiqari (2020) adumbrate the calls by scholars for the inclusion of qualitative research into the field of epidemiology and scientific research in general, as have other scholars (Agar, 2003; Popay, 2003; Silva and Fraga, 2012; Sale and Thielke, 2018; Knottnerus et al., 2020; Thompson and Schick-Makaroff, 2021). The authors argued the case for including qualitative research within epidemiology while highlighting the lack of qualitative approaches within social epidemiology. Consequently, Bannister-Tyrrell and Meiqari (2020) argue from philosophical standpoints for qualitative approaches. In their work, the authors cited the work of Popay (2003), identifying two (2) key frameworks that can be utilised by qualitative research integrating into epidemiology. These are the enhancement model and the epistemological model.

In the enhancement model, qualitative data are an explanatory add on of quantitative data, which can be argued is the most common utilisation of qualitative research in the field of epidemiology. The epistemological model, on the other hand, argues for qualitative research to be considered an equal partner. Additionally, Bannister-Tyrrell and Meiqari (2020) articulated the possible reasons for the underutilisation of qualitative approaches in the field of epidemiology, such as perceived value, funding opportunities and a lack of engagement with epidemiological literature by qualitative research, among others. The discussion of these issues could potentially pave the way for a better integration of qualitative approaches within the field of epidemiology. Popar (2003) argues that "[I]f epidemiology is to fulfil its full potential to contribute to improved population health and reduction of health inequalities then it must extend its methodological gaze to include qualitative research methodologies" (p. 62). An example of such application can be seen in the work of Gregory and Way (2009). The authors utilised grounded theory to gain further insight into the experiences of patients with end-stage renal disease undergoing haemodialysis. Semi-structured interviews were conducted among 44 consenting adults, which were then followed by another set of interviews six to eight weeks after the first phase of interviews. Data collected were analysed in line with the principles of grounded theory to generate a substantive theory of living with end-stage renal disease and haemodialysis (LESRD-H). Overall, the study informed the development of a clinical monitoring tool called the Patient Perception of Haemodialysis Scale (PPHS). The scale comprised 64 items and underwent quantitative psychometric analysis that showed its validity and reliability (Gregory and Way, 2009).

HIV/AIDS: A Key Social Epidemiological Issue

Key to social epidemiology is the concept of social determinants and their role in the transmission and progression of infectious diseases (Poundstone et al., 2004). This approach moves away from the focus on the individual to acknowledging the role social factors play in the epidemiology of HIV/AIDS. To fully conceptualise the challenge of HIV/AIDS from a social epidemiological perspective, the major social determinants beyond a predominant focus on the individual need to be considered primarily within the African context. This context is argued to be significantly different from the rest of the world. Consequently, the importance of integrating a theoretical framework through which to analyse this issue becomes very important.

There are several theories of social epidemiology reported in the literature. The major theories have been discussed in the work of (Krieger, 2001). The principal model that has previously dominated public health studies on HIV/AIDS has focused on the individual behavioural patterns and characteristics of the individual. Here, the focus was almost entirely on individual lifestyle choices, devoid of any external influence or factors (Krieger, 2001; Poundstone et al., 2004). To fully understand HIV/AIDS, especially within the African context, there needs to be a social epidemiological perspective adopted in discussing the condition. This approach will transcend the rather microscopic outlook of a very complicated condition by delineating all the multiple layers associated with it. These layers have been presented at the individual, social and structural levels (Poundstone et al., 2004).

The socio-ecological model (SEM) offers a comprehensive framework to delineate the complexities associated with living with this condition within the contextual setting of Africa. Additionally, the model holds promise in offering insight relevant to capturing the social dimensions key to social epidemiology. In an attempt to update the model, Baral et al. (2013) proposed the "modified social ecological model (MSEM)", which, they argued, will capture the multi-level domains of HIV and inform epidemiological studies related to HIV. It is the SEM and how it offers a lens towards understanding what it means to live with HIV/AIDS in Africa that the chapter now addresses.

The Socio-Ecological Model, HIV/AIDS and Social Epidemiology

The SEM is a useful theoretical model that helps to provide insight into the complexities of various factors in conceptualising health issues at multiple levels (Scarneo et al., 2019). The model was developed by Urie Bronfenbrenner in the 1970s to understand human development and became a theory in the 1980s (Kilanowski, 2017). The now widely applied model, especially in health studies, is predicated on the assumption that the individual is not the only variable at play when dealing with health issues. It posits that other environmental factors at several levels play a role in the individual in a corresponding way that one cannot detach the individual from the environment (Salihu et al., 2015).

In the case of HIV/AIDS, the SEM model will argue that the individual is not isolated from the environment, and the state of a person with HIV/AIDS will entail an interaction between the individual, the group/community and the physical, social and political environments. Although it is likely to find various variations of the SEM within the wider literature (Poundstone et al., 2004; Baral et al., 2013; Kaufman et al., 2014; Salihu et al., 2015; Scarneo et al., 2019), for example, Scarneo et al. (2019) outline the following levels for the model – intrapersonal, interpersonal, organisational, environmental and policy (p. 356). On the other hand, Salihu et al. (2015) put forward the following levels as constituents of the model: intrapersonal characteristics, interpersonal processes, institutional factors, community features and public policy (p. 87). For the purpose of this work, we will consider the complexities of living with HIV/AIDS in Africa using the SEM, which is conceptualised into the following levels:

- The individual level
- Interpersonal relationships or groups
- Community
- Societal levels

The Individual Level

Discussions, interventions and public health messaging on HIV/AIDS in the past have predominantly been dominated by a focus on the individual level (Baral et al., 2013). Public health messaging emphasised individual behavioural modifications and a focus on the biological aspects of living with the condition. Several public health campaigns on condom use, abstinence or adherence to medication are examples of how much focus on the epidemiology of HIV/AIDS has been individual-centred. It is worth highlighting that the focus on the individual from a public health perspective cannot be discounted. The focus on the individual has resulted in significant progress made in tackling HIV/AIDS, such as HIV testing and the administration of antiretroviral treatment, among others (Hedges, 2021).

However, the focus on the individual level has been attributed to the cost and difficultly of investigating pertinent issues at multiple levels (Kaufman et al., 2014). Additionally, the presence of the viral agent in the disease cycle feeds into the agent-host-environment epidemiological triad, which places a lot of focus on this level at the expense of others. Globally, there is now a consensus that, despite the importance of these individual-focused approaches, they are not sufficient to address this health challenge. Consequently, a multifaceted or multi-level approach recognises that an individual level tied to the wider determinants of health is vital in addressing HIV/AIDS (Kaufman et al., 2014).

At the individual level, variables such as knowledge/information, attitudes, perceptions, behaviours, beliefs and lived experiences are key to addressing HIV/AIDS. There have been several studies that have explored these variables within the African context (Gardner, 2013; De Wet et al., 2019; Estifanos et al., 2021; Hedges, 2021). Several of these studies have reported high levels of knowledge around issues relating to HIV/AIDS among African populations when viewed at the individual level. Knowledge can be described as one of the most important factors at the individual level when dealing with HIV/AIDS from a social epidemiological perspective. This is because knowledge of HIV/AIDS is key to preventing further transmission of the disease, and it is the first step in ensuring modifications needed to curb the spread of the disease are adhered to among affected populations. This is not an argument stating that knowledge of HIV/AIDS equals complete prevention (Mthembu et al., 2019). Mthembu et al. (2019) reported in their qualitative South African study that many of their student population – university students aged 18–24 years – were knowledgeable about the risks associated with HIV/AIDS. However, findings from their 20 in-depth interviews and a focus group showed this population engaged in risky behaviours such as unprotected sexual intercourse. Similar findings have also been reported among adolescents (Duby et al., 2021). Furthermore, there have also been several reports of misconceptions about the condition. For instance, Tarkang et al., (2019) found misconceptions such as that HIV can be transmitted by witchcraft or handshake among their study population. Some of these misconceptions can be argued to transcend the individual level and can be situated more at the community or societal level, more specifically cultural practices.

The Interpersonal Level

The SEM describes the interpersonal level as the one closest to the individual and impacts the individual level the most. It entails all the interactions and relationships linked to the individual that can exert influence on the individual (Kilanowski, 2017). Friends, families, peers, sexual partners and social support have all been grouped into this level (Kaufman et al., 2014; Salihu et al., 2015; Mitchell et al., 2021).

Family and family networks in the discussion related to HIV/AIDS can be very complicated, depending on who is being affected. For example, if the breadwinner of the family becomes affected by this condition, it could significantly impact the family structure, especially in areas where there is little or no formal healthcare or government support available to help these affected individuals or their families. The role of family and friends in the prevention and management of HIV/AIDS for those that have been affected by HIV/AIDS has been widely reported (Li et al., 2006). The bulk of health care delivery for these individuals lies within the interpersonal domain, as many affected by this condition remain at home with occasional contact with formal health care providers or home-based interventions and, in some cases, a complete absence of formal healthcare, with the care being provided solely by the people at the interpersonal level (Kipp et al., 2007).

The role of the family and family networks is one of the first barriers that impacts the willingness of individuals affected by HIV/AIDS to disclose their status, which is the first step in preventing the spread of the condition. A systematic review of factors influencing HIV disclosure among people with the condition in Nigeria identified family dynamics and the consequences of disclosure central to the interpersonal level, such as divorce, loss of relationships, accusation of infidelity, stigma and physical abuse, among several others (Adeoye-Agboola et al., 2016). The findings of the study, while broadly articulating factors that influence HIV disclosure, outlined several factors that lie within the interpersonal domain.

In most African settings, with little to non-existent support from the wider state, there is a huge amount of responsibility placed on the immediate family, friends and social support available to the individual. A similar finding has been reported in a study by Madiba et al., (2021) with the importance of family and friends as keys to disclosure. In the South African study of 28 interviews conducted among people living with HIV/AIDS, the findings showed the role of the interpersonal level in all six themes generated from the study. For example, in one of the themes of *Disclosure to Receive Appropriate Care* discussed in the study, participants were reported to have disclosed their HIV status to family members for the support they needed. In addition to the role of family and friends in disclosure and the provision of support, there is also an influence on adherence to antiretroviral treatment (Anyaike et al., 2019; Damulira et al., 2019).

Anyaike et al. (2019), in their Nigerian study on adherence to antiretroviral therapy, found a statistically significant association between support from friends and family and the adherence of individuals to antiretroviral treatment. The study also reported a significant relationship between disclosure of illness to friends and family and adherence to treatment, further highlighting the role of this group in the epidemiology of HIV/AIDS. A recent qualitative study (Mokwele et al., 2023) further underscores this position with the findings reporting that the support from family and friends was one of the main reasons young adults (21–34 years) in the South African study commenced and continued antiretroviral treatment. It is worth mentioning that there is a gender imbalance in the role played by family and friends for individuals affected by HIV/AIDS, as women most of the time bear the burden of providing care (Kipp et al., 2007). There are other broader structural issues that further impact the role of women within African societies that would be explored further under the societal level.

A large ethnographic study of 414 interviews and 136 field observations was conducted in three SSA countries – Nigeria, Tanzania and Uganda – on the success of adherence in SSA (Ware et al., 2009). The study reported findings from their ethnographic data showed that adherence to antiretroviral treatment was prioritised over several economic challenges, with the role of treatment "partners" or "supporters" (more than half of these were women) and family and friends being key in the provision of relevant resources (p. 40). Additionally, the study highlighted the role of people outside the interpersonal level in the management of HIV/AIDS. It is to this level that we now turn to our discussion.

The Community Level

Associated with the interpersonal level is the community level. This level extends beyond the immediate, closer interactions as seen in the interpersonal level to more about contact such as work settings, places of worship or religious settings and the neighbourhood (Kilanowski, 2017). This domain covers a larger group and integrates social capital, including healthcare services, cultural norms, economic sources and livelihoods, all of which play a key role within this domain (Baral et al., 2013; Kaufman et al., 2014). The role of the community in the epidemiology of HIV/AIDS has been widely reported, with several studies advocating for the need to plan interventions at community levels (Merten et al., 2010; van de Ruit, 2019; Mitchell et al., 2021). What happens at the community level plays a key role in the experiences of people living with HIV/AIDS. Unlike the previous two levels we have considered, the community level, although close to the individual, can also be outside the reach of the individual, with affected persons having little or no agency over the workings at this level. For example, while an individual with HIV/AIDS can seek direct engagement with a friend or family member should the need arise, things are more complicated at the community level, especially when such engagement revolves around cultural norms. Consequently, one is overseen by a layer that significantly impacts their experiences but to which they are rather passive actors than active stakeholders. In the ethnographic study by Mattes (2014) among 13 children receiving antiretroviral treatment in Tanzania, findings highlighted the influence of community. All children in the study carefully tried to preserve their HIV health status among only family members and people they trusted (interpersonal level) and not the community to avoid being discriminated or stigmatised (Mattes, 2014).

The community level is also crucial, as it is the level next to that of society, which is crucial in discussing the wider determinants of health as key aspects of social epidemiology. By implication, if there is a failing societal level, as seen in many African countries, a robust community level can mitigate some of the major fallouts as a result of the failure at the societal level. This has been the story of how HIV/AIDS have been largely managed in many African countries with many interventions and health programmes targeted at community levels, such as those with community health workers and also those from various international and/or non-governmental organisations (van de Ruit, 2019). The crumbling of a societal structure first impacts the community, which could then cascade downward to the individual if a robust community level is absent. Baral et al. (2013) argue that the community could enhance health and well-being or be a source of stigma.

Stigma operates more commonly at the community level, although it is also observed at the interpersonal level and can limit various crucial aspects of HIV prevention, treatment and care provision (Baral et al., 2013). Yuh et al. (2014) extensively covered the issue of stigma among people with HIV/AIDS in Africa. The authors defined stigma as "…labelling a person or group and connecting the label to undesirable behaviour" (Yuh et al., 2014, p. 582). They further alluded to the high levels of stigma in Africa associated with HIV/AIDS, with no adequate response to this issue.

At the community level, cultural or cultural norms have been offered as key contributing factors to the epidemiology of HIV/AIDS in Africa, with little or no cognisant of broader determinants (Sovran, 2013). The work of Sovran (2013) adumbrates major cultural practices broadly practiced within African settings that have been associated with HIV/AIDS. The author argues that many of these cultural practices have been *over-implicated* in the prevalence of HIV/AIDS. For cultural practices within Africa, there is little doubt that there are cultural norms that further propagate the spread of HIV within communities and the wider society, especially cultural norms that subvert the role of women in making key decisions such as those related to sexual health (Somefun, 2019; Toefy et al., 2019). There are also cultural practices within African communities that have been identified to act as protective factors or reduce the transmission of HIV. For instance, male circumcision and religious practices such as those that prescribe moral behaviours such as monogamy and abstinence from sexual relationships until marriage. Conversely, there are also religious practices that have correspondingly negative outcomes, such as opposition to the use of protective measures like condoms. Consequently, it could be argued that there is a complex relationship between epidemiology, HIV/AIDS and cultural practices within communities in SSA. An ethnographic study on the effects of traditional healing practices on HIV/AIDS management in South Africa found both beneficial and detrimental practices by traditional healers in the management of HIV/AIDS (Ndou-Mammbona, 2022). This complex relationship within this level further highlights the role of the societal level in the epidemiology of HIV/AIDS.

The Societal Level

Due to our recent understanding of the wider determinants of health and their roles in the health and well-being of societies, an argument could be made that the societal or situational level may be the most important domain when discussing the epidemiology of HIV/AIDS in SSA. Most health interventions targeting certain groups tend to oversimplify complex behaviours and overlook the social determinants in which people live (Corcoran, 2024). The relevance of this level and the wider social factors further inform the need for a social epidemiological outlook on the issue of HIV/AIDS within the SSA setting. For Poundstone et al.

(2004, p. 24), the structural factors from a social epidemiological perspective of HIV/AIDS include "war and militarization", "demographic changes", "structural violence and discrimination", "legal structures" and "policy environment". Several studies have independently considered the impact of these factors on the epidemiology of HIV and/or AIDS. Paying attention to these structures moves the discussion and interventions from being predominantly considered at an individual level to addressing the root causes associated with exposures for those without the condition and management for those with this condition.

A clear link between societal factors and the epidemiology of HIV/AIDS could be deduced from the prevalence and incidence of the condition being predominant among the most deprived or poorest communities in SSA. An estimated 26.0 million [23.6–28.8 million] people were living with HIV in 2023", (WHO, 2004, p. 3).

A little argument is needed to make the case for the need of a robust healthcare system in the prevention and management of HIV/AIDS, which is something most SSA countries lack.

According to Poundstone et al. situational factors comprise of the following: the policy environment, legal structures, structural violence and discrimination, demographic changes and war and militarisation, that is, the environment in which people live and work. A useful concept to consider is Bourdieu's symbolic violence:

> The most personal is the most impersonal, that many of the most intimate dramas the deepest malaises, the most singular suffering that men and women can experience find their roots in the objective contradictions, constraints and double binds inscribed in the structure of the labour market, the school system and housing or in the mechanics of economics and social inheritance.
> *Bourdieu and Wacquant (1992, p. 201)*

Violence is symbolic, although it must also be acknowledged that many people live in fear of actual violence being perpetrated.

Policies can disadvantage many people; for example, the structure of a society can disadvantage women and ensure they are in a subordinate position. Many countries have anti-homosexual legislation. In terms of AIDS/HIV infection, it can mean that many people are reluctant to come forward for treatment. Structural violence and discrimination are also reflected in the attitudes of people, resulting in racism, discrimination against women and other groups.

Qualitative research around the structural factors would largely explore individual experiences. An example of this is the work of Dugassa (2009), who considered women's health and violations of human rights in the context of AIDS/HIV and, in doing so, considered how these factors can interact with health. She argued that lack of freedom can affect choices in life; the experience of AIDS/HIV can have different trajectories in someone who is affluent compared to those who are socially and economically disadvantaged.

Dugassa (2009) outlines the human rights violations affecting many women in Africa: lack of sexual freedom, neglect of health issues and lack of access to education, to name a few. All contribute to a higher risk of infection and a lack of effective treatment. She gives the example of Oromo men in Ethiopia conscripted by the government to the army. Many of the men died, leaving impoverished widows who turned to sex work. The government did not think that many would survive and neglected health education around HIV and AIDS. The soldiers used sex workers, and when they returned home, infected their wives, unwitting spreading HIV infection. These examples can be replicated in different situations but illustrate the point of how structural factors can, in a very real way, affect the course and outcome of diseases.

The Work of Paul Farmer

It is useful to discuss the work of the physician and anthropologist Dr Paul Framer (1959–2022) (Farmer, 2004a, 2004b). He was a physician and anthropologist, and through his anthropological studies, he came to appreciate the interplay of the wider social determinants of health and the health status of individuals. Paul carried out ethnographic studies of AIDS sufferers in Haiti and highlighted their experience and how the structural factors greatly exacerbated their position. Ethnography was, as he ably demonstrated, a very powerful tool to illustrate and illuminate the plight of many people and how the illness trajectory could differ so greatly depending on circumstances, infrastructure, and income.

Farmer was not content to only highlight the ways in which the biological could interact with societal and socio-political factors that exacerbate illnesses. He also took practical steps to mitigate these wider factors; he emphasised the importance of reducing social inequalities as part of the treatment package, and he set up several schemes. In 1987, he founded Partners in Health which has as its slogan "we believe quality health care is a universal human right around the world; we fight injustice by providing care first to those who need it most" (Partners in Care, 2024). He founded, in partnership with the Cummings Foundation and the Bill and Melissa Gates foundation, the Global Health University in Buttaro, Rwanda, which trains a new generation in these principles.

Conclusion

This chapter considers the ways in which qualitative research can enhance and illuminate the experiences of individuals and groups. This is particularly relevant when looking at health and illness. It can tell the story of the illness experience of individuals and their illness trajectory, thus illuminating many of the problems and inequalities in the contemporary universe. It can also look at the wider determinants of health and tell the story of the individual against these factors and the ways in which particular outcomes can be inevitable. These points were illustrated through consideration of the individual level, interpersonal relationships, the community level and the wider factors occurring at a societal level.

References

Adeoye-Agboola, D.I., Evans, H., Hewson, D. and Pappas, Y. (2016) 'Factors influencing HIV disclosure among people living with HIV/AIDS in Nigeria: a systematic review using narrative synthesis and meta-analysis'. *Public Health* 136, pp. 13–28. doi: 10.1016/j.puhe.2016.02.021.

Agar, M. (2003) 'Toward a qualitative epidemiology'. *Qualitative Health Research* 13(7), pp. 974–986. doi: 10.1177/1049732303256886.

Anyaike, C., Atoyebi, O.A., Musa, O.I., Bolarinwa, O.A., Durowade, K.A., Ogundiran, A. and Babatunde, O.A. (2019) 'Adherence to combined Antiretroviral therapy (cART) among people living with HIV/AIDS in a Tertiary Hospital in Ilorin, Nigeria'. *Pan African Medical Journal* 32(1). Available at: https://www.ajol.info/index.php/pamj/article/view/207962 (Accessed: 29 September 2023).

Bannister-Tyrrell, M. and Meiqari, L. (2020) 'Qualitative research in epidemiology: theoretical and methodological perspectives'. *Annals of Epidemiology* 49, pp. 27–35. doi: 10.1016/j.annepidem.2020.07.008.

Baral, S., Logie, C.H., Grosso, A., Wirtz, A.L. and Beyrer, C. (2013) 'Modified social ecological model: a tool to guide the assessment of the risks and risk contexts of HIV epidemics'. *BMC Public Health* 13, p. 482. doi: 10.1186/1471-2458-13-482.

Berkman, L.F., Kawachi, I. and Glymour, M.M. (2014) *Social epidemiology*. Oxford University Press, Oxford, United Kingdom.

Bourdieu, P. and Wacquant, L.J. (1992) *An invitation to reflexive sociology* (Vol. 106, p. 97). Cambridge: Polity.

Corcoran, N. (2024) *Health promotion: the basics*. Oxford: Routledge.

Creswell, J.W. (2018) *Qualitative inquiry & research design: choosing among five approaches* (4th ed.). London: SAGE Publications.

Creswell, J.W. and Creswell, J.D. (2017) *Research design: qualitative, quantitative, and mixed methods approaches*. SAGE Publications, USA.

Damulira, C. et al. (2019) 'Examining the relationship of social support and family cohesion on ART adherence among HIV-positive adolescents in southern Uganda: baseline findings'. *Vulnerable Children and Youth Studies* 14(2), pp. 181–190. doi: 10.1080/17450128.2019.1576960.

Denzin, N.K. and Lincoln, Y.S. (2011) *The SAGE handbook of qualitative research*. SAGE.

De Wet, N., Akinyemi, J. and Odimegwu, C. (2019) 'How much do they know? An analysis of the accuracy of HIV knowledge among youth affected by HIV in South Africa'. *Journal of the International Association of Providers of AIDS Care (JIAPAC)* 18, p. 2325958218822306. doi: 10.1177/2325958218822306.

Duby, Z., Jonas, K., McClinton Appollis, T., Maruping, K., Dietrich, J. and Mathews, C. (2021) '"Condoms are boring": navigating relationship dynamics, gendered power, and motivations for condomless sex amongst adolescents and young people in South Africa'. *International Journal of Sexual Health* 33(1), pp. 40–57. doi: 10.1080/19317611.2020.1851334.

Dugassa, B.F. (2009) 'Women's rights and women's health during HIV/AIDS epidemics: the experience of women in sub-Saharan Africa'. *Health Care for Women International* 30(8), pp. 690–706. doi: 10.1080/07399330903018377.

Estifanos, T.M., Hui, C., Tesfai, A.W., Teklu, M.E., Ghebrehiwet, M.A., Embaye, K.S. and Andegiorgish, A.K. (2021) 'Predictors of HIV/AIDS comprehensive knowledge and acceptance attitude towards people living with HIV/AIDS among unmarried young females in Uganda: a cross-sectional study'. *BMC Women's Health* 21(1), p. 37. doi: 10.1186/s12905-021-01176-w.

Farmer, P. (2004a) An anthropology of structural violence. *Current Anthropology* 45(3), pp. 305–325.

Farmer, P. (2004b) *Pathologies of power: Health, human rights, and the new war on the poor* (Vol. 4). University of California Press.

Gardner, J. (2013) The experiences of HIV-positive women living in an African Village: perceptions of voluntary counseling and testing programs. *Journal of Transcultural Nursing* 24(1), pp. 25–32. doi: 10.1177/1043659612462404.

Geertz, C. (2008) 'Thick description: toward an interpretive theory of culture'. In Oakes, T., & Price, P. L. (Eds.). *The Cultural Geography Reader* (pp. 41–51). London: Routledge.

Gregory, D.M. and Way, C.Y. (2009) 'Qualitative research in clinical epidemiology'. *Methods in Molecular Biology* 473, pp. 203–215. doi: 10.1007/978-1-59745-385-1_12.

Hedges, K. (2021) 'Maasai girls' experiences of Ukimwi ni Homa (AIDS is a fever): idioms of vulnerability and HIV risk in East Africa'. *Human Organization* 80(4), pp. 332–342.

Kaufman, M.R., Cornish, F., Zimmerman, R.S. and Johnson, B.T. (2014) 'Health behavior change models for HIV prevention and AIDS care: practical recommendations for a multi-level approach'. *Journal of Acquired Immune Deficiency Syndromes (1999)* 66(Suppl 3), pp. S250–S258. doi: 10.1097/QAI.0000000000000236.

Kilanowski, J.F. (2017) 'Breadth of the socio-ecological model'. *Journal of Agromedicine* 22(4), pp. 295–297. doi: 10.1080/1059924X.2017.1358971.

Kipp, W., Tindyebwa, D., Rubaale, T., Karamagi, E. and Bajenja, E. (2007) 'Family caregivers in Rural Uganda: the hidden reality'. *Health Care for Women International* 28(10), pp. 856–871. doi: 10.1080/07399330701615275.

Knottnerus, B.J., Bertels, L.S. and Willems, D.L. (2020) 'Qualitative approaches can strengthen generalization and application of clinical research'. *Journal of Clinical Epidemiology* 119, pp. 136–139. doi: 10.1016/j.jclinepi.2019.11.002.

Krieger, N. (2001) 'Theories for social epidemiology in the 21st century: an ecosocial perspective'. *International Journal of Epidemiology* 30(4), pp. 668–677. doi: 10.1093/ije/30.4.668.

Li, L., Wu, S., Wu, Z., Sun, S., Cui, H. and Jia, M. (2006) 'Understanding family support for people living with HIV/AIDS in Yunnan, China'. *AIDS Behaviour* 10(5), pp. 509–517. doi: 10.1007/s10461-006-9071-0.

Madiba, S., Ralebona, E. and Lowane, M. (2021) 'Perceived stigma as a contextual barrier to early uptake of HIV testing, treatment initiation, and disclosure; the case of patients admitted with AIDS-related illness in a rural hospital in South Africa'. *Healthcare* 9(8), p. 962. doi: 10.3390/healthcare9080962.

Mattes, D. (2014) '"Life is not a rehearsal, it's a performance": an ethnographic enquiry into the subjectivities of children and adolescents living with antiretroviral treatment in northeastern Tanzania'. *Children and Youth Services Review* 45, pp. 28–37. doi: 10.1016/j.childyouth.2014.03.035.

Merten, S., Kenter, E., McKenzie, O., Musheke, M., Ntalasha, H. and Martin-Hilber, A. (2010) 'Patient-reported barriers and drivers of adherence to antiretrovirals in sub-Saharan Africa: a meta-ethnography'. *Tropical Medicine & International Health* 15(s1), pp. 16–33. doi: 10.1111/j.1365–3156.2010.02510.x.

Mitchell, E. et al. (2021) 'A socio-ecological analysis of factors influencing HIV treatment initiation and adherence among key populations in Papua New Guinea'. *BMC Public Health* 21, p. 2003. doi: 10.1186/s12889-021-12077-w.

Mokwele, T., Peu, D. and Moeta, M. (2023) 'Support needs of young adults on antiretroviral therapy in Capricorn District, Limpopo province'. *Health SA Gesondheid* 28. doi: 10.4102/hsag.v28i0.2125.

Mthembu, Z., Maharaj, P. and Rademeyer, S. (2019) '"I am aware of the risks, I am not changing my behaviour": risky sexual behaviour of university students in a high-HIV context'. *African Journal of AIDS Research* 18(3), pp. 244–253. doi: 10.2989/16085906.2019.1655075.

Ndou-Mammbona, A.A. (2022) 'The effects of traditional healing on HIV and AIDS management: an ethnographic study'. *South African Family Practice* 64(1), p. 5559. doi: 10.4102/safp.v64i1.5559.

Popay, J. (2003) 'Qualitative research and the epidemiological imagination: a vital relationship'. *Gaceta Sanitaria* 17(Supl.3), pp. 58–63. doi: 10.1157/13057793.

Poundstone, K.E., Strathdee, S.A. and Celentano, D.D. (2004) 'The social epidemiology of human immunodeficiency virus/acquired immunodeficiency syndrome'. *Epidemiologic Reviews* 26(1), pp. 22–35. doi: 10.1093/epirev/mxh005.

Safdar, N., Abbo, L.M., Knobloch, M.J. and Seo, S.K. (2016) 'Research methods in healthcare epidemiology: survey and qualitative research'. *Infection Control and Hospital Epidemiology* 37(11), pp. 1272–1277. doi: 10.1017/ice.2016.171.

Sale, J.E.M. and Thielke, S. (2018) 'Qualitative research is a fundamental scientific process'. *Journal of Clinical Epidemiology* 102, pp. 129–133. doi: 10.1016/j.jclinepi.2018.04.024.

Salihu, H.M., Wilson, R.E., King, L.M., Marty, P.J. and Whiteman, V.E. (2015) 'Socioecological model as a framework for overcoming barriers and challenges in randomized control trials in minority and underserved communities'. *International Journal of MCH and AIDS* 3(1), pp. 85–95.

Scarneo, S.E. et al. (2019) 'The socioecological framework: a multifaceted approach to preventing sport-related deaths in high school sports'. *Journal of Athletic Training* 54(4), pp. 356–360. doi: 10.4085/1062–6050–173-18.

Silva, S. and Fraga, S. (2012) 'Qualitative research in epidemiology'. doi: 10.5772/32986.

Somefun, O.D. (2019) 'Religiosity and sexual abstinence among Nigerian youths: does parent religion matter?' *BMC Public Health* 19, p. 416. doi: 10.1186/s12889-019-6732-2.

Sovran, S. (2013) 'Understanding culture and HIV/AIDS in sub-Saharan Africa'. *Sahara J* 10(1), pp. 32–41. doi: 10.1080/17290376.2013.807071.

Tarkang, E.E., Lutala, P.M. and Dzah, S.M. (2019) 'Knowledge, attitudes and practices regarding HIV/AIDS among senior high school students in Sekondi-Takoradi metropolis, Ghana'. *African Journal of Primary Health Care and Family Medicine* 11(1), pp. 1–11. doi: 10.4102/phcfm.v11i1.1875.

Thompson, S. and Schick-Makaroff, K. (2021) 'Qualitative research in clinical epidemiology'. In Parfrey, P.S. and Barrett, B.J. (eds.) *Clinical epidemiology: practice and methods. Methods in molecular biology* (pp. 369–388). New York: Springer. Available at: https://doi.org/10.1007/978-1-0716-1138-8_20 (Accessed: 21 September 2023).

Toefy, Y., Skinner, D. and Thomsen, S.C. (2019) 'What do you mean i've got to wait for six weeks?!' Understanding the sexual behaviour of men and their female partners after voluntary medical male circumcision in the Western Cape. *PLoS One* 10(7), p. e0133156. doi: 10.1371/journal.pone.0133156.

van de Ruit, C. (2019) 'Unintended consequences of community health worker programs in South Africa'. *Qualitative Health Research* 29(11), pp. 1535–1548. doi: 10.1177/1049732319857059.

von dem Knesebeck, O. (2015) 'Concepts of social epidemiology in health services research'. *BMC Health Services Research* 15(1), p. 357. doi: 10.1186/s12913-015-1020-z.

Ware, N.C. et al. (2009) 'Explaining adherence success in sub-Saharan Africa: an ethnographic study'. *PLoS Medicine* 6(1), p. e11. doi: 10.1371/journal.pmed.1000011.

Whyte, W.F. (2012) *Street corner society: the social structure of an Italian slum.* University of Chicago Press, Chicago, Illinois, USA.

World Health Organisation (2024) *HIV statistics, globally and by WHO region.* World Heath Organisation.

Yuh, J.N., Ellwanger, K., Potts, L. and Ssenyonga, J. (2014) 'Stigma among HIV/AIDS patients in Africa: a critical review'. *Procedia - Social and Behavioral Sciences* 140, pp. 581–585. doi: 10.1016/j.sbspro.2014.04.474.

PART 2

Exploring Contexts, Challenges, and Inequalities in Infectious and Chronic Diseases across Africa

5

SOCIO-STRUCTURAL FACTORS INFLUENCING MALARIA EPIDEMIOLOGY

Philip Emeke Anyanwu, Adilson De Pina and Vivian Osuchukwu'

Introduction

Malaria has been a major global health issue for centuries. Its burden goes beyond the discovery of the causal parasite in the 19th century by Alphonse Laveran in Algeria.[1] It is a life-threatening disease caused by Plasmodium parasites transmitted to people through the bites of infected female Anopheles mosquitoes.[2] Of the Plasmodium parasite species, only five have been identified to cause malaria in humans. These include *Plasmodium falciparum, Plasmodium vivax, Plasmodium malariae, Plasmodium ovale* and *Plasmodium knowlesi*. Among these five species, *P. falciparum* and *P. vivax* cause the most malaria cases globally; *P. falciparum* is the most common species causing malaria morbidity and mortality, especially in the sub-Saharan Africa region where most malaria infections occur.[3]

In 2020, an estimated 241 million malaria cases and 657,000 deaths occurred in 85 malaria-endemic countries; about 95% (228 million) of the cases and 92% (602,000) of the deaths were in the WHO African Region.[3] The number of malaria cases has seen fluctuations globally, especially in the WHO African Region. The region has seen a consistent reduction in malaria burden in the last two decades, with the number of cases dropping from 368 per 1,000 population at risk in 2,000 to 222 per 1,000 population in 2019.[3] However, in 2020, the direction of malaria incidence changed with an increase in the number of cases to 232 per 1,000 people. A similar trend is seen in malaria deaths in the WHO African Region (840,000 in 2000, 534,000 in 2019 and 602,000 in 2020). These changes in malaria burden have been attributed to factors such as antimalarial resistance and the disruptive impact of the COVID-19 pandemic on malaria response in the WHO African Region.[3]

DOI: 10.4324/9781003467601-7

Also, the persistent, relatively high burden of malaria in Africa is partly explained by environmental and socioeconomic factors that drive the transmission and determine the outcome of malaria infection. The link between economic development and malaria is well established.[4,5] The pattern of global malaria distribution is consistent with the theory of epidemiologic transition.[6] The intrinsic relationship between malaria and poverty remains a significant factor in sustaining this preventable and treatable disease.

This chapter discusses the role of socio-structural factors in the uneven distribution of malaria risk, the adoption of preventive measures, treatment-seeking behaviours, illness experiences and outcomes from malaria infection within and between endemic countries. It also covers contemporary issues such as antimalarial resistance. We present evidence from Nigeria (a high malaria-endemic country) and Cabo Verde (currently at the pre-certification stage towards achieving an elimination status) on the contributions of socio-structural factors in malaria epidemiology in Africa.

Environmental and Sociocultural Factors in Malaria Risk

The determinants of malaria risk go beyond biological factors. Environmental factors play an essential role in malaria risk. Contextual environmental factors, such as living in a tropical country endemic to malaria, put one at risk of malaria infection.[7] As of 2020, 85 countries were still malaria-endemic[3]; most of these countries have the enabling climatic factors (high temperature, humidity and rainfall) for the Anopheles mosquitoes that transmit malaria to survive and multiply. For instance, Nigeria, the country with the highest malaria burden (26.8% and 27% of global malaria cases and deaths in 2020),[3] has a tropical climate with a mean annual temperature of about 27°C. Among endemic populations, malaria infection risk is directly proportional to the vector population and exposure to mosquito bites.

The geographical location of a population impacts its economic activities; this interaction can influence malaria risk and the success of control programmes. For instance, located in the middle of the Atlantic, Cabo Verde's position is considered strategic in connecting Africa, Europe and America. Its openness and positioning between the different ideological and political currents have earned the country good acceptance by the international community and trade. However, these features of Cabo Verde have impacted its efforts to achieve malaria elimination, as the number of reported malaria cases since 2010 has been mostly imported cases.[8]

In addition to contextual factors, compositional factors also play a role in determining malaria risk and epidemiology. The characteristics of populations, such as levels of education, income, culture and concentration, can influence understanding of the aetiology of malaria and its prevention, treatment, and control. Inaccurate knowledge and perception of malaria aetiology—such as high consumption of fatty food, exposure to the sun and spiritual forces as causes of malaria—are driven by social constructions, mostly common in those at lower levels of the socioeconomic gradient.[9,10]

Culture also influences malarial risk related to prevention and treatment-seeking behaviours by shaping norms, practices and perceptions about illnesses, recognition of illness and decisions on where to seek treatment.[11] The multiple symptoms associated with malaria influence beliefs around its aetiology; this is seen in instances where communities share multiple beliefs on what causes malaria.[12] The cultural belief that attacks from spiritual forces cause malaria exists in Nigeria. There are different dimensions to this belief in the spiritual aetiology of malaria: the first dimension involves a belief in sole causation (i.e. malaria is only caused by spiritual attacks); the second dimension draws on multiple causations (i.e. malaria can be caused by spiritual attacks as well as the malaria parasite transmitted through mosquito bites, for example); and the third dimension sees malaria as a gateway for spiritual attacks. For example, some of the participants in a qualitative study by Anyanwu et al.[12] believed that spiritual forces can "pass through malaria" and explain some of their "mysterious" oral symptoms, such as bitter taste. Although not a common symptom, bitter taste is an established clinical oral symptom of malaria.[13,14] The influence of sociocultural factors on malaria causality translates to behaviours that determine levels of infection risk in a population.

Inequalities in Malaria Diagnosis and Treatment

Early diagnosis and treatment of malaria remain a critical aspect of malaria control. The World Health Organisation recommends that all suspected malaria cases be confirmed using parasite-based diagnostic testing before treatment.[7] Tests before treatment are important in controlling the overuse of antimalarials by ensuring malaria medications are only used in cases where treatment is indicated. In addition, diagnostic testing before treatment is more cost-effective in the long term than presumptive treatment. Consequently, the need for a confirmatory test for malaria before treatment informed the Test, Treat and Track strategy rolled out by the WHO in 2012. The available parasite-based diagnostic tests for malaria are microscopy, rapid diagnostic tests (RDTs) and polymerase chain reaction. The availability and use of these diagnostic tests in suspected malaria cases are patterned in endemic populations by social and economic factors, health system policies and performance and the level of malaria endemicity.

The cost of malaria diagnostic tests is a significant factor in their use, aiding the practice of presumptive diagnosis. The average cost of diagnosis by RDT is between USD1 and 2 per test, with microscopy slightly cheaper.[10,15] This is substantial, especially in Nigeria and Cabo Verde, where 40% and 35%, respectively, live below the national poverty lines.

In Nigeria, presumptive malaria diagnosis is common in public and private health facilities and among drug retailers and pharmacies. The high rate of presumptive diagnosis and treatment of malaria in Nigeria calls for major action. This trend is partly because of the National Policy on Malaria in Nigeria, which still recommends malaria treatment for suspected fever cases. The study by Mangham et al.[16] on the treatment of uncomplicated malaria at public health facilities and medicine retailers in southeastern Nigeria found that very few health facilities in the region offered malaria microscopy testing. The study also reported that among all health facilities—both public health facilities and retail outlets—surveyed, none offered RDTs. The findings from other studies on antimalarial use in Nigeria highlight the intensity of presumptive diagnosis and treatment. Some of these studies, like Onwujekwe et al.[17] and Uzochukwu et al.,[18] have shown that treatment through medicine outlets is mainly based on a presumptive diagnosis, with most of the patients treated classified as cases where antimalarial treatment is not indicated. Other factors, such as a population's level of malaria endemicity, also contribute to presumptive diagnosis and treatment.

Presumptive malaria diagnosis tends to be more prevalent in highly endemic countries compared to those at the pre-elimination stage. For instance, in Cabo Verde, between 2010 and 2019, all 814 cases of malaria were confirmed by RDT and/or microscopy.[8,19,20] With the number of malaria cases as low as approximately 30 per year in Cabo Verde, the cost of malaria diagnosis through microscopy and RDT is substantially low compared to a highly endemic setting like Nigeria, where the number of cases per year can be up to 70 million.

Similar to diagnosis, inequalities exist in malaria treatment-seeking behaviour. Socioeconomic factors have always played a role in malaria treatment-seeking.[21] Income level as a socioeconomic factor reflects financial abilities, which can determine treatment-seeking behaviours such as choosing a health facility for treatment[22] and the use of diagnostic tests prior to treatment.[21] Income and education level have repeatedly been reported to affect adherence to malaria treatment guidelines, especially among those of low income.[23–25] Education level as a socioeconomic factor can determine access to adequate information needed to make an informed malaria treatment decision.[26]

Inequalities in physical infrastructures, such as the location of health facilities and road networks, can affect malaria treatment-seeking behaviours by determining access, the source of treatment and the availability of healthcare professionals.[27] In addition, the location of a facility can influence its usage and the characteristics/demographies of its users. These physical factors could be the effects of political forces on the population.

The importance of good access to health facilities in promoting prompt malaria seeking behaviour is seen in Cabo Verde, where about 64% of malaria patients will present in a formal health facility within 24 hours of the onset of malaria symptoms; this increases to 88% in 48 hours. Despite the good treatment-seeking behaviour of the Cabo Verdean population, there is still more to do to achieve 100% of patients promptly seeking treatment at the health facilities; this is important in the timely treatment of malaria to prevent further transmission and crucial in the country's achievement and sustainability of an elimination status.[28]

Artemisinin-based combination therapies (ACTs) have been the first-line treatment for malaria. However, the choice of the combination drug differs across populations depending on the level of resistance to the second drug. For instance, in the WHO African region, Artemether-lumefantrine, artesunate-amodiaquine, artesunate-pyronaridine and dihydroartemisinin-piperaquine are the recommended first-line treatments for malaria. Each malaria-endemic country in this region will have one of these as its national first-line therapy.[3] Using the recommended antimalarials helps to reduce wastage and unnecessary costs by ensuring that drugs that the Plasmodium parasites in the population are sensitive to are used in malaria treatment. Nevertheless, whether to use recommended ACTs or not can be influenced by the interaction of different factors, most importantly socioeconomic.

When treatment is sought for malaria infection, socioeconomic inequalities can determine the quality of treatment received and outcomes. In settings like Nigeria, where the out-of-pocket health system is adopted, healthcare costs are relatively high, and healthcare expenditure accounts for most household domestic spending. Appropriate treatments become challenging for households with low incomes. The adoption of treatment options for cost-coping, such as the mixing of drugs (the practice of combining different drugs to treat malaria. "Mixing" involves the combination of single doses from each of the included drugs to form a mixed dose)[29] affects treatment outcomes by increasing the likelihood of experiencing treatment failure and the development of antimalarial resistance. The adoption of this cost-coping practice is unequally distributed in the Nigerian population, particularly higher among those in lower-income and rural settlements.

The cost of malaria treatment also drives other risky behaviours, such as stopping the treatment to save the medications for future use and sharing antimalarial courses among two or more people. In most cases of sharing antimalarials with others, all parties involved do not get a complete treatment course.[12] These practices have implications for the development and spread of antimalarial resistance, which is currently an important threat to malaria control.

The Role of Socio-Structural Factors in Malaria Prevention

The transmission mechanism of malaria is an integral aspect of the infection. The *Plasmodium* parasite has a complex life cycle, parts of which are spent in a human host (asexual reproductive stage) and a mosquito host (sexual reproductive stage).[30] Therefore, for a successful life cycle and transmission of the infection, the parasite requires both human and mosquito hosts. Hence, most of the preventive measures are centred around interrupting the completion of the two stages of the plasmodium life cycle.

Malaria preventive measures are usually centred on vector control by reducing the vector population and personal protection from the vector (mosquito bites). The currently used malaria preventive measures can be broadly categorised into two: those that involve the use of preventive tools (insecticide-treated nets (ITN), indoor residual spraying (IRS) with insecticide, use of nets on windows and doors and malaria prophylaxis, among others) and those that do not (hence are centred mainly on human behaviours. Examples: avoiding stagnant water around the home; avoiding staying or sleeping outside at night; wearing long-sleeved shirts and trousers at night times; and closing doors and windows at night time). It is important to understand the human behaviour and socio-structural context in which malaria behaviours occur to prevent and control malaria effectively.[31] A major barrier to using malaria preventive tools is the financial cost of acquiring them.[32] This issue is more pronounced in the highly endemic areas where almost the entire population is constantly at risk of malaria infection; therefore, affording these preventive tools all year round becomes a challenge for those of low income levels.

As in most malaria-endemic countries, socio-structural factors play a role in malaria preventive behaviours in Nigeria. To put this into perspective, let's look at some of the contextual issues faced by the Nigerian population. Most parts of Nigeria have limited social infrastructures, such as electricity and a poor drainage system. With the high temperature in Nigeria all year round, sweating at night is a common challenge. This issue is further exacerbated by the unsteady electricity power supply, which limits the use of temperature control devices such as electric fans and air conditioners, especially at night times. Consequently, some of the measures used to cope with the heat include opening doors and windows at night time for ventilation or sleeping out in the open.[12] Although these behaviours help reduce the issue of sweating at night, they increase exposure to mosquito bites and malaria transmission. A similar mechanism is seen in relation to the interaction between socio-structural factors, the climate and the use of ITNs as a malaria preventive tool. One of the most reported reasons for inconsistency in the use of ITNs is sweating when sleeping under the bednets, especially on a hot night with no electricity to power fans and air conditioners.[12] The ability to afford and run private electricity generators through the night partly explains the differences in ITN use for malaria prevention, consistently higher among the least deprived.[33]

Knowledge and understanding of the cause of a disease condition play a significant role in shaping societal perceptions, which can subsequently reflect in their preventive and treatment-seeking behaviours for the disease. Although knowledge of the causation and preventability of malaria is moderate to high in most endemic areas, the rate of wrong perceptions on the cause of malaria is still concerning and affects efforts to prevent malaria. For instance, perceiving spiritual forces as a sole or contributory cause of malaria can affect the use of preventive measures against mosquito bites. Furthermore, the distribution of these perceptions by social factors contributes to the inequalities in malaria prevention, infection and outcomes. Also, the perception of spiritual attack as a cause of malaria is significantly associated with education level and type of settlement (urban/rural).[9] On perceptions regarding prevention, a study in Cabo Verde showed that even though most respondents believe that malaria is preventable, the perception of low risk or severity can lead to inaction in preventing the infection at the individual level.[28] This shifts the burden of malaria prevention to local health facilities already tasked with malaria treatment.

Threats to Sustainable Malaria Control: Climate Change and Antimicrobial Resistance

The sustainability of efforts to control diseases refers to the ability to retain the effectiveness of strategies and tools used to reduce morbidity and mortality due to the condition. With increased focus on achieving elimination at the country level and global eradication of malaria, the need for sustainable malaria control approaches has become necessary.

Socio-structural factors, such as cultural beliefs and constructions around public health strategies and tools for controlling infectious diseases, can threaten the optimal application of such tools in disease control and eradication. This has been seen in poliomyelitis, where social constructions in some African countries around the polio vaccine deterred uptake, hindering polio eradication efforts. The recent improvements in malaria vaccine development and the WHO's recommendation for widespread use of the RTS,S/AS01 (RTS,S) malaria vaccine among children in Sub-Saharan Africa and other regions with moderate to high *P. falciparum* malaria transmission are expected to facilitate malaria eradication and elimination. However, the sustainability of the impact of this primary preventive measure for malaria control can be threatened by social constructions and beliefs. The need to sustain the effectiveness of malaria vaccines is further amplified by the fact that vaccines, in the long term, are a cheap preventive tool and one of the few primary preventive tools for malaria that do not rely on vector control. Vector control tools, such as IRS, can be expensive as they require recurrent spending.

A consolidated effort is required to achieve global malaria elimination. A high level of malaria endemicity in one country can threaten malaria eradication achievements in other countries. For instance, in Cabo Verde, malaria importation from neighbouring countries has been a critical pathway for reintroducing malaria to areas with zero local transmission, continuously threatening this population's sustainability of control efforts.

Climate change is also a threat to the sustainability of malaria control efforts. Changes in temperature, rainfall, and humidity can lead to parasite and vector readaptation, reintroducing malaria in areas that have achieved elimination. Similarly, extreme weather patterns increase the rates and patterns of rainfall and severe flooding, providing breeding grounds for mosquito vectors.

The development and spread of resistance to insecticides and antimalarials by mosquito vectors and Plasmodium parasites, respectively, is a major threat to sustainable malaria control. Insecticide resistance by malaria vectors threatens vector control strategies; this is crucial to the sustainability of current achievements.[34] Most malaria control's success is attributed to effective prevention through ITNs and IRS and treatment using ACTs. The extensive use of insecticides drives selection pressure on malaria vectors. Weak quality control, monitoring and evaluation of insecticide concentrations in malaria-endemic countries are also factors in insecticide resistance.

The development of resistance to antimalarials is not a new phenomenon. As far back as 1844 and 1910, there were reports of quinine resistance, although these reports were not supported by clear evidence. After the introduction of chloroquine, the first report of resistance against it (1957 in Asia) emerged rapidly. The spread of chloroquine resistance led to its replacement with sulphadoxine-pyrimethamine (SP) as the first-line drug in many countries in Asia, South America, and Africa. However, resistance to SP also emerged soon after its introduction.[35] These resistance developments were first reported and confirmed in Southeast Asia, then spread widely to the Sub-Saharan Africa region. The use of ACTs has contributed to the recent reduction in the global malaria burden since 2000. However, resistance to artemisinin in Southeast Asia and Africa is a significant challenge to sustaining recent achievements in malaria control. With no ideal candidate as a replacement drug for first-line treatment, resistance to artemisinin poses a considerable threat to global efforts to control and eradicate malaria.

Conclusion

Achieving malaria elimination requires a biopsychosocial approach to health. As a disease of poverty, understanding the socio-structural factors influencing malaria epidemiology in Africa is crucial for designing strategies to control malaria and optimising existing malaria control efforts. Sustainable malaria control requires a focus on the social determinants of malaria infection risk, prevention, and treatment. Given that the extent of the impact of sociostructural factors can differ based on the level of malaria endemicity in a population, interventions should be tailored to each population's health needs and context.

References

1. Harrison, G. A. *Mosquitoes, Malaria, and Man: A History of the Hostilities since 1880.* (Dutton, 1978).
2. World Health Organisation. Fact Sheet about Malaria. (2021).
3. World Health Organization. World Malaria Report 2021. (2021).
4. Rudasingwa, G. & Cho, S.-I. Determinants of the Persistence of Malaria in Rwanda. *Malaria Journal* **19**, 36 (2020).
5. Teklehaimanot, A. & Mejia, P. Malaria and Poverty. *Annals of the New York Academy of Sciences* **1136**, 32–37 (2008).
6. Sanders, J. W., Fuhrer, G. S., Johnson, M. D. & Riddle, M. S. The Epidemiological Transition: The Current Status of Infectious Diseases in the Developed World versus the Developing World. *Science Progress* **91**, 1–37 (2008).
7. World Health Organization. World Malaria Report 2016. (2016).
8. DePina, A. J. *et al.* Updates on Malaria Epidemiology and Profile in Cabo Verde from 2010 to 2019: The Goal of Elimination. *Malaria Journal* **19**, 380 (2020).
9. Anyanwu, P. *Contributory Role of Socioeconomic Factors in the Development and Spread of Antimalarial Drug Resistance.* (University of Sunderland, 2017).
10. Batwala, V., Magnussen, P., Hansen, K. S. & Nuwaha, F. Cost-effectiveness of Malaria Microscopy and Rapid Diagnostic Tests versus Presumptive Diagnosis: Implications for Malaria Control in Uganda. *Malaria Journal* **10**, 372 (2011).
11. Colvin, C. J. *et al.* Understanding Careseeking for Child Illness in Sub-Saharan Africa: A Systematic Review and Conceptual Framework Based on Qualitative Research of Household Recognition and Response to Child Diarrhoea, Pneumonia and Malaria. *Social Science & Medicine* **86**, 66–78 (2013).
12. Anyanwu, P. E., Fulton, J., Evans, E. & Paget, T. Exploring the Role of Socioeconomic Factors in the Development and Spread of Antimalarial Drug Resistance: A Qualitative Study. *Malaria Journal* **16**, 203 (2017).
13. Lasisi, T. J., Duru, M. E. & Lawal, B. B. Salivary Secretion and Composition in Malaria: A Case-control Study. *Nigerian Journal of Physiological Sciences* **30**, 119–123 (2015).
14. Shuai, Y. *et al.* Oral Manifestations Related to Malaria: A Systematic Review. *Oral Diseases* **27**, 1616–1620 (2021).
15. Du, Y.-Q. *et al.* Cost-effectiveness Analysis of Malaria Rapid Diagnostic Test in the Elimination Setting. *Infectious Diseases of Poverty* **9**, 135 (2020).
16. Mangham, L. J. *et al.* Treatment of Uncomplicated Malaria at Public Health Facilities and Medicine Retailers in Southeastern Nigeria. *Malaria Journal* **10**, 155 (2011).
17. Onwujekwe, O. *et al.* Where Do People from Different Socioeconomic Groups Receive Diagnosis and Treatment for Presumptive Malaria, in Southeastern Nigeria? *Annals of Tropical Medicine and Parasitology* **99**, 473–481 (2005).
18. Uzochukwu, B. S. C. *et al.* Examining Appropriate Diagnosis and Treatment of Malaria: Availability and Use of Rapid Diagnostic Tests and Artemisinin-based Combination Therapy in Public and Private Health Facilities in South East Nigeria. *BMC Public Health* **10**, 486 (2010).
19. DePina, A. J. *et al.* Spatiotemporal Characterisation and Risk Factor Analysis of Malaria Outbreak in Cabo Verde in 2017. *Tropical Medicine and Health* **47**, 3 (2019).
20. DePina, A. J. *et al.* Achievement of Malaria Pre-Elimination in Cape Verde According to the Data Collected from 2010 to 2016. *Malaria Journal* **17**, 236 (2018).

21. Uzochukwu, B. S. & Onwujekwe, O. E. Socio-Economic Differences and Health Seeking Behaviour for the Diagnosis and Treatment of Malaria: A Case Study of Four Local Government Areas Operating the Bamako Initiative Programme in South-East Nigeria. *International Journal of Equity in Health* **3**, 6 (2004).
22. Kiwanuka, S. N. *et al.* Access to and Utilisation of Health Services for the Poor in Uganda: A Systematic Review of Available Evidence. *Transactions of the Royal Society of Tropical Medicine and Hygiene* **102**, 1067–1074 (2008).
23. Beer, N. *et al.* Adherence to Artesunate-Amodiaquine Combination Therapy for Uncomplicated Malaria in Children in Zanzibar, Tanzania. *Tropical Medicine & International Health* **14**, 766–774 (2009).
24. Cohen, J. L., Yavuz, E., Morris, A., Arkedis, J. & Sabot, O. Do Patients Adhere to Over-the-Counter Artemisinin Combination Therapy for Malaria? Evidence from an Intervention Study in Uganda. *Malaria Journal* **11**, 83 (2012).
25. Onyango, E. O. *et al.* Factors Associated with Non-adherence to Artemisinin-based Combination Therapy (ACT) to Malaria in a Rural Population from Holoendemic Region of Western Kenya. *BMC Infectious Diseases* **12**, 143 (2012).
26. Hanson, K. *et al. The Economics of Malaria Control Interventions.* https://apps.who.int/iris/handle/10665/43004 (2004).
27. Chuma, J., Okungu, V. & Molyneux, C. Barriers to Prompt and Effective Malaria Treatment among the Poorest Population in Kenya. *Malaria Journal* 90
28. DePina, A. J. *et al.* Knowledge, Attitudes and Practices about Malaria in Cabo Verde: A Country in the Pre-Elimination Context. *BMC Public Health* **19**, 850 (2019).
29. Anyanwu, P. E., Fulton, J. & Evans, E. Socioeconomic Inequalities in the Adoption of Antimalarial Resistance-Promoting Behaviours: A Quantitative Study of the Use of Mixed Drugs for Malaria Treatment. *Journal of Public Health and Disease Prevention* **1**, (2018). url={https://api.semanticscholar.org/CorpusID:189800529}
30. Huijben, S. Experimental Studies on the Ecology and Evolution of Drug-Resistant Malaria Parasites. PhD thesis University of Edinburgh (2010) . available at https://era.ed.ac.uk/bitstream/handle/1842/3945/Huijben2010.pdf?sequence=1 accessed 29th June 2024.
31. Mwenesi, H. A. Social Science Research in Malaria Prevention, Management and Control in the Last Two Decades: An Overview. *Acta Tropica* **95**, 292–297 (2005).
32. Choonara, S., Odimegwu, C. O. & Elwange, B. C. Factors Influencing the Usage of Different Types of Malaria Prevention Methods during Pregnancy in Kenya. *African Health Sciences* **15**, 413–419 (2015).
33. Essé, C. *et al.* Social and Cultural Aspects of 'Malaria' and Its Control in Central Côte d'Ivoire. *Malaria Journal* **7**, 224 (2008).
34. Birkholtz, L.-M., Bornman, R., Focke, W., Mutero, C. & de Jager, C. Sustainable Malaria Control: Transdisciplinary Approaches for Translational Applications. *Malaria Journal* **11**, 431 (2012).
35. Talisuna, A. O., Bloland, P. & D'Alessandro, U. History, Dynamics, and Public Health Importance of Malaria Parasite Resistance. *Clinical Microbiology Reviews* **17**, 235–254 (2004).

6

VACCINE ACCEPTANCE IN AFRICA DURING THE COVID-19 PANDEMIC

Judith Eberhardt and Jonathan Ling

Introduction

The COVID-19 pandemic has had a profound global impact. As of 31 March 2022, over 483 million people had been infected, and more than 6.1 million people had died due to COVID-19.[1] However, the World Health Organization (WHO) estimates that the total number of excess deaths that were directly and indirectly attributable to COVID-19 in 2020 alone amounted to at least 3 million.[2] The total number of excess deaths worldwide due to the COVID-19 pandemic between 1 January 2020 and 31 December 2021 was estimated to be 18.2 million.[3] The pandemic brought with it unprecedented challenges, and although many of its impacts were similar between continents, some of these were, and continue to be, unique to Sub-Saharan Africa (SSA). Vaccinating the population of SSA against COVID-19 presents one such challenge.

This chapter focuses on the effect of COVID-19 on SSA. It explores the vaccination roll-out in SSA and the barriers and facilitators to vaccine uptake. An overview of research evidence on SSA on vaccine hesitancy is provided. Finally, we examine how social epidemiology can be used to explain and address COVID-19 vaccine uptake before exploring potential future directions in vaccine acceptance and uptake across SSA, not just in relation to COVID-19 but also for vaccination efforts more broadly in this region.

COVID-19 in Sub-Saharan Africa

The African continent was the last to be affected by the COVID-19 pandemic. Initially, cases were brought in from Europe and the USA rather than from the country of origin, China. Community transmissions were therefore the main driver

DOI: 10.4324/9781003467601-8

of infections.[4] Africa recorded its first case of COVID-19 in Egypt in February 2020. By April 2021, there were 4.5 million infections, over 121,000 fatalities, and around 4.1 million recoveries.[5] In SSA, South Africa was worst-affected by COVID-19, with more than 1.5 million infections, over 54,000 fatalities, and approximately 1.5 million recoveries by April 2021.[5] Although overall SSA has reported relatively few fatalities, a number of issues have affected its response to the pandemic, which means that COVID-19 is likely to have profound and long-term effects across the region.

Responses to the Pandemic

Early on in the pandemic, a unified African strategy was established by health ministers from across African nations.[6] This strategy focused on three elements – preventing COVID-19 transmission, avoiding deaths, and minimising social and economic harm. This included a travel ban for countries with ongoing outbreaks and local restrictions on travel and gatherings. Furthermore, countries were faced with the challenge of rolling out mass testing and securing personal protective equipment (PPE) for healthcare staff, ventilators, and hand sanitiser. In response to this challenge, the African Union and the Africa Centre for Disease Control (CDC) launched the Partnership to Accelerate COVID-19 Testing (PACT) and deployed 1 million community health workers to help with contact tracing. In 2021, the Africa CDC collaborated with WHO and other organisations to make 120 million rapid diagnostic tests available.[6] Furthermore, local manufacturing of items such as hand sanitiser, PPE, and ventilators has been on the rise in African countries. These efforts have contributed to lower death rates in Africa than in Europe or the USA. Furthermore, 80% of people with COVID-19 had mild or no symptoms, which is most likely attributable to the greater number of young people in Africa compared to Europe or North America. Kuehn additionally points out that Africa's past experience with infectious disease outbreaks most likely facilitated a rapid response to COVID-19.[6]

However, responses across SSA were variable, with misconceptions about COVID-19 influencing decision-making at both national and local policy and community levels. These include the beliefs that the temperature in SSA is too warm for COVID-19 to spread and that the strong immune systems of Africans would mean that the virus would be relatively harmless.[7] Despite inconsistencies in surveillance across SSA, the speed at which reported COVID-19 cases rose across the region led to a reconsideration of these beliefs among many. Unfortunately, responses to heightened concerns were not uniformly met with consistently robust health protection policies across the region.

Countries differed in terms of their lockdown measures in relation to international travel and closures of establishments, ranging from limited restrictions or relatively relaxed measures (e.g., Tanzania[8] and Sierra Leone[9]) to comparatively stricter measures (e.g., South Africa, Nigeria,[10] and Uganda[11]). Haider and colleagues[12] described the differing lockdown measures of nine SSA countries – Ghana, Nigeria, South Africa, Sierra Leone, Sudan, Tanzania, Uganda, Zambia, and Zimbabwe – at the start of the pandemic. All countries suspended international passenger flights early on and restricted land and sea border crossings as well, apart from the passage of goods and commodities. However, only Nigeria and Ghana implemented lockdown measures, and then only in specific areas within the country. While most countries kept restrictions on international travel, the Tanzanian government began lifting restrictions and abolishing mandatory quarantine for international arrivals in May 2020, albeit with enhanced screening of passengers on arrival.

The countries studied also differed in terms of the closure of establishments. Apart from Sierra Leone and Tanzania, non-essential businesses, hospitality, and recreational establishments were closed, although shops and markets continued to sell food and essential commodities. Sierra Leone allowed all shops and businesses to stay open apart from during two very short periods of lockdown, and Tanzania implemented no closures of shops, religious congregations, government offices, parliamentary sessions, or hospitality. All countries closed schools, colleges, and universities and either prohibited or restricted public and private gatherings.[12] South Africa was particularly severely affected by the pandemic compared to the rest of SSA[13] and implemented comparatively strict measures, with a strict lockdown during the early months of the pandemic. Due to South Africa's previous public health campaigns targeting the spread of HIV/AIDS, the country was able to apply the knowledge gained from these campaigns to dealing with COVID-19.[10]

Varying responses to the pandemic will most likely have contributed to the differing degrees of impact of the pandemic on each country in SSA. However, in addition to countries' responses to the pandemic, there are a number of other factors affecting outcomes. Notable among these are socioeconomic factors, the spread of misinformation, and conspiracy beliefs.

Socioeconomic Factors

Although there have been encouraging efforts in recent years to address the socioeconomic problems that worsen health inequalities, there remain grave disparities in health status, both between and within countries.[14] While these issues influence public health globally, such health disparities had a significant effect on the COVID-19 response in SSA. For example, health disparities in Nigeria influence the distribution of water and hygiene services among socioeconomically disadvantaged groups, which in turn may lead to significant negative effects on public health outcomes during pandemics such as COVID-19.[15] Common issues are lack of access to handwashing facilities; for example, in the Democratic Republic of the Congo (DRC), more than three-quarters of the population have no access to such facilities. Water scarcity also has a substantial influence on health in general and is becoming more severe due to climate change.[15] SSA is one of the world's regions most affected by income inequality, and poverty is associated with poorer health and disparities in health status.[16]

Being socioeconomically disadvantaged is associated with poorer access to healthcare,[17] and this had particularly devastating effects in countries where health systems are already weak and ill-equipped to deal with the pandemic. Responses to the pandemic were slow in SSA and inadequate for the magnitude of the problem. Interventions are needed to improve and strengthen the resilience of health systems, although these need to be funded through local, national, and global engagement.[18]

Global responses to the pandemic with lockdowns, closure of borders, workplaces, and schools, self-isolation of infected individuals, and social distancing led to a transformation of life for most people. The pandemic is likely to have exacerbated existing inequalities in access to infrastructure for those living in poverty. For many of those living in extreme poverty, changing one's life in response to COVID-19 restrictions was impossible. Public health recommendations, such as those made in South Africa,[19] failed to take account of these inequalities and adapt the advice to local and/or national contexts. The COVID-19 pandemic has exposed healthcare system limitations that exist both in the global north and the global south; the shortage of hospital beds and medical equipment, inadequate supply chains, and insufficient national surveillance systems are all testaments to these limitations. However, both within and between societies in SSA, there is a grossly uneven distribution of the health, social, and economic risks associated with the pandemic, as well as the public health measures implemented in response to the COVID-19 pandemic.[20]

Apart from health inequalities as a result of this uneven distribution of pandemic-associated risks, there is a significant gap in global COVID-19 vaccine access, with SSA being left behind other regions. High- and middle-income countries have sufficient access to vaccines and are therefore in a far better position to protect their populations from illness, thereby ensuring their return to economic and social activity. SSA countries, however, have been opening up to this activity without sufficient protection through vaccines, leading to wider circulation of the virus and potentially a reinstatement of lockdowns, which will in turn impact economically and socially. This has the potential to lead to a 'great divide' between high- and low-income nations, deepening gaps between them and increasing global instability, economic uncertainty, and geopolitical tensions.[21]

Conspiracy Beliefs and Misinformation

Conspiracy beliefs – the idea that governments or other organisations are responsible for unusual or unexplained phenomena – in relation to COVID-19 have arisen and been perpetuated during the pandemic. Early in the pandemic, Ola-tunji and colleagues[22] recruited Nigerian undergraduates through social media to explore their beliefs related to COVID-19. They found high levels of conspiracy beliefs, with the COVID-19 infection viewed by some respondents as "an exaggeration by the government and media" and as a "Chinese biological weapon." When asked about trusted sources of information related to COVID-19, participants cited the Nigeria Centre of Disease Control as the most trusted source, while information from political leaders and social media was perceived as the least trustworthy. This mirrors data collected globally, where political leaders are consistently viewed as the most untrustworthy sources of COVID-19 information, followed by social media.[23]

Religion is an important aspect of life for many people living in SSA, with a large proportion of adherents active in their faith, such as through regular church or mosque attendance. Although religion may have been a source of comfort for many during the pandemic, faith leaders can play a positive role in public health education through their ability to connect with large congregations. Such congregations may be receptive to public health messaging from a trusted source and also hard to reach in other ways by traditional public health campaigns due to a lack of access to TV, radio, or poor literacy. That said, religion has not always had a positive effect; most obviously, large congregations may cause the rapid spread of COVID-19 within communities. Churches and religious leaders have also played a role in disseminating conspiracy beliefs, undermining confidence in vaccinations, and adopting directly anti-science rhetoric. In particular, Fosuh-Ankrah and Amoako-Gyampah[24] discuss the directly antagonistic stance taken by religious leaders towards governmental and WHO public health efforts to limit the spread of COVID-19.

A key hindrance to responding effectively to the pandemic in SSA has been misinformation related to COVID-19. Misinformation can come from a range of sources, including social and traditional media, politicians, and religious figures. Misinformation can take many forms, such as conspiracy theories (e.g., the virus is man-made and spread as a deliberate attempt by global companies to take control) or the use of unproductive[25] and/or potentially harmful products to cure COVID-19.[26,27] For example, one home-made preparation reported on social media to possess antimicrobial, antiviral, and antibacterial properties had no effect on COVID-19 but did cause severe vomiting, life-threatening low blood pressure, and acute liver failure.[28] Numerous cases of chloroquine (a medicine used to treat malaria) overdose were reported after news reports falsely claimed its efficacy for the treatment of COVID-19.[29]

Although misinformation can potentially lead to over-reactions, such as panic-buying, which can lead to food insecurity and interpersonal violence, an even greater risk is when people under-react. This can take many forms, including failing to maintain social distancing, declining to wear masks, and refusing vaccinations. Such behaviours in response to misinformation or 'fake news' can spread the virus rapidly within communities[27] and supplant official public health advice on COVID-19. Ahinkorah et al.[30] argue that the current socio-political climate in Africa has helped the spread of COVID-19 misinformation through politicians promoting nationalism and anti-immigration views through video messages, pictures, interviews, and newspapers to provide false claims for personal or political gain.[31] Misinformation has also been spread through social media, with provocative ('click bait') headlines promising cures for COVID-19 or promoting concerns about vaccines. Although these stories may only be written to drive advertising revenue for those operating the blogs, they have real-world consequences in terms of health behaviours and, ultimately, increasing the number of coronavirus cases.

If left unchecked, misinformation also spreads like a virus and has the potential to undermine public trust in wider public health activities, such as hand washing and vaccinations against non-COVID-19 diseases. WHO[32] has recently reported the first global increase in tuberculosis in more than a decade, which may be related to an increase in vaccine hesitancy generally, as a direct consequence of heightened reluctance to receive vaccination for COVID-19. Undermining trust in the efforts of governments, the WHO, and other organisations to combat COVID-19, therefore has a far wider potential to negatively affect population health.

Social media has a global reach. Although it has been a source of misinformation, it can also help spread accurate messaging, especially if delivered through a trusted channel (e.g., WHO, Centre for Disease Control). As most people in SSA who access the Internet do so through their phones, it is important that any messaging is optimised for small screens, is clear, and is just as easy to share as misinformation. Social media platforms also have a duty here by flagging, hiding, or removing misinformation and promoting information that has been fact-checked and comes from credible sources.[30] Numerous fact-checking websites have also been developed to investigate claims made related to COVID-19 (e.g. infotagion.com).

COVID-19 Vaccination in Sub-Saharan Africa

Large-scale global vaccination for COVID-19 began in December 2020, and by the end of February 2022, around 4.3 billion (56%) of the world population had been fully vaccinated.[33]

The rollout of COVID-19 vaccinations across nations led to a decrease in social distancing, fewer new cases, perhaps especially during the early stages of the rollout and in high-income countries, and a relaxation of government social distancing rules.[34]

Similar to the pandemic response in SSA, COVID-19 vaccination programmes varied between countries. The WHO[35] reports that over 40 African nations had vaccine deployment plans before the first vaccines arrived, and these nations tended to fare better than the countries with less developed or no plans. In its report, WHO presents the vaccination efforts of several SSA countries to illustrate this point. Botswana was one of only six African countries to reach the WHO global target of fully vaccinating 40% of its population by the end of 2021 and used emergency operation centres to handle operational issues, for example, coordinating the transport of vaccines. Ethiopia demonstrated efficiency in using 80% of its available vaccines, which was partly achieved by employing a reverse logistics system to return vaccine doses from areas where they were underutilised and redistributing them to where they were needed, thus preventing doses from expiring. Ghana prioritised the elderly, the vulnerable, and those at risk of exposure on the job (such as people working in healthcare) for vaccination. Furthermore, innovative methods, such as drones, were used to reach remote communities. WHO's report emphasises that African countries are overall experienced at mass vaccination as part of controlling diseases such as polio and Ebola, and that these experiences and the existing infrastructure to support mass vaccination were helpful in planning and coordinating the rollout of COVID-19 vaccination. For example, South Sudan used vaccine accountability tools developed for polio vaccination campaigns to track the distribution and use of COVID-19 vaccines. Countries that had had Ebola outbreaks already had the facilities to store vaccines at very cold temperatures – a requirement of storing Ebola vaccines that proved useful for some types of COVID-19 vaccine. Furthermore, countries like Liberia and the DRC set up vaccination sites in places where people typically congregate, such as churches and markets, and repurposed prisons, military areas, and mining sites for COVID-19 vaccination.[35]

However, the United Nations[36] reported in February 2022 that although there was improved coverage of vaccine supplies on the African continent, countries were struggling to expand the COVID-19 vaccine rollout, with only 11% of the population fully vaccinated. Africa had received more than 587 million doses up to that point, largely through the United Nations-backed COVAX facility as well as through bilateral deals and the African Union. There was an urgent need to increase vaccine rollout sixfold. With 6 million people vaccinated weekly at that point, the number needed to increase to 36 million to reach the target of vaccinating 70% of Africa's population against COVID-19. Thus, much work remains to be done to build capacity for a faster, more efficient, and sustained COVID-19 vaccination programme on the African continent. Such efforts are further hampered by vaccine hesitancy in parts of the population, which is discussed in the following section.

Vaccine Hesitancy

The World Health Organisation has listed vaccine hesitancy as one of its ten threats to global health.[37] In order to prevent outbreaks of infectious diseases, vaccine coverage of 95% of the population needs to be reached and maintained.[38,39]

Many people have doubts about the need for immunisation or its safety and will either seek alternative vaccination schedules, delay, or refuse vaccines outright.[40] Vaccine hesitancy refers to a *"delay in acceptance or refusal of vaccination despite the availability of vaccination services."*[41] This makes it difficult to maintain high levels of vaccine coverage. Identifying the reasons for vaccine hesitancy or refusal is therefore critical to increasing the uptake of vaccinations.

Vaccine hesitancy is complex and specific to context; it varies across time, place, and vaccines.[41] It is influenced by factors such as complacency, convenience, and confidence[41] and can be associated with alternative or religious belief systems, lifestyle choices, or prior experience of adverse reactions.[42]

General vaccine hesitancy has been on the rise in some SSA countries, such as Nigeria.[43] In relation to COVID-19 vaccination specifically, hesitancy has been contributing to the slow uptake of vaccines in nations where large proportions of the populations remain unvaccinated, including South Africa, Tanzania, and the DRC.[44] The prevalence of COVID-19 vaccine hesitancy has been examined in SSA countries, finding acceptance of the vaccine to range from moderate to very high. One study using telephone surveys conducted in late 2020 examined six SSA nations: Burkina Faso, Ethiopia, Malawi, Mali, Nigeria, and Uganda. Acceptance rates ranged from 64.5% in Mali – lower than the vaccination rate required to reach herd immunity – to 97.9% in Ethiopia.[45] A study in Zambia conducted in late 2020 with parents who were having their children vaccinated for measles and rubella found a high acceptability of the COVID-19 vaccination of their children, but uncertainty and hesitancy about being vaccinated themselves.[46]

Although these studies were conducted prior to the wider availability of COVID-19 vaccines and respondents' answers were therefore hypothetical, other more recent studies yielded similar findings in terms of COVID-19 vaccine hesitancy. An anonymous Ghanaian survey conducted in February 2021 with over 2,300 adults found that 51% of urban-dwelling adults over 15 years of age were likely to get vaccinated for COVID-19 if made available to the general public. However, 21% stated they were unlikely to take the vaccine, and 28% were undecided.[47]

As stated previously, factors affecting vaccine hesitancy are complex. Looking at childhood immunisations, a study in Nigeria discovered that while partial immunisation was the result of factors such as maternal availability and a lack of knowledge, parental disapproval had a stronger influence on non-immunisation.[48] In some SSA countries, religion also contributes towards parents' hesitancy to vaccinate their children. For example, members of Zimbabwe's Apostolic Church voiced their concern that vaccinating their children may lead to conflict with their religious leaders.[49] Barriers towards vaccination are thus multifaceted, and physical, psychological, and social factors interact to produce vaccine hesitancy.

A significant practical barrier to vaccination has been the lack of availability of COVID-19 vaccination in many SSA countries. Physical access to vaccination facilities is a critical prerequisite for COVID-19 vaccine uptake. Difficulties accessing vaccination can prevent significant numbers of people from getting vaccinated, thereby hindering efforts to tackle the pandemic. Indeed, it has been argued that COVID-19 vaccine hesitancy in SSA has been exaggerated,[50] and that there is a substantial appetite in the population for getting vaccinated, as a large-scale survey of 15 African countries conducted by the Africa Centres for Disease Control and Prevention (Africa CDC) has shown.[51] Poorly coordinated logistics, including difficulties in moving vaccines to remote areas, have slowed the rollout of the COVID-19 vaccines in many parts of SSA, not vaccine hesitancy.[50]

Older adults in SSA appear to be particularly affected by physical access problems. A study mapping older adults' access to the nearest healthcare facility in SSA countries through travel time found that many had low physical access to such facilities, which may lead to under-reporting of COVID-19 symptoms in this population group.[52] Access to COVID-19 vaccination is thus likely to be the most important problem to solve in relation to vaccine uptake.

In addition to practical barriers, psychological barriers had the potential to hinder COVID-19 vaccination even when vaccines were easily and readily accessible. These psychological barriers are arguably more difficult to overcome, as they usually involve a complex interplay of cognitive, affective, and psychosocial factors. There is some SSA research that has examined such factors. For example, in the Zambian study described above, individuals' perceptions of the severity of COVID-19 and the efficacy of the vaccine were the strongest predictors of adults' vaccination intentions. Vaccine safety and efficacy were the strongest predictors of intent to vaccinate children.[46] Safety concerns over vaccines are a reliable predictor of the intention to get vaccinated.[53]

Psychological barriers are often rooted in the information sources that people seek out when making decisions about vaccination. A survey conducted in the spring of 2021 with around 2,500 individuals from SSA countries – Cameroon, Ghana, Kenya, Mozambique, Nigeria, South Africa, and Tanzania – showed that information influenced COVID-19 vaccine hesitancy and refusal. Those who relied on television and information from family and/or friends were more likely to hesitate to get the COVID-19 vaccine than those who had been vaccinated. However, social media use played the strongest role in COVID-19 vaccine hesitancy and refusal, as social media users were almost twice more likely to hesitate and three times more likely to refuse vaccination than non-users.[54]

Social media can play an important role in the dissemination of conspiracy beliefs, and using Facebook and YouTube for news increases conspiracy beliefs, both general and COVID-19 specific.[55] These beliefs appear to affect vaccine acceptance in some SSA countries. A systematic review on vaccine hesitancy in the global south[56] reports findings from African countries where there was the perception that the population was being used as test subjects for the development of vaccines. In South Africa, for example, concerns that teenagers are being used for testing the human papillomavirus vaccine have been reported.[57] Findings from Mozambique show a reluctance to be treated as 'guinea pigs' in relation to vaccination.[58] This mistrust may, in part, stem from historical events. For example, tests carried out by Pfizer during an outbreak of meningitis in 1996 in Nigeria may have contributed to suspicion in relation to Western health measures and played a role in a boycott of the polio vaccine.[59] Medical mistrust and conspiracy beliefs are sometimes fuelled by local differences, which impact people's attitudes towards the COVID-19 vaccine. For example, in the DRC, years of war and Ebola outbreaks have led to distrust in the leadership and in products from the West, and COVID-19 vaccine hesitancy may also affect individuals' acceptance of other vaccines.[44]

COVID-19 vaccine hesitancy in SSA is thus the product of a number of factors relating to physical, psychological, and social barriers to vaccination. Thus far, little effort has been made to integrate these factors into a model or framework in an attempt to holistically explain and predict COVID-19 vaccine acceptance. The following section outlines efforts to understand COVID-19 vaccine hesitancy using a social cognition model.

Applying Social Epidemiology to COVID-19 Vaccine Acceptance in Sub-Saharan Africa

In the context of COVID-19 vaccine acceptance in SSA, social epidemiology is crucial to understanding why certain groups may be more hesitant to receive vaccines. Applying concepts in social epidemiology, such as social inequalities and social relationships, offers valuable insights into the barriers and facilitators of vaccine acceptance in this diverse region, as well as develop strategies to address these.

Socioeconomic Status and COVID-19 Vaccine Acceptance

Socioeconomic status is a significant determinant of health outcomes, including vaccine acceptance. It encompasses not only income but also educational attainment, occupational status, and other related factors. In the context of COVID-19 vaccination in SSA, SES plays a crucial role.

Individuals from lower socioeconomic backgrounds often face barriers to healthcare services, including vaccination programmes. These barriers can be financial, such as the inability to afford transportation to vaccination sites or take time off work to get vaccinated. They can also be informational, with individuals lacking access to reliable and understandable information about vaccines.[60,61]

Lower socioeconomic status has also been associated with greater exposure to COVID-19 due to living conditions and occupational factors. Individuals in lower-income jobs might not have the option to work from home or socially distance at work, increasing their risk of contracting the virus. Despite being at greater risk, these individuals are often less likely to get vaccinated due to the barriers mentioned above.

Hesitation towards COVID-19 vaccination is more prevalent in wealthier households, among individuals living in urban environments, females, and those with higher levels of education. On the other hand, there is less hesitancy in larger households and among individuals who are heads of their households. The primary reasons for this hesitancy include worries about the vaccine's side effects, its safety and effectiveness, and evaluations of COVID-19 risk. However, these reasons are likely to vary over time.[62]

Cultural and Belief Systems

Cultural factors and belief systems profoundly impact vaccine acceptance in the SSA. The region is characterised by diverse cultures and practices, each with its own views on health and illness. Cultural norms, practices, and misconceptions can shape vaccination attitudes.

Some communities may hold traditional beliefs that conflict with modern medicine or vaccines. This can result in vaccine hesitancy or refusal. Cultural beliefs and attitudes significantly influence health behaviours, including vaccine acceptance, in SSA. In some communities, traditional beliefs about disease causation and treatment may conflict with biomedical understandings of vaccination, leading to vaccine hesitancy or outright refusal.[63] For instance, some cultural beliefs may attribute illness to supernatural causes rather than biological pathogens.[63] In such contexts, vaccines, which are based on the biomedical model of disease, may not be seen as relevant or effective. Additionally, some traditional health practices may involve treatments incompatible with vaccination, further contributing to hesitancy.[63]

Fear of side effects is another common concern that can deter individuals from getting vaccinated. This fear can be exacerbated by misinformation or a lack of information about vaccines. For example, rumours or misconceptions about vaccines causing infertility or other serious health problems can spread rapidly in communities, leading to widespread hesitancy.[64]

Religious or philosophical objections to vaccination can also play a role. Some religious groups may oppose vaccination on theological grounds, while others may object to specific vaccines due to the use of animal-derived ingredients or other ethical concerns.[63]

Addressing these cultural beliefs and attitudes is crucial for increasing COVID-19 vaccine acceptance in the SSA. This requires culturally sensitive communication strategies that respect local beliefs and values while providing accurate and understandable information about vaccines. It also involves building trust with communities through transparency, accountability, and engagement.[65]

Mistrust in healthcare providers or pharmaceutical companies can also contribute to vaccine hesitancy. This mistrust can stem from historical abuses in medical research or perceived inequities in healthcare provision. It can also be fuelled by conspiracy theories about the motives of those promoting vaccination.[65]

Social Networks and Peer Influence

In terms of social relationships, social networks and peer influence have played a significant role in shaping COVID-19 vaccination decisions in the SSA. Individuals are often influenced by the attitudes and behaviours of their family, friends, and community members.[60,66] Family and community discussions can either promote or hinder the COVID-19 vaccination. When trusted individuals endorse vaccines and share positive experiences, it can increase acceptance. Conversely, COVID-19 vaccine hesitancy within a social network can lead to the spread of doubts and reluctance.[60,66]

Leveraging the influence of social networks for positive change through community-led interventions can be an effective strategy to enhance vaccine acceptance in SSA. Community health workers and trusted community leaders can serve as vaccination advocates.[60,66]

Misinformation and Social Media

The spread of misinformation and rumours, especially through social media, has become a significant challenge to COVID-19 vaccine acceptance. False information can stoke fear and uncertainty, leading to vaccine hesitancy.[66] In SSA, where access to information is improving but still unevenly distributed, countering misinformation is crucial. False narratives that suggest vaccines are unsafe, ineffective, or harmful can deter individuals from getting vaccinated.[67]

Thus, effective communication strategies are essential to combat misinformation. Culturally sensitive and community-specific messaging, disseminated through trusted channels, can help address vaccine hesitancy and promote accurate information about vaccines.

Applying Social Epidemiology to Increasing COVID-19 Vaccine Acceptance in SSA

Increasing COVID-19 vaccine acceptance in SSA requires a multi-faceted, social epidemiology-informed approach that addresses the various barriers to vaccination identified in the region. Firstly, improving access to healthcare services is crucial. This includes enhancing the healthcare infrastructure, particularly in rural and remote areas, and ensuring that vaccination services are available and accessible to all. This could involve mobile vaccination clinics or community-based vaccination initiatives.[68]

Secondly, providing accurate and understandable information about vaccines is essential. Misinformation and misconceptions about vaccines can fuel vaccine hesitancy. Therefore, public health campaigns that provide clear and factual information about the safety and efficacy of vaccines can help to dispel these misconceptions.[63]

Thirdly, engaging with communities is key. This involves understanding and respecting local cultural beliefs and values and working with community leaders to promote vaccination. Community engagement can also help to build trust in healthcare providers and the healthcare system more broadly.[69]

Lastly, addressing socioeconomic barriers to vaccination is important. This could involve financial incentives for vaccination or policies that make it easier for individuals in lower-income jobs to get vaccinated.[70]

In sum, applying social epidemiology to the study of COVID-19 vaccine acceptance in SSA provides valuable insights into the complex interplay of social determinants, cultural beliefs, healthcare access, social networks, misinformation, and government policies. Recognising the multifaceted nature of vaccine acceptance in the region is essential to developing effective strategies for improving vaccination rates. Increasing COVID-19 vaccine coverage and acceptance in SSA requires a comprehensive approach that addresses access to healthcare services, misinformation about vaccines, cultural beliefs and attitudes, and socioeconomic barriers to vaccination.

Future Directions

Beyond the focus on COVID-19 vaccination in SSA, it is essential to broaden our perspective and address various other vaccination challenges faced by the region. While increasing COVID-19 vaccine uptake remains a high priority, there are other types of vaccination programmes that require attention. According to the WHO, the most common vaccine-preventable diseases in SSA are rotavirus, pneumococcal diseases, measles, and rubella.[71] Practical, psychological, and social barriers are prevalent across the spectrum of vaccinations, and a multifaceted approach should be taken to address them. To promote equitable access to vaccines, several strategies have been proposed. These include donating surplus vaccine doses, advocating for waivers of intellectual property rights, sharing manufacturing expertise, supporting regional vaccine production, and bolstering local health systems.[72] Applying these strategies could help improve access to a variety of vaccines, not just COVID-19 vaccines.

In Ghana and Kenya, vaccination reminders combined with small cash incentives increased childhood routine immunisation coverage.[73,74] Cash and in-kind incentive programmes were also effective in Nigeria.[75] The utility of such approaches when applied to the COVID-19 vaccination should be evaluated.

Hossain et al.[50] point to useful examples of successful vaccination campaigns in low- and middle-income nations. For example, polio was eradicated in Nigeria by joining forces with religious leaders to promote immunisations, and Rwanda vaccinated 93% of girls against HPV with the help of local leaders. Similarly, engaging religious and community leaders in the drive to vaccinate the population for COVID-19 may help uptake.

A rapid review of perceptions of the COVID-19 vaccine in South Africa[76] concludes that approaches to improve uptake should be developed with the guidance of affected groups through the use of participatory methods. The authors report that following the results of a survey indicating high levels of vaccine hesitancy, staff in a South African vaccination centre conducted a series of focus groups with staff to identify themes related to vaccine acceptance. These data were used to design a series of interventions. This unpublished research found that addressing concerns was not only about providing the facts but also required a deeper engagement with these concerns. People were more receptive when information was delivered by trusted individuals with the necessary knowledge and skills.[76]

Conversely, to increase the uptake of other vaccines in SSA, it is crucial to utilise knowledge gained from studying barriers to COVID-19 vaccination. Practical barriers in relation to vaccine supply and access also need to be addressed. Social epidemiological factors in terms of aspects such as socioeconomic status and social relationships need to be factored into vaccination strategies. At the community level, the influence of religious and community leaders needs to be harnessed in efforts to increase vaccine uptake. As vaccine acceptance and uptake are complex phenomena, it will take a complex, multifaceted approach to address them.

Conclusions

This chapter has overviewed the effect of COVID-19 on SSA, exploring barriers and facilitators to vaccine uptake. We have argued for the need to apply social epidemiology concepts to COVID-19 vaccine acceptance in SSA in light of the complex social factors governing vaccine uptake in the region. The complex nature of vaccine acceptance and uptake, coupled with the unique challenges SSA has faced as part of the COVID-19 pandemic, will require creative, multifaceted approaches to address this problem. Such efforts could improve vaccination efforts not only for COVID-19 but also for other vaccines in the SSA region.

References

1. Worldometer. COVID-19 coronavirus pandemic, https://www.worldometers.info/coronavirus/ (accessed 31 March 2022).
2. World Health Organization. COVID-19 responsible for at least 3 million excess deaths in 2020, https://www.who.int/news-room/spotlight/the-impact-of-covid-19-on-global-health-goals#:~:text=COVID%2D19%20responsible%20for%20at,more%20than%201.8%20million%20worldwide. (2021).
3. Wang H, Paulson KR, Pease SA, et al. Estimating excess mortality due to the COVID-19 pandemic: a systematic analysis of COVID-19-related mortality, 2020–21. *The Lancet*. DOI: 10.1016/S0140–6736(21)02796-3.
4. Lone SA, Ahmad A. COVID-19 pandemic – an African perspective. *Emerging Microbes & Infections* 2020; 9: 1300–1308.
5. Agwanda B, Dagba G, Opoku P, et al. Sub-Sahara Africa and the COVID-19 pandemic: reflecting on challenges and recovery opportunities. *Journal of Developing Societies* 2021; 37: 502–524.
6. Kuehn BM. Africa succeeded against COVID-19's first wave, but the second wave brings new challenges. *JAMA* 2021; 325: 327–328.
7. Ryder H, Lynch L. COVID-19 is only slowly reaching Africa. That's no surprise, https://www.theafricareport.com/24160/covid-19-is-only-slowly-reaching-africa-thats-no-surprise/ (2020, accessed 24 March 2022).
8. Deutsche Welle. Tanzania under fire from WHO for lackluster response to COVID-19 pandemic, https://www.dw.com/en/tanzania-under-fire-from-who-for-lackluster-response-to-covid-19-pandemic/a-53304699 (2020, accessed 24 March 2022).
9. Grieco K, Yusuf Y. Sierra Leone's response to COVID-19, https://www.opml.co.uk/files/Publications/A2241-maintains/final-2707-sierra-leone-covid-rapid-study-4-.pdf?noredirect=1 (2020, accessed 24 March 2022).
10. Obahor S, Dunning H. How African countries are dealing with the COVID-19 pandemic, https://www.imperial.ac.uk/news/232655/how-african-countries-dealing-with-covid-19/ (2021, accessed 24 March 2022).
11. Biryabarema E. Uganda re-imposes lockdown to beat back COVID-19 case surge, https://www.reuters.com/world/africa/uganda-re-imposes-lockdown-beat-back-covid-19-case-surge-2021-06-06/ (2021, accessed 24 March 2022).
12. Haider N, Osman AY, Gadzekpo A, et al. Lockdown measures in response to COVID-19 in nine sub-Saharan African countries. *BMJ Global Health* 2020; 5: e003319.
13. Galal S. Number of coronavirus (COVID-19) cases in the African continent as of March 02, 2022, by country, https://www.statista.com/statistics/1170463/coronavirus-cases-in-africa/ (2022, accessed 24 March 2022).
14. Omotoso KO, Koch SF. Assessing changes in social determinants of health inequalities in South Africa: a decomposition analysis. *International Journal of Equity Health* 2018; 17: 181.
15. Okoi O, Bwawa T. How health inequality affect responses to the COVID-19 pandemic in Sub-Saharan Africa. *World Development* 2020; 135: 105067.
16. Marmot M. Achieving health equity: from root causes to fair outcomes. *The Lancet* 2007; 370: 1153–1163.
17. Soors W, Dkhimi F, Criel B. Lack of access to health care for African indigents: a social exclusion perspective. *International Journal for Equity in Health* 2013; 12: 91.

18. Tessema GA, Kinfu Y, Dachew BA, et al. The COVID-19 pandemic and healthcare systems in Africa: a scoping review of preparedness, impact and response. *BMJ Global Health* 2021; 6: e007179.

19. De Groot J, Lemanski C. COVID-19 responses: infrastructure inequality and privileged capacity to transform everyday life in South Africa. *Environment and Urbanization* 2021; 33: 255–272.

20. Jensen N, Kelly AH, Avendano M. The COVID-19 pandemic underscores the need for an equity-focused global health agenda. *Humanities and Social Sciences Communications* 2021; 8: 15.

21. Mamo LT, Andersen H. Africa without vaccines: inequity sets the world on course for a great divide, https://institute.global/advisory/africa-without-vaccines-inequity-sets-world-course-great-divide (2021, accessed 29 March 2022).

22. Olatunji O, Ayandele O, Ashirudeen D, et al. 'Infodemic' in a pandemic: COVID-19 conspiracy theories in an african country. *Social Health and Behavior* 2020; 3: 152–157.

23. Nolsoe E. Global survey: which sources of information do people trust on COVID-19?, https://yougov.co.uk/topics/politics/articles-reports/2021/02/08/global-survey-which-sources-information-do-people- (2021, accessed 24 March 2022).

24. Fosu-Ankrah JF, Amoako-Gyampah AK. Prophetism in the wake of a pandemic: Charismatic Christianity, conspiracy theories, and the Coronavirus outbreak in Africa. *Research in Globalization* 2021; 3: 100068.

25. Mian A, Khan S. Coronavirus: the spread of misinformation. *BMC Medicine* 2020; 18: 89.

26. Oxford Analytica. Misinformation will undermine coronavirus responses. *Expert Briefings*. Epub ahead of print 2020. DOI: 10.1108/OXAN-DB250989.

27. Pennycook G, McPhetres J, Zhang Y, et al. Fighting COVID-19 misinformation on social media: experimental evidence for a scalable accuracy-nudge intervention. *Psychological Science* 2020; 31: 770–780.

28. Frenkel S, Alba D, Zhong R. Surge of virus misinformation stumps Facebook and Twitter. The New York Times, https://www.nytimes.com/2020/03/08/technology/coronavirus-misinformation-social-media.html (2020, accessed 24 March 2022).

29. Busari S, Adebayo B. Nigeria records chloroquine poisoning after Trump endorses it for coronavirus treatment, https://edition.cnn.com/2020/03/23/africa/chloroquine-trump-nigeria-intl/index.html (2020, accessed 24 March 2022).

30. Ahinkorah BO, Ameyaw EK, Hagan JE, et al. Rising above misinformation or fake news in Africa: another strategy to control COVID-19 spread. *Frontiers Communication* 2020; 5: 45.

31. Oxford Analytica. Tech may curb virus profiteering, not disinformation. *Expert Briefings*. Epub ahead of print 2020. DOI: 10.1108/OXAN-DB251502.

32. World Health Organization. Tuberculosis deaths rise for the first time in more than a decade due to the COVID-19 pandemic, https://www.who.int/news/item/14-10-2021-tuberculosis-deaths-rise-for-the-first-time-in-more-than-a-decade-due-to-the-covid-19-pandemic (2021, accessed 24 March 2022).

33. Our World in Data. Coronavirus (COVID-19) vaccinations, https://ourworldindata.org/covid-vaccinations (2022, accessed 28 February 2022).

34. Auld MC, Toxvaerd F. The great covid-19 vaccine rollout: behavioural and policy responses. *NIER* 2021; 257: 14–35.

35. World Health Organization. Key lessons from Africa's COVID-19 vaccine rollout, https://www.afro.who.int/news/key-lessons-africas-covid-19-vaccine-rollout (2021, accessed 29 March 2022).

36. United Nations. Africa needs to ramp up COVID-19 vaccination rate six-fold, https://news.un.org/en/story/2022/02/1111202 (2022, accessed 29 March 2022).

37. World Health Organization. Ten threats to global health in 2019, https://www.who.int/news-room/spotlight/ten-threats-to-global-health-in-2019 (2019, accessed 18 February 2022).

38. Lane S, MacDonald NE, Marti M, et al. Vaccine hesitancy around the globe: analysis of three years of WHO/UNICEF joint reporting form data-2015–2017. *Vaccine* 2018; 36: 3861–3867.

39. Hancock D. Vaccine hesitancy: a serious threat to global health. *Journal of Health Visiting* 2019; 7: 112–115.

40. Luyten J, Bruyneel L, van Hoek AJ. Assessing vaccine hesitancy in the UK population using a generalized vaccine hesitancy survey instrument. *Vaccine* 2019; 37: 2494–2501.

41. MacDonald NE. Vaccine hesitancy: definition, scope and determinants. *Vaccine* 2015; 33: 4161–4164.

42. Larson HJ, Cooper LZ, Eskola J, et al. Addressing the vaccine confidence gap. *The Lancet* 2011; 378: 526–535.

43. de Figueiredo A, Simas C, Karafillakis E, et al. Mapping global trends in vaccine confidence and investigating barriers to vaccine uptake: a large-scale retrospective temporal modelling study. *The Lancet* 2020; 396: 898–908.

44. Mallapaty S. Researchers fear growing COVID vaccine hesitancy in developing nations. *Nature* 2022; 601: 174–175.

45. Kanyanda S, Markhof Y, Wollburg P, et al. Acceptance of COVID-19 vaccines in sub-Saharan Africa: evidence from six national phone surveys. *BMJ Open* 2021; 11: e055159.

46. Carcelen AC, Prosperi C, Mutembo S, et al. COVID-19 vaccine hesitancy in Zambia: a glimpse at the possible challenges ahead for COVID-19 vaccination rollout in sub-Saharan Africa. *Human Vaccines & Immunotherapeutics* 2022; 18: 1–6.

47. Acheampong T, Akorsikumah EA, Osae-Kwapong J, et al. Examining vaccine hesitancy in Sub-Saharan Africa: a survey of the knowledge and attitudes among adults to receive COVID-19 vaccines in Ghana. *Vaccines* 2021; 9: 814.

48. Babalola S. Maternal reasons for non-immunisation and partial immunisation in northern Nigeria: reasons for non-immunisation and partial immunisation. *Journal of Paediatrics and Child Health* 2011; 47: 276–281.

49. Machekanyanga Z, Ndiaye S, Gerede R, et al. Qualitative assessment of vaccination hesitancy among members of the apostolic church of Zimbabwe: a case study. *Journal of Religion and Health* 2017; 56: 1683–1691.

50. Hossain A, Aziimwe S, Ivers L. Claims of vaccine hesitancy in African countries are at odds with the reality on the ground, https://www.statnews.com/2021/12/21/claims-of-vaccine-hesitancy-in-african-countries-are-at-odds-with-the-reality-on-the-ground/.

51. Africa Centers for Disease Control and Prevention. COVID 19 vaccine perceptions: A 15 Country Study, https://africacdc.org/download/covid-19-vaccine-perceptions-a-15-country-study/.

52. Geldsetzer P, Reinmuth M, Ouma PO, et al. Mapping physical access to health care for older adults in sub-Saharan Africa and implications for the COVID-19 response: a cross-sectional analysis. *The Lancet Healthy Longevity* 2020; 1: e32–e42.

53. Karafillakis E, Larson HJ. The benefit of the doubt or doubts over benefits? A systematic literature review of perceived risks of vaccines in European populations. *Vaccine* 2017; 35: 4840–4850.

54. Levi Osuagwu U, Mashige K, Ovenseri-Ogbomo G, et al. *The impact of information sources on COVID-19 Vaccine hesitancy and resistance in Sub- Saharan Africa.* 2022. Epub ahead of print 22 February 2022. DOI: 10.21203/rs.3.rs-1385351/v1.

55. Stecula DA, Pickup M. Social media, cognitive reflection, and conspiracy beliefs. *Frontiers in Political Science* 2021; 3: 647957.

56. de Souza Amorim Matos CC, Gonçalves BA, Couto MT. Vaccine hesitancy in the global south: towards a critical perspective on global health. *Global Public Health* 2021; 17: 1–12.

57. Wiyeh AB, Cooper S, Jaca A, et al. Social media and HPV vaccination: unsolicited public comments on a Facebook post by the Western Cape Department of Health provide insights into determinants of vaccine hesitancy in South Africa. *Vaccine* 2019; 37: 6317–6323.

58. Démolis R, Botão C, Heyerdahl LW, et al. A rapid qualitative assessment of oral cholera vaccine anticipated acceptability in a context of resistance towards cholera intervention in Nampula, Mozambique. *Vaccine* 2018; 36: 6497–6505.

59. Jegede AS. What led to the Nigerian boycott of the polio vaccination campaign? *PLoS Medicine* 2007; 4: e73.

60. Deml MJ, Githaiga JN. Determinants of COVID-19 vaccine hesitancy and uptake in sub-Saharan Africa: a scoping review. *BMJ Open* 2022; 12: e066615.

61. Kunyenje CA, Chirwa GC, Mboma SM, et al. COVID-19 vaccine inequity in African low-income countries. *Front Public Health* 2023; 11: 1087662.

62. Wollburg P, Markhof Y, Kanyanda S, et al. 2023. The evolution of COVID-19 vaccine hesitancy in Sub-Saharan Africa: evidence from panel survey data. In *BMC proceedings (Vol. 17, No. Suppl 7, p. 8)*. London: BioMed Central.

63. Kanyanda S, Markhof Y, Wollburg P, et al. Acceptance of COVID-19 vaccines in sub-Saharan Africa: evidence from six national phone surveys. *BMJ Open* 2021; 11: e055159.

64. Ackah M, Ameyaw L, Salifu MG, et al. COVID-19 vaccine acceptance among health care workers in Africa: a systematic review and meta-analysis. *PLOS ONE* 2022; 17: e0268711.

65. Azanaw J, Endalew M, Zenbaba D, et al. COVID-19 vaccine acceptance and associated factors in 13 African countries: a systematic review and meta-analysis. *Frontiers in Public Health*; 10, https://www.frontiersin.org/articles/10.3389/fpubh.2022.1001423 (2023, accessed 28 October 2023).

66. Osuagwu UL, Mashige KP, Ovenseri-Ogbomo G, et al. The impact of information sources on COVID-19 vaccine hesitancy and resistance in sub-Saharan Africa. *BMC Public Health* 2023; 23: 38.

67. Singh K, Lima G, Cha M, et al. Misinformation, believability, and vaccine acceptance over 40 countries: takeaways from the initial phase of the COVID-19 infodemic. *PLoS ONE* 2022; 17: e0263381.

68. Eick M. European Union provides fresh funding to support COVID-19 vaccination in sub-Saharan Africa, https://www.unicef.org/esa/press-releases/european-union-

provides-fresh-funding-support-covid-19-vaccination-sub-saharan (accessed 28 October 2023).

69. Ajeigbe O, Arage G, Besong M, et al. Culturally relevant COVID-19 vaccine acceptance strategies in sub-Saharan Africa. *The Lancet Global Health* 2022; 10: e1090–e1091.

70. Miner CA, Timothy CG, Percy K, et al. Acceptance of COVID-19 vaccine among sub-Saharan Africans (SSA): a comparative study of residents and diasporan dwellers. *BMC Public Health* 2023; 23: 191.

71. World Health Organization. Immunization. *WHO | Regional Office for Africa*, https://www.afro.who.int/health-topics/immunization (2023, accessed 1 November 2023).

72. Ghebreyesus TA. Five steps to solving the vaccine inequity crisis. *PLOS Glob Public Health* 2021; 1: e0000032.

73. Levine G, Salifu A, Mohammed I, et al. Mobile nudges and financial incentives to improve coverage of timely neonatal vaccination in rural areas (GEVaP trial): a 3-armed cluster randomized controlled trial in Northern Ghana. *PLoS ONE* 2021; 16: e0247485.

74. Gibson DG, Ochieng B, Kagucia EW, et al. Mobile phone-delivered reminders and incentives to improve childhood immunisation coverage and timeliness in Kenya (M-SIMU): a cluster randomised controlled trial. *The Lancet Global Health* 2017; 5: e428–e438.

75. ID Insight. Impact of conditional cash transfers on routine childhood immunizations in North West Nigeria, https://files.givewell.org/files/DWDA%202009/NewIncentives/IDinsight_Impact_Evaluation_of_New_Incentives_Final_Report.pdf (2020, accessed 23 February 2022).

76. Roldan de Jong T. Rapid review: perceptions of COVID-19 vaccines in South Africa. *Social Science in Humanitarian Action (SSHAP)*. Epub ahead of print 2021. DOI: 10.19088/SSHAP.2021.021.

7

SOCIAL DETERMINANTS OF MATERNAL HEALTH IN SUB-SAHARAN AFRICA

Ahmed Ali Hassan

Introduction

Compared to other regions of the world, Sub-Saharan Africa (SSA) has the lowest ratings for wellbeing and the lowest satisfaction with healthcare (Deaton et al., 2015). The World Bank's data regarding SSA for 2019 showed a gross domestic product (GDP) of 1.803 trillion United States dollars, a population of 1.107 billion, and a life expectancy at birth of 62.627 years (World Bank, 2022). Although population in SSA are suffering from poor healthcare and its devastating consequences, maternal and under-five children are more vulnerable to morbidity and mortality. Maternal and child health are major public health concerns in SSA (Batist et al., 2019; Hailu et al., 2021; Monden and Smits, 2013; Tesema et al., 2021; WHO, 2019). Across the globe, the highest rates of maternal mortality as well as under-five mortality (Morden et al., 2013; WHO, 2019) occurred in SSA. For example, according to the World Health Organization (WHO, 2019) estimation of maternal mortality for 2017, SSA alone accounted for about 66% (196,000), giving a maternal mortality ratio of 542/100,000 live births (WHO, 2019). In SSA, among 398,574 mothers under the age of 50 years, 27% suffered at least one child death (Hailu et al., 2018).

The prevalence of adverse birth outcomes (e.g., stillbirth, preterm birth, low birth weight, and complications related to caesarean section (CS) in SSA was high (Dikete, 2019; Tamirat, 2021). Although high rates of CS were reported in high-income countries (HICs), for example, in the United Kingdom (26.2%) (Wise, 2018) and the United States (US) (31.7%) (Martin et al., 2021), maternal and perinatal deaths were high following CS in SSA. This could indicate the poor provision of healthcare services in SSA. Hence, child health depends

DOI: 10.4324/9781003467601-9

on maternal health, especially under-five years age (Bado and Susman, 2016; Monden and Smits, 2013). This chapter highlights both maternal and child health. Unlike biomedical risk factors, in SSA less attention was paid to the influence of social determinants of health (SDH) on maternal health, namely educational, socio-economic, and socio-cultural factors (Batist, 2019). In addition, researchers in SSA reported the key role that social context plays in inequalities in women and children's chances of survival (Macassa et al., 2011). Lack of well-addressing social epidemiology and health could be the reason why many African countries did not meet the millennium development goals (MDGs) (e.g., Goal5 regarding maternal mortality) (Adgoy, 2018). Unfortunately, the existing literature shows this pattern will continue with sustainable development goals (SDGs), (e.g., MDG3) (Adde et al., 2020). Therefore, for SSA to meet the SDGs by 2030, especially SDG3 target 1: reduce the global maternal mortality ratio below 70/100,000 live births, and SDG3 target 2 end preventable deaths of newborns and children under-five years of age, all countries aim to reduce neonatal mortality to at least as low as 12/1,000 live births and under-five mortality to at least as low as 25/1,000 live births. Since the first issuing of the WHO commission's SDH report (WHO, 2008) in 2008, many reports have been issued for regions such as the European region in 2017 (WHO, 2017) and the Eastern Mediterranean Region in 2021 (WHO, 2021), but no report has been dedicated to the Africa region. Therefore, aiming to improve maternal and early-years health, this chapter is aimed at addressing influence of SDH on maternal health in SSA. To achieve this, social determinants of maternal health need to be well understood, and accordingly, appropriate solutions need to be taken. The authors believe the good start in achieving so is to be proactive rather than reactive. To be proactive in predicting maternal and child health by understanding the social contexts and putting appropriate preventive measures accordingly. By doing so, the SDGs can be achieved, especially those related to maternal and child health (Aheto, 2019; Liu et al., 2016; Katsinde, 2016) in SSA and across the globe.

Operational Definitions

Sub-Saharan Africa

The World Bank categorizes SSA into four regions (WB, 2024):

- Central Africa (Angola, Burundi, Central African Republic, Chad, Congo, Democratic Republic of the Congo, Republic of Rwanda),
- Eastern Africa (Comoros, Eritrea, Ethiopia, Kenya, Madagascar, Mauritius, Seychelles, Somalia, South Sudan, Sudan, Tanzania, and Uganda),
- Southern Africa (Botswana, Eswatini, Lesotho, Malawi, Mozambique, Namibia, South Africa, Zambia, Zimbabwe), and

- Western Africa (Benin, Burkina Faso, Cabo Verde, Cameroon, Cote d'Ivoire, Equatorial Guinea, Gabon, Gambia, Ghana, Guinea, Guinea-Bissau, Liberia, Mali, Mauritania, Niger, Nigeria, Sao Tome and Principe, Senegal, Sierra Leone, Togo).

Social Determinants of Health

The WHO defines SDH as the conditions in which people are born, grow, work, live, and age, and the wider set of forces and systems shaping the conditions of daily life (WHO, 2009). These forces and systems include, but are not limited to, economic policies and systems, development agendas, policies, political systems, cultural and societal norms, and values (WHO, 2009).

Education and Maternal Health in Sub-Saharan Africa

As education is a driving force for nation sustainability, the United Nations (UN) gives more attention to education in both the MDGs (MDG2: achieve universal primary education) and the SDGs (MDG4: quality education). Education is considered a key driver because it influences all SDH, such as work, income, and access to healthcare. Although education is a basic human right for both girls and boys, educational gender inequality does exist in the SSA (Baten et al., 2021). In the literature, the benefits of education on maternal health are documented in many regions, and SSA is not an exception (Bado et al., 2016). The bidirectional association between education and health is well documented by researchers. For example, education influences health in many ways, such as:

Improving Maternal Health

Education helps women in many ways: it gives women more employment opportunities as it equips them with the necessary working skills; it empowers women to make decisions regarding health and marriage; and it improves women's access to healthcare services, for example, prenatal care and vaccination. In Africa, the educational status of adolescents, mothers, and fathers was associated with adolescent pregnancy (Kassa et al., 2018). On the other hand, a rise in the rate of unemployment is correlated with income inequality in SSA and its sub-regions (Gimba et al., 2021). In SSA, women's and men's higher levels of education and increased household wealth are associated with a decrease in physical and/or sexual intimate partner violence (IPV); however, in the case of only women's employment, women earning more than their partners are associated with an increase in IPV (Stöckl, 2021). Other study suggested that eliminating violence against women in SSA requires a comprehensive approach rather than addressing household poverty wealth status alone (Bamiwuye et al., 2014).

Adequate birth spacing (24–59 months) is linked to better health outcomes for both mothers and babies (Ajayi and Somefun.2018. Inadequate birth spacing was reported in SSAs such as Chad (30.2%) and the Democratic Republic of Congo (DRC) (27.1%) (Ajayi and Somefun, 2018). In East SSA, inadequate birth spacing is associated with under-five mortality (Tesema et al., 2021). Unequal access and use of contraceptives, especially among parenting adolescent girls in SSA, may contribute to the short inter-pregnancy interval (IPI), as 27.12% of parenting adolescent girls used contraceptives (ranging from 5.10% in Chad to 70.0% in South Africa) (Ahinkorah, 2021a). There is a relatively low prevalence of modern contraceptive use (29.6%) among women with no intention to give birth in SSA (Ahinkorah et al., 2021b). The main factors associated with modern contraceptive use were young women's age, age at first sex, high level of education, media exposure, urban residence, medium community literacy level, and medium community socio-economic status (Londero et al., 2019). Compared to other geographic regions in SSA, women in Southern Africa had higher odds of modern contraceptive use (55.5%) (Ahimkorah et al., 2021a, 2021b). It is worth mentioning that both extreme maternal ages (i.e., <20 years and >35 years) have negative impacts on poor pregnancy outcomes (Londero et al., 2019), and this can be linked to SDH such as low access to healthcare services, especially in SSA (Mekonnen et al., 2019).

Clark reported that investing in adolescent girls will improve the future of maternal and child health in the SSA (Clark, 2013). Although education is strongly associated with health and wellbeing because it influences life expectancy, morbidity, health behaviours, employment, and income, it is one of the most neglected SDHs (Lancet Public Health, 2020).

Improving Access to Healthcare Services

Education improves access to healthcare services (Bado et al., 2016; Doctor et al., 2018). Among 29 SSA countries, women with at least primary education were two times more likely to deliver at healthcare facilities compared to women with no formal education (Doctor et al., 2018). In SSA, 66% of deliveries occurred in healthcare facilities, ranging from 23% in Chad to 94% in Gabon (Adde et al., 2020). The main determinants of healthcare facility delivery were urban residency, high maternal education, and high wealth status (Adde et al., 2020). In East SSA, access to healthcare and delivery at healthcare facilities are significantly associated with a lower risk of under-five mortality (Tesema et al., 2021). Poor maternal access to healthcare services is common among adolescents' pregnancy girls across SSA countries, and it is associated with a greater risk of adverse pregnancy outcomes (Kassa et al., 2018; Mekonnen et al., 2019).

Improving Under-five Health

The governmental policies taken by the SSA on women's education contributed to a decline in under-five mortality rates (Bado et al., 2016). Maternal education is associated with reduced infant and under-five mortality in SSA, especially among girls (Chewe et al., 2020; Monden and Smits, 2013; Tesema et al., 2021). Education increases maternal awareness about infant and child health and hygiene. In Malawi and Uganda, for each additional year of maternal education, under-five mortality has a 10% and 16.6% lower probability of dying, respectively (Andnamo and Monden, 2019). On the contrary, a lack of maternal education is associated with both child morbidity and mortality (Andamo and Monden, 2019; Monden and Smits, 2013). It is worth mentioning that COVID-19 puts a heavy burden on already limited healthcare resources, such as in the SSA. According to UNESCO's (2020) estimation, SSA students, especially female students, are at greater risk of not returning to education due to the COVID-19 pandemic (UN & UNESC, 2020). According to the International Monetary Fund (IMF), digitalizing SSA is a real hope for those students to continue their education (Cangul et al., 2020).

It can be concluded that parental education is a key factor in achieving SDG3 targets 1 and 2; however, more research is required to explore the mechanisms by which education influences maternal and child health.

Maternal Employment Status and Maternal Health in Sub-Saharan Africa

The education of women is not the end of the story; educated women need to be connected to the workforce in Africa. Unfortunately, in the last few decades, women's labour force participation rates have stagnated in SSA (Backhaus and Lochinger, 2021). As a result, persistent gender gaps in labour force participation and pay do exist in the SSA (Gender, 2013). For example, the gender pay gap is 30% in SSA in comparison to the global average (24%) (Gender, 2013). This widening gender gap in labour supply may be attributed to a lack of education and early motherhood in SSA. Not to mention the possibility of further widening of the existing gender inequalities for women and girls (e.g., healthcare, income, education) within SSA by the COVID-19 pandemic (Ahinkorah et al., 2021b; Mashige et al., 2021).

In addition to the low employment rates of women compared to men in the SSA, employed women face many challenges, especially among young, employed women of them: majority of employed women work in vulnerable working environment (Chakravarty et al., 2017), are low paid (Gender, 2013), and work in the informal economy (Malta et al., 2019). Such employment conditions will put women at a greater risk of falling into poverty compared to men.

Maternal employment status influences child health. The influence of maternal employment on child health depends on the nature of the occupation and the residential and regional context (Akinyemi et al., 2018). Both formal and informal maternal employment in low- and middle-income countries (LMICs), including SSA, is associated with improved infant and young child feeding through improved dietary diversity and feeding frequency (Oddo and Ickes, 2018).

In Nigeria, both infant and child mortality among employed women was higher compared to unemployed women (Akinyemi et al., 2018). Although children of unemployed parents have the greatest risks of death during infancy, a father's occupation alone did not show any independent relationship with infant and child mortality (Akinyemi et al., 2018). Child mortality among unemployed parents could be explained by the risk of poverty and a lack of payment for basic child needs such as food and access to healthcare services.

To advance women's economic empowerment in SAA, Chichester et al. (2017) revealed six practical areas: gender-sensitive workplaces and benefits, leadership and advancement, education and training, freedom from harassment and violence, entrepreneurship and business linkages, and inclusive communities.

Socio-Economic Status and Maternal Health in Sub-Saharan Africa

In SSA, wealth distribution inequality remains one of the strongest barriers to healthcare coverage (Wehrmeister et al., 2020). Women in the richest wealth quintile were 68% more likely to occur in health facilities compared to women in the lowest wealth quintile (Doctor et al., 2018). Variations of wealth-related inequalities were common within countries and between the four regions of SSA (highest for West Africa and lowest for Southern Africa) (Wehrmeister et al., 2020). Interestingly, absolute income was not a predictor of healthcare coverage, as this was observed in the South with about 70% coverage compared to the Central and West with 40% for the same income (Wehrmeister et al., 2020). Likewise, UNICEF revealed that economic poverty alone is not an adequate measure of children's overall wellbeing. A multidimensional approach to child health is required to improve understanding, monitoring, and policy effectiveness (UNICEF, 2007). In Africa, average income exerts a negligible contemporaneous effect on women's health outcomes (Dominic et al., 2020). This indicates that income alone is not enough to have a healthy nation.

Despite the presence of conflict, economic hardship, and political instability in most SSA countries, there is success in reducing wealth-related inequalities in the coverage of essential health services (UNICEF, 2007). Although corruption is correlated with income inequality (Manu, 2021) and reduction in corruption in the short run and long run shows reducing inequality in SSA (Gimba et al., 2021), the governmental anti-corruption efforts are not satisfactory (Duri, 2020).

Socio-Political, Cultural Issues, and Maternal Health in Sub-Saharan Africa

Theisen and colleagues revealed maternal healthcare service delivery is affected by ethno-political favouritism in SSA (Theisen et al., 2020). Political instability and poor governance quality negatively impact infant mortality and maternal mortality in SSA (Iheonu et al., 2019). Political determinants were reported as a main cause of SSA lagged nation in achieving targets for the MDGs, especially maternal and under-five mortality (Atti et al., 2017). Over the past decades, lack of job opportunities, poverty, economic inequality, climate change, political instability, armed conflict, and food insecurity have represented the main determinants of international migration from SSA to Europe and the US (Onafeso, 2020; Sadiddin et al., 2019; Sumata, 2021). Unfortunately, much migration from SSA is forced migration (Naudé, 2010; Onafeso, 2020), and it is associated with the health penalty (Ginsburg et al., 2021). It seems that without focusing on strengthening countries' political, economic, and social capacities, it will be difficult for SSA to achieve the SDGs in SSA. On the other hand, the burden of mental health problems such as depression, anxiety disorders, emotional and behavioural difficulties, posttraumatic stress, and suicidal behaviour among youth is under-addressed in SSA (Jorns-Presentati et al., 2021). Silva et al. (2016) highlighted the importance of social factors (i.e., low education, not living with a partner, lack of social support, female gender, low income, low socioeconomic status, unemployment, financial strain, and perceived discrimination) in the initiation and maintenance of mental illness and the need for political action and effective interventions to improve the conditions of everyday life to improve the population's mental health.

In summary, in a region characterized by armed conflict, political instability, and poverty (Iheonu et al., 2019; Munezero et al., 2021; Nyoni et al., 2022; Sumata, 2021), it is common to find a high prevalence of mental problems, especially among children and adolescents. Such mental problems in children and adolescents can lead to significant impairment and disability and high social and financial costs for the children, their families, and society (Nyoni et al., 2022).

Access to Healthcare and Maternal Health in Sub-Saharan Africa

In Africa, women's health outcomes depend on healthcare service utilization; therefore, to utilize health service, healthcare services need to be accessible and well equipped with healthcare workers, equipment, and drugs (Dominic et al.,

2020). For example, for a long time, researchers have reported the critical shortage of healthcare workers (e.g., midwives, nurses, and doctors) and its implications on maternal and child health in SSA (Gerein et al., 2006; Naicker et al., 2009). In addition to that, the COVID-19 pandemic has overwhelmed health systems across the globe, especially in regions with weak healthcare systems such as Africa (Tessema et al., 2021). In SSA, the increase in life expectancy and reduction in infant mortality can be accelerated by paying more attention to education, healthcare access, and access to clean water (Chewe et al., 2020). According to Dominic et al. (2020), in the SSA, women's access to healthcare facilities is determined by (Deaton et al., 2015) service availability, (World Bank, 2022) service utilization/affordability, and (Tessema et al., 2021) service decision ability. Deficits in prenatal care visits (<4) are more prevalent among poorer women in comparison to 'surpluses' (>4) that are concentrated among the rich (Obse, 2021). The main SDH associated with prenatal care 'deficits' and 'surpluses' in SSA include wealth status, education status, and area of residency (Obse, 2021). A systematic review conducted by Okedo-Alex and others reported in SSA that adequate prenatal care is influenced by parent education, maternal employment, socioeconomic status, urban residence, older maternal age, being married, having healthcare insurance, and Christian religion (Okedo-Alex, 2019). Despite the substantial contribution of childhood vaccination for reducing morbidity and mortality among children and the global progress in vaccination coverage, poor and high inequality in vaccination coverage continues to persist in SSA (Babo et al., 2022). According to a recent analysis of Demographic and Health Survey data for 25 SSA, 56.5%, 35.1%, and 8.4% of children received full vaccination, incomplete vaccination, and were unvaccinated, respectively (Bobo et al., 2022). In addition, inequality in unvaccinated children was disproportionately concentrated among disadvantaged subgroups, with full vaccination coverage ranging from 24% in Guinea to 93% in Rwanda. Increased vaccination coverage was associated with high maternal education, higher household wealth, adequate prenatal care, delivery at healthcare facilities, and media exposure (Bobo et al., 2022). A similar childhood vaccination rate and determinant factors were identified in SSA. For example, Fenta et al. (2021) reported the prevalence of full childhood vaccination coverage among children aged 12–23 months in SSA was 59.40%, and it was associated with high parent education, healthcare facility delivery, adequate prenatal care, higher household wealth status, media exposure, and proximity to healthcare facilities. A recent systematic review showed the main identified barriers to childhood vaccination in SSA were child gender, beliefs, and socio-cultural factors (Bangura et al., 2020).

Educated women are more likely to have health insurance coverage, to seek healthcare services (Amu, 2021), and to seek vaccination services (73). Accessibility to healthcare services is a good opportunity for women to be educated about contraceptive methods and safe sex methods, especially in countries with a high prevalence of sexually transmitted infections such as HIV/AIDS. According to the WHO estimation, among 37.7 million (30.2–45.1 million) people living with HIV at the end of 2020, more than two thirds of whom (25.4 million) are in the WHO African Region (WHO, 2021). The HIV/AIDS epidemic in SSA has a significant negative effect on education, the workforce (Coulibaly, 2005), economic growth (Lovász and Schipp, 2009), and sustainable development (Odugbesan and Rjoub, 2020). Achieving sustainable development in the presence of a high prevalence of HIV/AIDS in SSA is very challenging (Odugbesan and Rjoub, 2020). Correa-Agudelo et al. (2021) reported a positive association between maternal anaemic, malaria, and HIV.

In SSA, low healthcare access can be attributed to many reasons, including:

1 The overall relatively low prevalence of health insurance coverage among women of reproductive age (Amu et al., 2021). The average health insurance was 8.5%, with cross-country variations ranging from 0.9% in Chad to 62.4% in Ghana (Amu et al., 2021).
2 The overall health expenditure, from 46 SSA countries, covering the period 2000–2015 showed that health expenditure was associated with a positive and significant impact on health outcomes, (i.e., a 1% increase in health expenditure per capita resulted in a 0.5% reduction in under-five mortality, a 0.35% reduction in maternal mortality, and improved life expectancy by 0.06% (Nketiah-Amponsah, 2019). In addition, it revealed that health expenditures in SSA countries represent only a small proportion of GDP in comparison to developed countries (Carrasco-Escobar et al., 2021).
3 There is existing armed conflict in the SSA. There is no doubt that armed conflict disrupts the healthcare system, especially the already weak one, as in the SSA. Unfortunately, most armed conflict exists in Africa. In conflict settings, individuals are forced to choose between fulfilling their basic needs and attending healthcare services (Munezero and Manoukian, 2021). For example, disruptions in the healthcare system by unanticipated events (e.g., armed conflict) and emerging pandemics (e.g., COVID-19) lead to overcome the achievement of some programmes such as malaria (Carrasco-Escobar et al., 2021; Guerra et al., 2020) and HIV (Jewell et al., 2020). Such disruptions of maintaining preventive measures and drug delivery could potentially lead to significant increases in morbidity and mortality in the region, especially among vulnerable groups (women and children) in SSA (Carrasco-Escobar, 2021; Guerra et al., 2020; Jewell et al., 2020).

Conclusions

The authors conclude that health, socioeconomic, and gender inequalities do exist in SSA, and the COVID-19 pandemic is worsening the existing situation.

Such a situation has a significant negative impact on maternal and child health. Lack of access to education, employment, health, and other factors are generally considered to contribute to women's empowerment in SSA. Among SDH, education is a key driver of maternal and child health in SSA. Therefore, SSA countries must prioritize quality education, as addressing education, especially among young girls and boys and at an early stage of life, will significantly reduce inequalities in workforce and healthcare service utilization and, as a consequence, accelerate progress to meet the SDGs. We hope that this chapter inspires researchers to address impact of SDH on maternal and child health in SSA and across the globe.

Recommendations

The main goal of this chapter is to improve maternal and child health in SSA and similar regions by highlighting the SDH with more focus on education, employment, and access to healthcare. Improving maternal and child health is a key to for any nation's sustainability, as both mother and child represent the core of the SDGs. We are providing the below recommendations, aiming to achieve our main goal:

1 Expansion of healthcare insurance coverage, especially to younger women of reproductive age, rural women, and remote areas.
2 Solving the armed conflict should be a priority in Africa. A good starting point is dealing with the root causes of such conflicts.
3 Enforcement of existing policies and development of new policies if needed to (1) provide high-quality education for all, (2) close the gender gaps in labour force participation and pay, (3) encourage investing in increasing and improving women employment and working conditions, (4) improve access to healthcare services (prenatal care and vaccination), and (4) tackle health, social, and environmental problems such as age of marriage, malaria, HIV/AIDS, violence, gender, corruption, mental health, and climate change.

References

Adde KS, Dickson KS, Amu H. Prevalence and determinants of the place of delivery among reproductive age women in sub–Saharan Africa. *PLoS One*. 2020;15(12): e0244875.

Adgoy ET. Key social determinants of maternal health among African countries: a documentary review. *MOJ Public Heal*. 2018;7(3):140–144.

Aheto JMK. Predictive model and determinants of under-five child mortality: evidence from the 2014 Ghana demographic and health survey. *BMC Pub Health*. 2019;19(64). 1–10.

Ahinkorah BO, Budu E, Aboagye RG, Agbaglo E, Arthur-Holmes F, Adu C, et al. Factors associated with modern contraceptive use among women with no fertility intention in sub-Saharan Africa: evidence from cross-sectional surveys of 29 countries. *Contracept Reprod Med.* 2021a;6(1):1–13.

Ahinkorah BO, Hagan JE, Ameyaw EK, Seidu A-A, Schack T. COVID-19 pandemic worsening gender inequalities for women and girls in Sub-Saharan Africa. *Front Glob Women's Heal.* 2021b;2(July):686984.

Ahinkorah BO, Obisesan MT, Seidu AA, Ajayi AI. Unequal access and use of contraceptives among parenting adolescent girls in sub-Saharan Africa: a cross-sectional analysis of demographic and health surveys. *BMJ Open.* 2021c;11(9):e051583.

Ajayi AI, Somefun OD. Patterns and determinants of short and long birth intervals among women in selected sub-Saharan African countries. *Medicine (Baltimore).* 2020;99(19):e20118.

Akinyemi JO, Solanke BL, Odimegwu CO. Maternal employment and child survival during the era of sustainable development goals: insights from proportional hazards modelling of Nigeria birth history data. *Ann Glob Heal.* 2018;84(1):15–30.

Amu H, Seidu AA, Agbaglo E, Dowou RK, Ameyaw EK, Ahinkorah BO, et al. Mixed effects analysis of factors associated with health insurance coverage among women in sub-Saharan Africa. *PLoS One.* 2021;16(3 March):1–15.

Andriano L, Monden CWS. The causal effect of maternal education on child mortality: evidence from a Quasi-experiment in Malawi and Uganda. *Demography.* 2019;56(5):1765–1790.Atti E, Gulis G. Political determinants of progress in the MDGs in Sub-Saharan Africa. *Glob Public Health.* 2017;12(11):1351–1368.

Backhaus A, Loichinger E. Female labour force participation in sub-Saharan Africa: a cohort analysis [Internet]. WIDER Working Paper. 2021. Available from: http://dx.doi.org/10.35188/unu-wider/2021/998-3

Bado AR, Susuman AS. Women's education and health inequalities in under-five mortality in selected sub-saharan African countries, 1990–2015. *PLoS One.* 2016;11(7):1–18.

Bamiwuye SO, Odimegwu C. Spousal violence in sub-Saharan Africa: does household poverty-wealth matter? *Reprod Health.* 2014;11(45):1–10.

Bangura JB, Xiao S, Qiu D, Ouyang F, Chen L. Barriers to childhood immunization in Sub-Saharan Africa: a systematic review. *PMC Public Heal.* 2020;20(1108).

Baten J, de Haas M, Kempter E, Meier zu Selhausen F. Educational gender inequality in Sub-Saharan Africa a long-term perspective. *Popul Dev Rev.* 2021;47(3):813–849.

Batist J. An intersectional analysis of maternal mortality in Sub-Saharan Africa: a human rights issue. *J Glob Health.* 2019;9(1):1–4.

Bobo FT, Asante A, Woldie M, Dawson A, Hayen A. Child vaccination in sub-Saharan Africa: increasing coverage addresses inequalities. *Vaccine.* 2022;40(1):141–150.

Cangul M, Diouf MA, Esham N, Gupta PK, Li Y, Mitra P, et al. Digitalization in Sub-Saharan Africa. Sub-Saharan Africa Regional Economic Outlook, April 2020. Reg Econ Outlook Sub-Saharan Africa [Internet]. 2020;(April):1–19. Available from: https://www.imf.org/~/media/Files/Publications/REO/AFR/2020/April/English/ch3.ashx?la=en

Carrasco -Escobar G, Fornace K, Benmarhnia T. Mapping socioeconomic inequalities in malaria in Sub-Sahara African countries. *Sci Rep.* 2021;11(1):1–8. Available from: https://doi.org/10.1038/s41598-021-94601-x

Chakravarty S, Das S, Vaillant J. Gender and property rights in Sub-Saharan Africa: a review of constraints and effective interventions [Internet]. 2017. Available from:

https://openknowledge.worldbank.org/bitstream/handle/10986/28905/WPS8245. pdf?sequence=1&isAllowed=y

Chewe M, Hangoma P. Drivers of health in sub-Saharan Africa: a dynamic panel analysis. *Heal Policy OPEN*. 2020;1:100013.

Chichester O, Pluess DJ, Lee M, Taylor A. Women's economic empowerment in Sub-Saharan Africa: recommendations for business action [Internet]. The Business of a Better World. 2017. Available from: https://www.bsr.org/reports/BSR_Womens_ Empowerment_Africa_Main_Report.pdf

Clark S. Improving the future of maternal and child health in [Internet]. 2013. Available from: https://www.mcgill.ca/isid/files/isid/pb_2013_18_clark.pdf

Correa -Agudelo E, Kim HY, Musuka GN, Mukandavire Z, Miller FDW, Tanser F, et al. The epidemiological landscape of anemia in women of reproductive age in sub-Saharan Africa. *Sci Rep*. 2021;11(1):1–10.

Coulibaly I. *The impact of HIV/AIDS on the labour force in Sub-Saharan Africa: a preliminary assessment*. Geneva: International Labor Office; 2005.

Deaton A, Tortora R. People in Sub-Saharan Africa rate their health and health care among lowest in world. *Health Aff (Millwood)*. 2015;34(3):519–527.

Dikete M, Coppieters Y, Trigaux P, Englert Y, Simon P. An analysis of the practices of caesarean section in sub-Saharan Africa: a summary of the literature. *Arch Community Med Public Heal*. 2019;5(2):77–86.

Doctor HV, Nkhana-Salimu S, Abdulsalam-Anibilowo M. Health facility delivery in sub-Saharan Africa: successes, challenges, and implications for the 2030 development agenda. *BMC Public Health*. 2018;18(765):1–12.

Dominic A, Ogundipe A, Ogundipe O. Determinants of women access to healthcare services in Sub-Saharan Africa. *Open Public Health J*. 2020;12(1):504–514.

Duri J. Sub-Saharan Africa: overview of corruption and anti-corruption. Bergen: U4 Anti-Corruption Resource Centre, Chr. Michelsen Institute (U4 Helpdesk Answer 2020:5). Available from: https://www.u4.no/publications/sub-saharan-africa-overview-of-corruption-and-anti-corruption.pdf

Fenta SM, Biresaw HB, Fentaw KD, Gebremichael SG. Determinants of full childhood immunization among children aged 12–23 months in sub-Saharan Africa: a multilevel analysis using Demographic and Health Survey Data. *Trop Med Health*. 2021;49(29) 1–12.

Gender P, In G, Participation F, Care U, Limits W, To P, et al. Fact sheet – Sub-Saharan Africa. 2013; Available from: https://www.unwomen.org/sites/default/files/Headquarters/ Attachments/Sections/Library/Publications/2015/POWW-2015-FactSheet-SubSaharanAfrica-en.pdf

Gerein N, Green A, Pearson S. The implications of shortages of health professionals for maternal health in Sub-Saharan Africa. *Reprod Health Matters*. 2006;14(27):40–50.

Gimba OJ, Seraj M, Ozdeser H. What drives income inequality in sub-Saharan Africa and its sub-regions? An examination of long-run and short-run effects. *African Dev Rev*. 2021;33(4):729–741.

Ginsburg C, Bocquier P, Menashe-Oren A, Collinson MA. Migrant health penalty: evidence of higher mortality risk among internal migrants in sub-Saharan Africa. *Glob Health Action*. 2021;14(1):1930655.

Guerra CA, Tresor Donfack O, Motobe Vaz L, Mba Nlang JA, Nze Nchama LO, Mba Eyono JN, et al. Malaria vector control in sub-Saharan Africa in the time of COVID-19: no room for complacency. *BMJ Glob Heal*. 2020;5(9):e003880.

Hailu BA, Ketema G, Beyene J. Mapping of mothers' suffering and child mortality in Sub-Saharan Africa. *Sci Rep.* 2021;11(1):1–11.

Hailu EM, Maddali SR, Snowden JM, Carmichael SL, Mujahid MS. Structural racism and adverse maternal health outcomes: A systematic review. *Health Place.* 2022 Nov;78:102923.

Iheonu CO, Agbutun SA, Omenihu CM, Ihedimma GI, Osuagwu VN. The impact of governance quality on mortality rates in Sub Saharan Africa. *African Popul Stud.* 2019;33(1):4655–4668.

Jewell BL, Mudimu E, Stover J, ten Brink D, Phillips AN, Smith JA, et al. Potential effects of disruption to HIV programmes in sub-Saharan Africa caused by COVID-19: results from multiple mathematical models. *Lancet HIV.* 2020;7(9):e629–e640.

Jorns-Presentati A, Napp AK, Dessauvagie AS, Stein DJ, Jonker D, Breet E, et al. The prevalence of mental health problems in sub-Saharan adolescents: a systematic review. *PLoS One.* 2021;16(5 May):1–23.

Kassa GM, Arowojolu AO, Odukogbe AA, Yalew AW. Prevalence and determinants of adolescent pregnancy in Africa: a systematic review and Meta-analysis. *Reprod Health.* 2018;15(1195):1–17.

Katsinde SM, Srinivas SC. Breast feeding and the sustainable development agenda. *Indian J Pharm Pract.* 2016;9(3):144–146.

Liu L, Oza S, Hogan D, Chu Y, Perin J, Zhu J, et al. Global, regional, and national causes of under-5 mortality in 2000–15: an updated systematic analysis with implications for the Sustainable Development Goals. *Lancet.* 2016;388(10063):3027–3035.

Londero AP, Rossetti E, Pittini C, Cagnacci A, Driul L. Maternal age and the risk of adverse pregnancy outcomes: a retrospective cohort study. *BMC Pregnancy Childbirth.* 2019;19:261.

Lovász E, Schipp B. The impact of HIV/AIDS on economic growth in Sub-Saharan Africa. *South African J Econ.* 2009;77(2):245–256.

Macassa G, Hallqvist J, Lynch JW. Inequalities in child mortality in Sub-Saharan Africa: a social epidemiologic framework. *Afr J Health Sci.* 2011;18(1–2):14–26.

Malta V, Kolovich L, Leyva AM, Tavares MM, Mendes Tavares M, Wiegand J, et al. Informality and gender gaps going hand in hand authorized for distribution [Internet]. 2019. Available from: https://www.imf.org/~/media/Files/Publications/WP/2019/WPIEA2019112.ashx

Manu C. Threshold effect of corruption on income inequality in Sub-Saharan Africa. *J Bus Stud Q.* 2021;10(3):11–26.

Martin J, Hamilton B, Osterman M, Driscoll A. Births: final data for 2019. *Natl vital Stat Rep.* 2021;70(2):1–51.

Mashige KP, Osuagwu UL, Ulagnathan S, Ekpenyong BN, Abu EK, Goson PC, et al. Economic, health and physical impacts of covid-19 pandemic in sub-saharan african regions: a cross sectional survey. *Risk Manag Healthc Policy.* 2021;14 (August):4799–4807.

Mekonnen T, Dune T, Perz J. Maternal health service utilisation of adolescent women in sub-Saharan Africa: a systematic scoping review. *BMC Pregnancy Childbirth.* 2019;19(366). doi:10.1186/s12884-019-2501-6.

Monden CWS, Smits J. Maternal education is associated with reduced female disadvantages in under-five mortality in sub-Saharan Africa and southern Asia. *Int J Epidemiol.* 2013;42(1):211–218.

Munezero E, Manoukian S. The social determinants of health and health seeking behaviour in populations affected by armed conflict: a qualitative systematic review. *Med Confl Surviv.* 2021;37(4):293–318.

Naicker S, Plange-Rhule J, Tutt RC, Eastwood JB. Shortage of healthcare workers in developing countries - Africa. *Ethn Dis.* 2009;19(1 Suppl.1):S1–60–4.

Naudé W. The determinants of migration from Sub- Saharan African countries. *J Afr Econ.* 2010;19(3):330–356.

Nketiah-Amponsah E. The impact of health expenditures on health outcomes in Sub-Saharan Africa. *J Dev Soc.* 2019;35(1):134–152.

Nyoni T, Ahmed R, Dvalishvili D. Poverty and children's mental, emotional, and behavioral health in Sub-Saharan Africa. *Child Behav Heal Sub-Saharan Africa.* 2022;4:19–39.

Obse AG, Ataguba JE. Explaining socioeconomic disparities and gaps in the use of antenatal care services in 36 countries in sub-Saharan Africa. *Health Policy Plan.* 2021;36(5):651–661.

Oddo VM, Ickes SB. Maternal employment in low- and middle-income countries is associated with improved infant and young child feeding. *Am J Clin Nutr.* 2018;107(3): 335–344.

Odugbesan JA, Rjoub H. Evaluating HIV/AIDS prevalence and sustainable development in sub-saharan africa: the role of health expenditure. *Afr Health Sci.* 2020;20(2):568–578.

Okedo-Alex IN, Akamike IC, Ezeanosike OB, Uneke CJ. Determinants of antenatal care utilisation in sub-Saharan Africa: a systematic review. *BMJ Open.* 2019;9(10):e031890.

Onafeso OD. Analysis of climate change induced forced migration in Sub-Saharan Africa. *Analele Univ Bucuresti Geogr Univ Bucharest – Geogr Ser.* 2020;69(1):153–174.

Sadiddin A, Cattaneo A, Cirillo M, Miller M. Food insecurity as a determinant of international migration: evidence from Sub-Saharan Africa. *Food Secur.* 2019;11(3):515–530.

Silva M, Loureiro A, Cardoso G. Social determinants of mental health: a review of the evidence. *Eur J Psychiatry.* 2016;30(4):259–292.

Stöckl H, Hassan A, Ranganathan M, Hatcher AM. Economic empowerment and intimate partner violence: a secondary data analysis of the cross-sectional demographic health surveys in Sub-Saharan Africa. *BMC Womens Health.* 2021;21(1):1–13.

Sumata C. A framework for understanding migration from Sub-Saharan Africa: transnational and global perspectives. 2021. Available from: https://www.elgaronline.com/view/edcoll/9781789903454/9781789903454.00022.xml

Tamirat K S, Sisay MM, Tesema GA, Tessema ZT. Determinants of adverse birth outcome in Sub-Saharan Africa: analysis of recent demographic and health surveys. *BMC Public Health.* 2021;21(1):1–10.

Tessema G A, Kinfu Y, Dachew BA, Tesema AG, Assefa Y, Alene KA, et al. The COVID-19 pandemic and healthcare systems in Africa: a scoping review of preparedness, impact and response. *BMJ Glob Heal.* 2021;6(12):e007179.

Tesema G A, Teshale AB, Tessema ZT. Incidence and predictors of under-five mortality in East Africa using multilevel Weibull regression modeling. *Arch Public Heal.* 2021;79(1):1–13.

Theisen O M, Strand H, Østby G. Ethno-political favouritism in maternal health care service delivery: micro-level evidence from sub-Saharan Africa, 1981–2014. *Int Area Stud Rev.* 2020;23(1):3–27.

The Lancet Public Health. Education: a neglected social determinant of health. *Lancet Public Heal.* 2020;5(7):e361.

UNICEF, I., 2007. An overview of child well-being in rich countries. *Innocenti Report Card, 7*, p.2007.

United Nations Educational S and CO. UNESCO Covid-19 education response: how many students are at risk of not returning to school? advocacy paper. 2020 [Internet]. Available from: https://education4resilience.iiep.unesco.org/en/resources/2020/unesco-covid-19-education-response-how-many-students-are-risk-not-returning-school

Wehrmeister FC, Fayé CM, da Silva ICM, Amouzou A, Ferreira LZ, Jiwani SS, et al. Wealth-related inequalities in the coverage of reproductive, maternal, newborn and child health interventions in 36 countries in the African region. *Bull World Health Organ.* 2020;98(6):394–405.

Wise J. Alarming global rise in caesarean births, figures show. *BMJ.* 2018;363:k4319. doi: 10.1136/bmj.k4319.

World Bank. FOCUS : Sub-Saharan Africa [Internet]. 2024. Available from: https://open knowledge.worldbank.org/pages/focus-sub-saharan-africa

World Bank. Sub-Saharan Africa [Internet]. 2022. Available from: https://data.world-bank.org/region/sub-saharan-africa

World Health Organization. Closing the gap in a generation: health equity through action on the social determinants of health. Final Report of the Commission on Social Determinants of Health, 2008.

World Health Organization. HIV/AIDS [Internet]. 2021. pp. 1–5. Available from: https://www.who.int/news-room/fact-sheets/detail/hiv-aids

World Health Organization. New report provides groundbreaking insights into the state of health inequities in the Eastern Mediterranean Region [Internet]. 2021. Available from: http://www.emro.who.int/media/news/new-report-reveals-groundbreaking-insights-into-the-state-of-health-inequities-in-the-region.html

World Health Organization. Review of social determinants and the health divide in the WHO European Region. Final report [Internet]. 2017. Available from: https://iris.who.int/handle/10665/108636.

World Health Organization. Social determinants of health. 2009. Available from: https://www.paho.org/en/topics/social-determinants-health

World Health Organization. Trends in maternal mortlaity 2000 to 2017. *Sex Reprod Heal* [Internet]. 2019;1–12. Available from: https://iris.who.int/handle/10665/327596

8

DISEASES OF THE WEST

Vivian Osuchukwu and Erhauyi Meshach Aiwerioghene

Introduction

> Today, getting people to lead healthy lifestyles and adopt healthy behaviours faces opposition from forces that are not so friendly.
>
> *Margaret Chan, former Director-General of the World Health Organization (2006–2017)*

In recent decades, Africa has been undergoing a transformation in its disease burden. As economies grow and urbanization accelerates, the continent is facing a shift from communicable diseases to non-communicable diseases (NCDs). The disease of the West, commonly referred to as the disease of affluence, is a term used to describe the negative health consequences that are associated with a high-income lifestyle as seen in the developed world. These consequences can include obesity, heart disease, stroke, diabetes, and certain types of cancer (Van de Poel et al., 2009).

The disease of the West is becoming increasingly common in Africa due to a number of factors, including (a). A shift towards a more Westernized diet, which is high in processed foods, sugary drinks, and red meat. (b). A decline in physical activity, as people spend more time sitting at desks or driving cars. (c). Increased exposure to environmental pollutants, such as air pollution and second-hand smoke.

The disease of the West can have a significant impact on health and well-being and can lead to premature death, disability, and reduced quality of life. It also has the ability to weaken the healthcare system of any country. The disease of the West is a complex issue, but it is one that can be addressed through a combination

DOI: 10.4324/9781003467601-10

of individual and societal changes. By taking steps to promote healthy lifestyles, we can help improve the health of people in Africa and around the world.

Some examples of the common diseases of the West in Africa include cardiovascular diseases (CVDs), obesity, diabetes, and certain cancers like breast and prostate. The manifestation of the diseases of the West/Affluence in Africa is evident in the continuous increase in prevalence of these diseases as well as the increase in their morbidity and mortality rates. For instance, the obesity prevalence rate in South Africa rose from 13% to 22% in 1998 and 2016, respectively (Tugendhaft et al., 2016). Also, in 2020, the death rate from heart diseases in Africa rose and is considered the leading cause of death in Africa, accounting for about 18% of all deaths in Africa. This current increase in the prevalence of the diseases of the West and their mortality in Africa is of great concern and calls for urgent attention.

This chapter will create awareness of the diseases of the West and their common risk factors, discuss why these diseases are present in Africa (epidemiological transition) and are currently increasing in prevalence and mortality (trend), discuss some diseases of the West common in Africa (CVDs, diabetes, obesity, and breast and prostate cancers) and their impact on individuals, communities, and countries at large, identify measures to tackle these diseases, and finally provide a summary of this chapter.

Common Risk Factors of Diseases of the West in Africa

This section explores the common risk factors contributing to the rise of diseases of West in Africa. These factors include unhealthy diets, physical inactivity, tobacco use, excessive alcohol consumption, and urbanization. The influence of cultural, social, and economic determinants on these risk factors is discussed, highlighting the interplay between traditional lifestyles and modern influences.

Shared Risk Factors

Shared risk factors are factors that increase the likelihood of developing two or more diseases. They can be modifiable or non-modifiable. Modifiable risk factors are mutable factors such as smoking, poor diet, and physical inactivity. However, non-modifiable risk factors are irreversible factors such as age, sex, and family history. Here are some common risk factors for the disease of the West in Africa:

Sedentary Lifestyle

It is a lack of regular physical activity. It is a major risk factor for many chronic diseases, including heart disease, stroke, type 2 diabetes, and some cancers.

Unhealthy Diet

This includes a diet high in processed foods, sugary drinks, and unhealthy fats. It also includes a diet low in fruits, vegetables, and whole grains.

Tobacco Use

This is the use of any tobacco product, including cigarettes, cigars, pipes, and smokeless tobacco. Tobacco use is a major risk factor for lung cancer, heart disease, stroke, and chronic obstructive pulmonary disease (COPD).

Excessive Alcohol Consumption

That is more than two glasses a day for men and one glass a day for women (Gunzerath et al., 2004). Excessive alcohol consumption can lead to many health problems, including liver disease, heart disease, stroke, and cancer.

Stress and Mental Health

This is the feeling of being overwhelmed or unable to cope with the demands of life. Stress can contribute to several health problems, including heart disease, high blood pressure, and depression.

Socioeconomic Factors and Disease Risk

Urbanization and Changing Lifestyles

Urbanization is the movement of people from rural areas to cities. In Africa, urbanization is rapid, and this can contribute to the risk of diseases of the West. This is because people in the city are more likely to have unhealthy diets, inactivity, and smoking. They will also be more vulnerable to air pollution.

Socioeconomic Disparities

Individuals with low and high socioeconomic status experience different levels of access to resources and opportunities. They are exposed to different levels of threat, deprivation, and adversity, and often follow different development paths (Kraus et al., 2012). There are several socioeconomic disparities that could be a contributory factor. We will discuss the most pervasive; income inequality, which is the gap between the rich and the poor. In Africa, income inequality is high, and this can contribute to the risk of diseases of the West. This is because low-income people are more likely to have unhealthy diets, inactivity, and smoking. They also may likely have less access to health care.

Epidemiological Transition of Diseases

In understanding the concept of epidemiological transition, it is very important to define it. According to WHO (2023), an epidemiological transition is a shift in disease patterns, from acute infectious and deficiency diseases associated with underdevelopment to chronic NCDs associated with modernization and advanced levels of development. In epidemiological transition, there is usually a change in the pattern of population distributions in relation to changes in patterns of mortality, fertility, life expectancy, and leading causes of death (McKeown, 2009).

Although the epidemiological transition is sometimes considered to be unidirectional, it could be a complex process where a reversal of the trend can occur. The complex process involves continuous transformation of processes in which diseases disappear and others appear or re-emerge (WHO, 2023). A good example of this complex process could be seen in global regions like Africa.

Africa is currently experiencing an epidemiological transition where both the unidirectional and complex processes are evident. In Africa, NCDs are projected to outpace communicable diseases due to their current increase in trend (unidirectional process of epidemiological transition) (Minja et al., 2022). On the other hand, some parts of Africa are battling with the emergence of new infectious diseases and an increase in previously controlled infectious diseases like tuberculosis and, at the same time, the emergence of NCDs (complex process of epidemiological transition).

The epidemiological transition could evolve because of demographic, biological, cultural, socioeconomic, technological, and environmental changes and modern medicines in several ways (Wahdan, 1996; WHO, 2023). Due to the epidemiological transition that is ongoing in the developing regions, these regions are faced with a double burden of disease.

Double Burden of Diseases in Africa

Africa is currently facing a double burden of disease as seen in other developing regions of the world (Agyei-Mensah & de-Graft Aikins, 2010). With a double burden of diseases in Africa, African countries are faced with continuous pressure from infectious diseases like malaria, and tuberculosis, while battling an increase in the prevalence of NCDs such as CVDs, and cancers, among others. Although with epidemiological transition, it is projected that NCDs will outpace communicable diseases in a short while, this might be the case in Africa in decades to come. The health systems of countries battling a double burden of diseases are weakened and under pressure due to this increase in the trend of NCDs (WHO, 2014; Zeltner et al., 2017).

This increase in trend has been attributed to globalization and economic change. Evidence from 2015 has shown that among NCDs currently trending in Africa, the ones associated with globalization and economic change (diseases of the West), accounted for 33.5% of all deaths as against 29.4% recorded in 2010. There is an estimation that the 'disease of the West' will continue to rise in Africa, with projected deaths exceeding deaths from most communicable diseases combined (Chikowore et al., 2021). This projection is a great worry because Africa is experiencing rapid growth in their economy (African Development Bank, 2023), which would lead to a continuous increase in the prevalence of 'diseases of the West'.

As the African economy grows, people move from rural to urban areas in search of greener pastures (Eyita-Okon, 2022). This process of urbanization exposes people to pollution, and changes in lifestyle and feeding. People tend to feed more on processed foods instead of whole foods and have easy access to alcohol and tobacco. Also, due to the busy work schedule of people living in the cities, engaging in physical activities becomes an issue. It is sad to note that these changes in lifestyle are risk factors for the 'diseases of the West'. Due to limited resources to manage diseases in regions like Africa, available funds are channelled to communicable diseases neglecting the dangers associated with the emerging NCDs (WHO, 2022a). The death rate from NCDs like the diseases of the West is likely to continue to rise due to negligence of the healthcare systems (Gobiṇa et al., 2022). There is a need to understand the diseases of the West common in Africa.

Common Diseases of the West in Africa

Cardiovascular Disease

Heart or blood vessel diseases are referred to as CVDs (NHS, 2022). Some researchers argue that CVD is not an actual disease in itself; rather, it is a lifestyle disease that is defined as a heart and blood vessel disease (Mohammadnezhad et al., 2016). In a functional body, there should be free blood flow to the heart, body, and brain but unfortunately, due to thrombosis and atherosclerosis, blood flow is limited for individuals suffering from CVDs. Thrombosis refers to a blood clot while atherosclerosis is the build-up of fatty deposits inside the artery, which makes the artery hard and narrow (WHO, 2023).

There are different diseases characterized as CVDs which include hypertension (high blood pressure), coronary heart disease, rheumatic heart disease, ischaemic heart disease, cardiomyopathies, atherosclerotic disease, high blood sugar, stroke, heart failure, and arrhythmia (Minja et al., 2022). Of all the above-listed CVDs, hypertension, stroke, cardiomyopathies, and rheumatic heart disease are the most common in Africa, especially in the Sub-Sahara regions (Mocumbi, 2012). CVD is one of the diseases of the West affecting people globally and with an increasing trend in developing regions like Africa.

CVDs Prevalence

There is a global increase in CVD prevalence. Currently, about 620 million people are living with CVDs, which is very high when compared to the prevalence report of 285 million in 1990, 350 million in 2000, and 430 million in 2010 (BHF, 2024). Globally, women account for 53% of the CVD prevalence and, hence, are at higher risk of developing CVD. Although CVD was formerly considered a disease of affluence affecting developed nations, developing nations have reported increased incidence and prevalence. Africa bears the brunt of the CVD burden in the world and records the highest risks of death from chronic diseases (Minja et al., 2022).

Of all the CVDs current in Africa, hypertension (high blood pressure) is the most prevalent. WHO (2022) reported an average estimation of a 27% prevalence rate for hypertension in Africa. Africa has recorded different prevalence rates based on the region, with regions like South and North Africa rating higher. For instance, South Africa has a record over 50% prevalence rate of hypertension (Wollum et al., 2018), while North Africa records 45.4% (Nejjari et al., 2013).

CVDs Mortality

CVDs are an established public health burden and the leading cause of global death (WHO, 2023). CVDs account for about one-third (32%) of global deaths (Roth, 2019; WHO, 2021), with an estimated 17.9 million CDV deaths in 2022 (WHO, 2022). Although global efforts are being made towards the reduction of deaths from CVDs in developed regions of the world (Sacco et al., 2016), the same cannot be said for developing regions like Africa (Gouda et al, 2019). Over three-quarters of CVD deaths take place in low- and middle-income countries. Out of the 17 million premature deaths (under the age of 70) due to noncommunicable diseases in 2019, 38% were caused by CVDs (Cappuccio et al., 2016; WHO, 2021). In Africa, the CVD burden has doubled in the last three decades, accounting for about 38.3% of deaths from NCDs (Gouda, 2019).

There are different disease types that are referred to as CVDs, and they include coronary heart disease, stroke, aortic disease, and peripheral arterial disease. Globally, coronary heart disease is the major cause of CVD global deaths (Monasta et al., 2019, followed by stroke (British Heart Foundation, 2023); but in Africa, stroke is historically recorded as the greatest contributor to these deaths (Mensah, 2015). The annual incidence rate of stroke in Africa is up to 316 per 100,000 individuals, which is within the highest incidence rates in the world, and the prevalence rate of 1,460 per 100,000 reported in one region of Nigeria, western Africa, is clearly among the highest in the world (Akinyemi et al., 2021). Evidence has shown that 38% of people suffering strokes are middle-aged (40–69), and the average age for a woman suffering a stroke has dropped from 75 to 73, and for men, it has dropped from 71 to 68 (Rudd, 2018). This reduction in the age of people suffering from CVD is evident in Sub-Saharan Africa, where the average stroke deaths were recorded among people of younger ages (Moran et al., 2013).

Risk Factors of Cardiovascular Diseases in Africa

The CVD death rate in Africa has been attributed to its risk factors. CVDs share the common lifestyle risk factors associated with diseases of the West, including alcohol intake, tobacco smoking, an unhealthy diet, and physical inactivity (WHO, 2023). Apart from these common lifestyle risk factors for the diseases of the West, there are other factors that could predispose someone to have CVDs, especially in Africa. These peculiar risk factors include hypertension, obesity and overweight, diabetes, high blood cholesterol, raised blood lipids, genetics, gender, age, ethnicity, and stress (Mehta et al., 2015; Murray et al., 2020; WHO, 2023). Some of the above-stated risk factors (age, genetics, gender, and ethnicity) are referred to as non-modifiable risk factors (Mohammadnezhad et al., 2016 This is because individuals have little or no control over them; hence, it may not be totally avoided. Of all the non-modifiable risk factors for CVDs, age plays a greater role in CVD prevalence and mortality rate.

Measures to Lower the Risk of CVDs

Despite the great burden of CVDs, there are ways to reduce the incidence and mortality of CVDs, especially in Africa. These ways include engaging in regular exercise, healthy eating, reducing alcohol intake and smoking, maintaining a healthy weight, and using medication (Grundy et al., 2019). In line with the recommendations for reducing CVD, more approaches, such as a good healthcare system in Africa, are very important.

Diabetes Mellitus: A Growing Concern

In Africa, diabetes is often seen as a disease of the West. This is because it is more common in people who have access to a Western diet and lifestyle, which is characterized by high levels of processed foods, sugary drinks, and physical inactivity. However, diabetes is increasingly becoming a problem for people of all socioeconomic backgrounds in Africa. This is due to several factors, which have been addressed under the common risk factors of diseases of the west in Africa. In 2021, an estimated 1 in 22 adults will have diabetes—24 million. The total number of people with diabetes is predicted to increase by 129% to 55 million by 2045, the highest increase of all IDF regions. In Africa alone, diabetes was responsible for 416,000 deaths in 2021 (IDF, 2021).

Types of Diabetes

Diabetes is a chronic disease that affects how your body metabolizes food into energy. There are two main types of diabetes: type 1 and type 2.

Type 1 diabetes is an autoimmune disease. This means that your immune system attacks and destroys the cells in your pancreas that produce insulin. Insulin is a hormone that helps the body use glucose for energy.

Type 2 diabetes is caused by a combination of genetic and lifestyle factors, such as being overweight or obese, having a family history of diabetes, or physical inactivity.

Challenges in Diagnosis and Management

Diabetes is becoming increasingly common in Africa, especially among the affluent. This is due to several factors, including (a) increased urbanization and westernization, which lead to changes in diet and lifestyle and (b) the rising prevalence of obesity. The challenges of diagnosing and managing diabetes in Africa are also different from those in developed countries. These challenges include: (a) high cost of medications and insulin; (b) lack of trained healthcare professionals, as a result of brain drain; (c). cultural beliefs and practices that may make it difficult to adhere to treatment. Despite these problems, it is important to diagnose and manage diabetes as soon as possible to prevent complications such as heart disease, stroke, blindness, and kidney disease.

Here are some of the specific types of diabetes that are more prevalent in Africa:

- **Gestational diabetes:** This is a type of diabetes that occurs during pregnancy. It is caused by the body's inability to produce enough insulin to meet the demands of pregnancy. Gestational diabetes usually goes away after the baby is born, but it increases the risk of developing type 2 diabetes later in life (McIntyre et al., 2019).
- **Maturity-onset diabetes of the young (MODY):** This is a rare genetic form of diabetes that usually starts in childhood or adolescence. MODY is caused by mutations in genes that control blood sugar levels (Gardner & Tai, 2012).
- **Latent autoimmune diabetes in adults (LADA):** This is a type of diabetes that is similar to type 1 diabetes, but it progresses more slowly. LADA is often misdiagnosed as type 2 diabetes (Jones et al., 2021).

The challenges of diagnosing and managing these types of diabetes in Africa are similar to those of type 1 and type 2 diabetes. However, there are some additional challenges, such as the lack of awareness of these types of diabetes among healthcare professionals. Most people who develop diabetes when they are older have type 2 diabetes, which contributes to the bias of the diagnosis (Thomas et al., 2019).

Cancer Incidence and Challenges

Breast Cancer: Beyond the Numbers

Breast cancer is the second leading cause of cancer deaths and the most common in women globally (Brinton et al., 2018; WHO, 2019). Breast cancer occurs as a result of an uncontrollable multiplication of the breast cells (WHO, 2024). Previously, breast cancer occurred only in developed nations and was considered a disease of the West/Affluence (WHO, 2019); the same cannot be said now due to the current increase in the trend of breast cancer in developing nations, making it a global health problem. Evidence has shown that the increase in breast cancer occurrence in Africa is attributed to globalization and the adoption of Western lifestyles by Africans. Breast cancer can be diagnosed via breast ultrasound, diagnostic mammogram, magnetic resonance imaging (MRI), and biopsy (NHS, 2016). In Africa, breast ultrasound and biopsy are the most common diagnosis approaches. It is unfortunate that in Africa, breast cancer is seen as a death sentence. The reason for this wrong perception of breast cancer in Africa is linked to the poor survival rate of less than 15% in this region (Onyia et al, 2023) unlike in countries like the UK, where 97.3% (survive at least one year) and 88.3% (survive five years and above) (Cancer Research UK, 2023). One of the factors that enhance the effective treatment of breast cancer is early diagnosis. Breast cancer has stages ranging from 0 to IV based on where the tumour is (Trayes & Cokenakes, 2021). Cases of breast cancer diagnosed at early stages have greater chances of survival (Akram et al., 2017). In Africa, most diagnoses take place at stage II, which is a contributing factor to the low survival rate of breast cancer in Africa (Osuchukwu et al., 2021). Managing breast cancer in Africa is challenging, and the current increase in its incidence and prevalence is worrisome.

Breast Cancer Prevalence and Incidence

The global prevalence of breast cancer is one in four cancer diagnoses (Globocan, 2020). Within the last five years, over 7.8 million women have been diagnosed with breast cancer globally, with 2.3 million new cases reported in 2020 (WHO, 2022). In developed nations such as the UK, about 55,900 cases of breast cancer are diagnosed annually (Cancer Research UK, 2023). This prevalence report from developed nations is high when compared to developing nations; nevertheless, there is an increase in the trend of breast cancer in developing nations, such as countries in Africa. In 2020, GLOBOCAN data recorded 186,598 cases of breast cancer in Africa. Although Africa recorded a lower incidence and prevalence of breast cancer, the mortality rate is higher when compared with developed nations (Sushma et al., 2017).

Mortality

It is established that breast cancer accounts for over 15% of cancer-related deaths, making it the most common cause of cancer deaths in women globally (WHO, 2020). Globally, the age standardized mortality rate (ASMR) of breast cancer is 12.9 (31) and, unfortunately, Africa records the highest ASMR in the world (Azubuike et al., 2018). As a result, it has been reported that 58% of breast cancer deaths will occur in developing regions like Africa (WHO, 2019). In 2020, the recorded number of deaths from breast cancer in Africa was 85,787 (Anyigba et al., 2021). This number of deaths is high when compared to developed nations like the UK, which recorded about 11,400 deaths from breast cancer in 2022 (Cancer Research UK, 2023). The developed nations are currently experiencing a decline in breast cancer mortality rates; the UK projected a 26% fall between 2014 and 2035 (Cancer Research UK, 2023); a reverse situation is experienced in Africa. The increase in breast cancer death rates in Africa is attributed to biological, socio-economic, environmental, racial disparity, cultural, and health equalities (Adeloye et al., 2018).

Risk Factors of Breast Cancer

Breast cancer, like some other diseases of the West, has some risk factors that increase a person's chance of developing the condition. Apart from the lifestyle risk factors associated with all the diseases of the West/Affluence (alcohol intake, tobacco smoking, physical inactivity, and unhealthy diet), there are other risk factors peculiar to breast cancer. These peculiar risk factors include being a woman, getting older, reproductive history, having dense breasts, genetic mutation, previous diagnosis, family history, use of combination hormone therapy, consumption of oral contraceptive pills, and prior treatment with radiation (WHO, 2019). In Sub-Saharan Africa, reproductive history (early menarche and menopausal status) and obesity are the most common recorded risk factors for breast cancer (Brandão et al., 2021).

Population at Higher Risk of Breast Cancer

Breast cancer occurs in both men and women, but the ratio of occurrence for men and women is 1:100, which means that women are 100 times more at risk of breast cancer than men (Siegel, 2017). Some of the reasons for the higher burden of breast cancer in women than in men are linked to the uncontrollable risk factors of breast cancer (WHO, 2020), such as being a woman and the presence of female hormones in older age. Evidence has shown that at least 12% of women globally will develop breast cancer at some point in their lives (Howlader et al., 2017).

Breast Cancer Treatment

There are different treatment options for breast cancer, ranging from surgery, chemotherapy, hormone therapy, immunotherapy, and radiotherapy (Mayo Clinic, 2022; WHO, 2019). The choice of treatment depends on the individual breast cancer case, but in Africa, surgery is the most common treatment option (Vanderpuye et al., 2017). The reason for this choice is that it is cheaper and a one-off treatment, except in cases of reoccurrence (Osuchukwu, 2022).

Prostate Cancer: Awareness and Barriers

The burden of prostate cancer in Africa is becoming enormous. Prostate cancer is a type of cancer that develops in the prostate gland, which is about the size of a walnut in men and produces the fluid that makes up sperm (Pernar et al., 2018).

Prostate cancer is considered a disease of the west in Africa. This is due to several factors, including:

- *Westernization of diets*: Eating more processed and red meat is associated with an increased risk of prostate cancer (Kolonel, 2001).
- *Lack of screening*: Awareness about prostate cancer is lacking in Africa, and many men are not screened for the disease. Studies show that men who are screened are more likely to die from the disease than men who are not screened and that African-American men lack knowledge about prostate cancer (Forrester-Anderson, 2005).
- *Financial barriers*: With out-of-pocket payments are the main form of health care payment in most African countries (Derkyi-Kwarteng et al., 2021). The cost of prostate cancer screening and treatment can be a stumbling block for many African men.

There are several barriers to raising awareness of prostate cancer in Africa. These include:

- *Cultural taboos*: There is a cultural taboo around discussing prostate cancer in some parts of Africa. This can make it difficult to talk about the disease and encourage men to get screened.

- *Lack of education*: Many men in Africa do not have enough education about prostate cancer. This can lead to them being unaware of the symptoms of the disease and the importance of getting screened.
- *Language barriers*: There are many languages spoken in Africa, and this can make it difficult to translate educational materials about prostate cancer into local languages.

Despite these barriers, many efforts are being made to raise awareness about prostate cancer in Africa. These include:

- *Public Awareness Campaign*: There are several public awareness campaigns about prostate cancer in Africa. These campaigns are used to educate men about the disease and the importance of screening.
- *Training of healthcare providers*: Healthcare providers in Africa are being trained to screen for and diagnose prostate cancer. This will help to ensure that more men, especially in rural areas, are diagnosed with the disease early, when it is more treatable.
- *Development of cancer registries*: Cancer registries are being developed in Africa to track the incidence and mortality of prostate cancer. This information will be used to improve the prevention, diagnosis, and treatment of the disease.

Raising awareness of prostate cancer in Africa is essential to reducing the burden of the disease. By overcoming the barriers to awareness, we can help more men in Africa get screened and diagnosed early and improve their chances of survival.

Obesity

Obesity, which was previously considered the disease of the West, is currently a public health problem that affects people in all regions of the world (Azeez, 2022). Obesity is defined as an abnormal or excessive accumulation of fat that is associated with increased health risk (Fruh, 2017). In diagnosing obesity, the body mass index (BMI) is commonly used. BMI is a measurement of weight in relation to height and is calculated by dividing a person's body mass (weight) by the square of their height (CDC, 2013). In establishing cases of obesity using BMI, any individual with a BMI value greater than or equal to 30.0 kg/m^2 is said to be obese (Osundolire, 2021). This aligns with the WHO definition of obesity as a BMI $> 30 \text{ kg/m}^2$ and overweight as a BMI $> 25 \text{ kg/m}^2$. Obesity is caused by an energy imbalance between calories consumed and calories expelled from the body. The problem of obesity is challenging considering that obesity is a risk factor for other diseases of the West such as CVDs, hypertension, and type

2 diabetes (Powell-Wiley et al., 2021). Obesity also affects the economies of nations via direct and indirect costs (Tremmel et al., 2017). Due to the availability of adequate economic resources in developed nations, managing obesity is not as challenging as it is in developing nations, where poverty is still the order of the day (Azeez, 2022). Although obesity was previously considered a disease of developed nations, developing regions of the world, like Africa, are currently battling obesity and overweight (Azeez, 2022). The continuous increase in obesity prevalence in Africa is attributed to increased globalization and the adoption of a western unhealthy lifestyle (Hruby & Hu, 2015). These attributed factors could determine the health of an individual. In social epidemiology, health determinants rather than just the disease cause are considered.

Prevalence of Obesity

Globally, obesity prevalence is on the rise, and a continuous increase is estimated (Agha & Agha, 2017; WHO, 2022b). There was a massive increase in global obesity prevalence between 1980 and 2019, from 6% to 15.7% in women and from 3.2% to 12.2% in men (Mathew et al., 2018). Currently, more than 650 million people aged 18 years and above are obese globally (Oguoma et al., 2021). This global rise in obesity prevalence is evident in Africa, where it is anticipated that childhood obesity will rise from 5% to 14% and obesity in women from 18% to 31% by the year 2035. As seen in breast cancer, women are at higher risk of obesity than men due to the higher percentage of body fat in women, which is biologically driven. In the absence of adequate measures to tackle obesity in Africa, it is estimated that by the end of 2023, one in five adults and one in ten children/teenagers will be obese (World Obesity Atlas, 2023). Obesity is a ticking time bomb in Africa that needs urgent attention and calls for worry, as some countries in Africa, like Nigeria, see obesity as a show of affluence rather than a disease condition.

Obesity Risk Factors and Health Determinants

The following are the risk factors for obesity: lack of physical activity, inadequate sleep, unhealthy eating behaviours, high amounts of stress, genetics and health conditions such as metabolic syndrome, medicines such as antidepressants, birth control, and antipsychotic medicines,CDC 2024. The health determinants for obesity in Africa include demographic (e.g., gender and age), socio-economic (e.g., income, education, and employment), lifestyle (e.g., sedentary lifestyle and poor diet), biological (genetic), and environmental factors (home and workplace). These factors could directly or indirectly determine the obesity status of a person. In using socioeconomic status, for example, obesity is common among people of higher socioeconomic status in Africa, which is a reverse situation in developed nations (Pampel et al 2012. Also, where a person lives and works could directly or indirectly determine their health (Bravemann and Gottlieb, 2014). In the case of obesity, having access to good meals and green space for exercise around where you live and work could contribute to obesity or not Consequences of Obesity

Obesity consequences include health, psychological, social, and economic consequences (CDC, 2023). Obesity is a risk factor for health conditions such as hypertension, type 2 diabetes, CVDs such as stroke and heart disease, sleep apnoea, breathing difficulty, body pain, osteoarthritis, different cancers, and gallbladder disease (Singh et al., 2013). The psychological consequences include anxiety, depression, low self-esteem, poor body image, and a low quality of life (Gatineau & Dent, 2011). The social consequences of obesity include isolation, discrimination, fewer friends, and lower employment. The economic consequences address the healthcare cost of obesity, which will include hospital admission and medication costs (Okunogbe et al., 2021; Vityala et al., 2022).

Obesity Preventive and Control Measures

In preventing and controlling obesity, different measures could be taken. These measures include dietary change, increased physical activity, a decreased sedentary lifestyle, health education, medication, weight loss surgery (liposuction), getting adequate sleep, and avoiding excessive stress (Ali, 2022).

Tackling Obesity in Africa

In order to address the problem of obesity in Africa, all hands must be on deck. A collective approach where individuals, communities, organizations, government, and non-government organizations (NGOs) play a role in addressing some of the risk factors for obesity is vital. For instance, the government could create safe and active transport systems, provide green places for physical activities, and establish policies to govern the food industry in terms of manufacturing healthy meals. Organizations like the food industry, on the other hand, will ensure that healthy foods are produced in line with established policies and made available for individuals for consumption. The NGO will work with the government in monitoring organizations' adherence to policies and the management of their infrastructure. Individuals will be encouraged to take charge of their health by utilizing all the available support for health promotion.

Tackling the Diseases of the West in Africa

Everyone deserves access to good health care, regardless of their income or social status. All nations must work to ensure that everyone has access to quality health care (WHO). Several approaches can be used to tackle these diseases of the West in Africa. We have highlighted some approaches that will fit well in the African region.

Multifaceted Approaches to Prevention

- *Promoting healthy lifestyles*: This includes encouraging people to eat a healthy diet, exercise regularly, and avoid smoking and excessive alcohol consumption.
- *Screening and early detection*: Early detection and treatment of chronic diseases can help to prevent complications and improve outcomes.
- *Public health interventions*: These interventions can include policies to reduce salt intake, promote breastfeeding, and improve sanitation.

Strengthening Healthcare Systems

- *Investing in human resources*: With the brain drain associated with healthcare professionals, is mostly rampant in West Africa (Aiwerioghene et al., 2021). Training more doctors, nurses, and other health workers will be a good measure to tackle issues relating to brain drain.
- *Improving infrastructure*: This includes building more hospitals and clinics and providing access to essential medicines and equipment.
- *Developing information systems*: The health information system (HIS) has proven to be an important aspect of managing healthcare delivery. This will help to track and monitor chronic diseases and improve the quality of care.
- *Strengthening community-based healthcare*: This will help to ensure that people have access to care, even in remote areas.

Policy and Advocacy

- *Taxing unhealthy foods and beverages*: This would make these products more expensive and encourage people to make healthier choices (Sacks et al., 2021).
- *Regulating the marketing of unhealthy products*: This would limit the advertising of unhealthy foods and beverages to children (Kelly et al., 2019).
- *Providing subsidies for healthy foods*: This would make healthy foods more affordable. In general, a healthy diet will usually cost more than 20% (Temple et al., 2011). As a result, low-income people are forced to choose unhealthy diets that are low in certain micronutrients (such as vitamin C and β-carotene) and high in energy density (Darmon & Drewnowski, 2008).
- *Encouraging physical activity*: This could be done by building more parks and recreation facilities and providing safe places for people to walk and bike.

Community Engagement and Empowerment

- *Community-based health education*: This would help people understand the risks of chronic diseases and how to prevent them (Merzel & D'Afflitti, 2003).
- *Support groups*: These groups could provide emotional support and practical advice to people with chronic diseases.
- *Advocacy*: Communities can advocate for policies and programmes that promote healthy lifestyles and prevent chronic diseases.

Future Perspectives and Challenges

The future of tackling the diseases of the West in Africa is promising. There is a growing awareness of the problem, and governments and other stakeholders are taking steps to address it. However, there are still a number of challenges that need to be overcome. These include:

Lack of resources: GDP allocated to healthcare is relatively low, leading to limited resources being invested in healthcare. In Sub-Saharan Africa, health spending as a share of GDP (%) in 2020 had an average of 4.92% spent on healthcare (WHO).

Inequity: The diseases of the West are disproportionately affecting the poor and marginalized.

Culture: In some cultures, in Africa, there is a stigma associated with chronic diseases, which can make it difficult for people to seek care (De-Graft Aikins et al., 2010).

Despite these challenges, there is hope that the diseases of the West can be tackled in Africa. By working together, we can create a healthier future for the continent.

Conclusion

'The Diseases of West in Africa' refers to the emergence of NCDs in African countries, traditionally associated with more affluent societies. These diseases, such as heart disease, diabetes, hypertension, and obesity, have been on the rise in Africa due to changing lifestyles, urbanization, and dietary shifts towards processed foods. Factors like increased sedentary behaviour, tobacco use, and excessive alcohol consumption have also contributed to this health challenge. The rise of NCDs in Africa presents a complex and growing public health concern, necessitating comprehensive strategies to address prevention, early detection, and management, given the limited healthcare resources available in many African nations. Rapid urbanization is leading to changes in diet and lifestyle. These changes are contributing to the increasing rates of CVDs, cancer, and diabetes. Adopting unhealthy lifestyles that are more common in developed countries. These unhealthy lifestyles include eating more processed foods, being more sedentary, and smoking more cigarettes. The rural part of Africa does not have access to adequate health care. This means that they are less likely to be diagnosed and treated on time. The diseases of the West are a major challenge to public health in Africa. They are responsible for millions of deaths each year, and they are a major drain on the economy. There is a need to raise awareness of these diseases and implement interventions to prevent them.

References

Adeloye, D., Sowunmi, O. Y., Jacobs, W., David, R. A., Adeosun, A. A., Amuta, A. O., et al. (2018). Estimating the incidence of breast cancer in Africa: a systematic review and meta-analysis. *Journal of Global Health*, 8(1): 010494.

African Development Bank. (2023). African Development Bank Group Report. Available at:https://www.afdb.org/en/news-and-events/press-releases/african-development-bank-group-report-2023-africa-remains-resilient-new-shocks-progress-and-financing-must-be-accelerated-61446.accessed 29/06/24

Agha, M. and Agha, R., 2017. The rising prevalence of obesity: part A: impact on public health. *IJS Oncology*, 2(7), p.e17.

Agyei-Mensah, S., & de-Graft Aikins, A. (2010). Epidemiological transition and the double burden of disease in Accra, Ghana. *Journal of Urban Health Bull New York Academy of Medicine*, 87, 879–897.

Aiwerioghene, E. M., Singh, M., & Ajmera, P. (2021). Modelling the factors affecting Nigerian medical tourism sector using an interpretive structural modelling approach. *International Journal of Healthcare Management*, 14(2), 563–575. https://doi.org/10.1080/20479700.2019.1677036

Akinyemi, R.O., Ovbiagele, B., Adeniji, O.A., Sarfo, F.S., Abd-Allah, F., Adoukonou, T., Ogah, O.S., Naidoo, P., Damasceno, A., Walker, R.W. and Ogunniyi, A., 2021. Stroke in Africa: profile, progress, prospects and priorities. *Nature Reviews Neurology*, 17(10), pp.634–656.

Akram, M., Iqbal, M., Daniyal, M., & Khan, A.U. (2017). Awareness and current knowledge of breast cancer. *Biological Research*, 50(1), 3

Ali, N., Mohanto, N.C., Nurunnabi, S.M., Haque, T. and Islam, F., 2022. Prevalence and risk factors of general and abdominal obesity and hypertension in rural and urban residents in Bangladesh: a cross-sectional study. *BMC Public Health*, 22(1), p.1707

Anyigba, C. A., Awandare, G. A., & Paemka, L. (2021). Breast cancer in sub-Saharan Africa: the current state and uncertain future. *Experimental Biology and Medicine (Maywood)*, 246(12), 1377–1387.

Azeez, T.A., 2022. Obesity in Africa: The challenges of a rising epidemic in the midst of dwindling resources. *Obesity Medicine*, 31, p.100397.

Azubuike, S.O., Muirhead, C., Hayes, L. and McNally, R., 2018. Rising global burden of breast cancer: the case of sub-Saharan Africa (with emphasis on Nigeria) and implications for regional development: a review. *World journal of surgical oncology*, 16, pp.1–13.

Brandão, M., Guisseve, A., Damasceno, A., Bata, G., Silva-Matos, C., Alberto, M., et al. (2021). Risk factors for breast cancer, overall and by tumor subtype, among women from Mozambique, Sub-Saharan Africa. *Cancer Epidemiology, Biomarkers and Prevention*, 30(6), 1250–1259.

Braveman P, Gottlieb L. The social determinants of health: it's time to consider the causes of the causes. Public Health Rep. 2014 Jan-Feb;129 Suppl 2(Suppl 2):19–31.

Brinton, L. A., Brogan, D. R., Coates, R. J., Swanson, C. A., Potischman, N., & Stanford, J. L. (2018). Breast cancer risk among women under 55 years of age by joint effects of usage of oral contraceptives and hormone replacement therapy. *Menopause*, 25(11), 1195–1200.

British Heart Foundation (2024). Global and circulatory Heart Diseases Factsheet. Available at https://www.bhf.org.uk/-/media/files/for-professionals/research/heart-statistics/bhf-cvd-statistics-global-factsheet.pdf?rev=e61c05db17e94 39a8c2e4720f6ca0a19&hash=6350DE1B2A19D939431D876311077C7B accessed 30/06/24.

British Heart Foundation (2023). Heart and Circulatory Statistics 2023. Available at https://www.bhf.org.uk/what-we-do/our-research/heart-statistics/heart-statistics-publications/cardiovascular-disease-statistics-2023

Cancer Research UK (2023). Breast cancer mortality statistics. Available at https://www.cancerresearchuk.org/health-professional/cancer-statistics/statistics-by-cancer-type/breast-cancer Accessed 01/07/2024

Cappuccio, F.P., Buchanan, L.A., Ji, C., Siani, A. and Miller, M.A., 2016. Systematic review and meta-analysis of randomised controlled trials on the effects of potassium supplements on serum potassium and creatinine. *BMJ open*, 6(8), p.e011716.

Centre for Disease Control and Prevention (2013). Body Mass Index: BMI for children and teens. https://en.m.wikipedia.org/wiki/body-mass-index

Centefor Disease Control and Prevention (CDC) (2023). How is breast cancer treated? https://www.cdc.gov/cancer/breast/basic_info/treatment.htm

Center for Disease Control and Prevention (CDC) (2024). Risk factors for Obesity available at https://www.cdc.gov/obesity/php/about/risk-factors.html accessed 01/02/2024

Chikowore, T., Kamiza, A. B., Oduaran, O. H., Machipisa, T., & Fatumo, S. (2021). Non-communicable diseases pandemic and precision medicine. Is Africa ready? *EBio Medicine*, 65, 103260.

Darmon, N., & Drewnowski, A. (2008). Does social class predict diet quality? *The American Journal of Clinical Nutrition*, 87(5), 1107–1117. https://doi.org/10.1093/ajcn/87.5.1107

De-Graft Aikins, A., Unwin, N., Agyemang, C., Allotey, P., Campbell, C., & Arhinful, D. (2010). Tackling Africa's chronic disease burden: from the local to the global. *Globalization and Health*, 6(1), 1–7. https://doi.org/10.1186/1744-8603-6-5

Derkyi-Kwarteng, A. N. C., Agyepong, I. A., Enyimayew, N., & Gilson, L. (2021). A narrative synthesis review of out-of-pocket payments for health services under insurance regimes: a policy implementation gap hindering universal health coverage in sub-Saharan Africa. *International Journal of Health Policy and Management*, 10(7), 443. https://doi.org/10.34172/ijhpm.2021.38

Eyita-Okon, E. (2022). Urbanization and human security in post-colonial Africa. *Frontier in Sustainable Cities*, 4, 917764.

Forrester-Anderson, I. T. (2005). Prostate cancer screening perceptions, knowledge and behaviors among African American men: focus group findings. *Journal of Health Care for the Poor and Underserved*, 16(4), 22–30. https://doi.org/10.1353/hpu.2005.0063

Fruh, S.M., 2017. Obesity: Risk factors, complications, and strategies for sustainable long-term weight management. *Journal of the American association of nurse practitioners*, 29(S1), pp.S3–S14.

Gardner, D. S., & Tai, E. S. (2012). Clinical features and treatment of maturity onset diabetes of the young (MODY). *Diabetes, Metabolic Syndrome and Obesity: Targets and Therapy*, 5, 101–108.

Gatineau, M., & Dent, M. (2011). *Obesity and mental health*. Oxford National Obesity Observatory.

GLOBOCAN (2020). New global cancer data. https://www.uicc.org/news/globocan-2020-new-global-cancer-data

Gobiņa, I., Avotiņš, A., Kojalo, U., Strēle, I., Pildava, S., Villeruša, A., & Briģis, Ģ. (2022). Excess mortality associated with the COVID-19 pandemic in Latvia: a population-level analysis of all-cause and non-communicable disease deaths in 2020. *BMC Public Health*, 22, 1109.

Gouda, H.N., Charlson, F., Sorsdahl, K., Ahmadzada, S., Ferrari, A.J., Erskine, H., Leung, J., Santamauro, D., Lund, C., Aminde, L.N. and Mayosi, B.M., 2019. Burden of non-communicable diseases in sub-Saharan Africa, 1990–2017: results from the Global Burden of Disease Study 2017. *The Lancet Global Health*, 7(10), pp.e1375–e1387.

Grundy, S.M., Stone, N.J., Bailey, A.L., Beam, C., Birtcher, K.K., Blumenthal, R.S., Braun, L.T., De Ferranti, S., Faiella-Tommasino, J., Forman, D.E. and Goldberg, R., 2019. 2018 AHA/ACC/AACVPR/AAPA/ABC/ACPM/ADA/AGS/APhA/ASPC/NLA/PCNA guideline on the management of blood cholesterol: executive summary: a report of the American College of Cardiology/American Heart Association Task Force on Clinical Practice Guidelines. *Circulation*, 139(25), pp.e1046–e1081.

Gunzerath, L., Faden, V. B., Zakhari, S., & Warren, K. W. (2004). National Institute on alcohol abuse and Alcoholism report on moderate drinking. *Alcoholism: Clinical and Experimental Research*, 28(6), 829–847. https://doi.org/10.1097/01.alc.0000128382.79375.b6

Howlader, N., Mariotto, A.B., Besson, C., Suneja, G., Robien, K., Younes, N. and Engels, E.A., 2017. Cancer-specific mortality, cure fraction, and noncancer causes of death among diffuse large B-cell lymphoma patients in the immunochemotherapy era. *Cancer*, 123(17), pp.3326-3334.

Hruby, A. and Hu, F.B., 2015. The epidemiology of obesity: a big picture. *Pharmacoeconomics*, 33, pp.673–689.

International Diabetes Federation (2021). https://diabetesatlas.org/idfawp/resource-files/2022/01/IDF-Atlas-Factsheet-2021_AFR.pdf

Jones, A. G., McDonald, T. J., Shields, B. M., Hagopian, W., & Hattersley, A. T. (2021). Latent Autoimmune Diabetes of Adults (LADA) is likely to represent a mixed population of autoimmune (type 1) and nonautoimmune (type 2) diabetes. *Diabetes Care*, 44(6), 1243–1251. https://doi.org/10.2337/dc20-2834

Kelly, B., Vandevijvere, S., Ng, S., Adams, J., Allemandi, L., Bahena-Espina, L., ... & Swinburn, B. (2019). Global benchmarking of children's exposure to television advertising of unhealthy foods and beverages across 22 countries. *Obesity Reviews*, 20, 116–128. https://doi.org/10.1111/obr.12840

Kolonel, L. N. (2001). Fat, meat, and prostate cancer. *Epidemiologic Reviews*, 23(1), 72–81. https://www.naturaleater.com/Science-articles/Fat-Meat-Prostate-Cancer.pdf

Kraus, M. W., Piff, P. K., Mendoza-Denton, R., Rheinschmidt, M. L., & Keltner, D. (2012). Social class, solipsism, and contextualism: how the rich are different from the poor. Psychological Review, 119(3), 546. https://doi.org/10.1037/a0028756

McKeown RE. (2009). The Epidemiologic Transition: Changing Patterns of Mortality and Population Dynamics. American Journal of Lifestyle Medicine. 2009 Jul 1;3(1 Suppl):19S–26S.

Mathew, H., Castracane, V. D., & Mantzoros, C. (2018). Adipose tissue and reproductive health. *Metabolism, 86*, 18–32.

Mayo Clinic (2022). Breast Cancer available at https://www.mayoclinic.org/diseases-conditions/breast-cancer/diagnosis-treatment/drc-20352475 accessed 01/07/2024

McIntyre, H. D., Catalano, P., Zhang, C., Desoye, G., Mathiesen, E. R., & Damm, P. (2019). Gestational diabetes mellitus. *Nature Reviews Disease Primers*, 5(1), 47. https://doi.org/10.1038/s41572-019-0098-8

Mensah, George A., Uchechukwu KA Sampson, Gregory A. Roth, Mohammed H. Forou-zanfar, Mohsen Naghavi, Christopher JL Murray, Andrew E. Moran, and Valery L. Feigin. "Mortality from cardiovascular diseases in sub-Saharan Africa, 1990–2013: a systematic analysis of data from the Global Burden of Disease Study 2013." *Cardio-vascular journal of Africa* 26, no. 2 H3Africa Suppl (2015): S6.

Merzel, C., & D'Afflitti, J. (2003). Reconsidering community-based health promotion: promise, performance, and potential. *American Journal of Public Health*, 93(4), 557–574. https://ajph.aphapublications.org/doi/full/10.2105/AJPH.93.4.557

Mehta, P.K., Wei, J. and Wenger, N.K., 2015. Ischemic heart disease in women: a focus on risk factors. *Trends in cardiovascular medicine*, 25(2), pp.140–151.

Minja, N.W., Nakagaayi, D., Aliku, T., Zhang, W., Ssinabulya, I., Nabaale, J., Amutu-haire, W., de Loizaga, S.R., Ndagire, E., Rwebembera, J. and Okello, E., 2022. Car-diovascular diseases in Africa in the twenty-first century: gaps and priorities going forward. *Frontiers in Cardiovascular Medicine*, 9, p.1008335.

Mocumbi, A.O., 2012. Lack of focus on cardiovascular disease in sub-Saharan Africa. *Cardiovascular diagnosis and therapy*, 2(1), p.74.

Mohammadnezhad, M., Mangum, T., May, W., Lucas, J.J. and Ailson, S., 2016. Common modifiable and non-modifiable risk factors of cardiovascular disease (CVD) among Pacific countries. *World Journal of Cardiovascular Surgery*, 6(11), pp.153-170.

Monasta, L., Abbafati, C., Logroscino, G., Remuzzi, G., Perico, N., Bikbov, B., Tam-burlini, G., Beghi, E., Traini, E., Redford, S.B. and Ariani, F., 2019. Italy's health performance, 1990–2017: findings from the global burden of disease study 2017. *The Lancet Public Health*, 4(12), pp.e645–e657.

Moran, G.M., Fletcher, B., Feltham, M.G., Calvert, M., Sackley, C. and Marshall, T., 2014. Fatigue, psychological and cognitive impairment following transient ischaemic attack and minor stroke: a systematic review. *European journal of neurology*, 21(10), pp.1258–1267.

Murray, C.J., Aravkin, A.Y., Zheng, P., Abbafati, C., Abbas, K.M., Abbasi-Kangevari, M., Abd-Allah, F., Abdelalim, A., Abdollahi, M., Abdollahpour, I. and Abegaz, K.H., 2020. Global burden of 87 risk factors in 204 countries and territories, 1990–2019: a system-atic analysis for the Global Burden of Disease Study 2019. *The lancet*, 396(10258), pp.1223–1249.

National Health Service (NHS) (2022). Breast cancer in women: diagnosis. https://www. nhs.uk/conditions/breast-cancer/

Nejjari, C., Arharbi, M., Chentir, M.T., Boujnah, R., Kemmou, O., Megdiche, H., Boulahrouf, F., Messoussi, K., Nazek, L. and Bulatov, V., 2013. Epidemiological Trial of Hypertension in North Africa (ETHNA): an international multicentre study in Algeria, Morocco and Tunisia. *Journal of Hypertension, 31*(1), pp.49–62.

NHS, England (2016). Clinical Guidelines for the Management of Breast Cancer available at https://www.england.nhs.uk/mids-east/wp-content/uploads/sites/7/2018/02/ guidelines-for-the-management-of-breast-cancer-v1.pdf. Accessed 01/06/2024

Oguoma, V.M., Coffee, N.T., Alsharrah, S., Abu-Farha, M., Al-Refaei, F.H., Al-Mulla, F. and Daniel, M., 2021. Prevalence of overweight and obesity, and associations with socio-demographic factors in Kuwait. *BMC public health, 21*, pp.1–13.

Okunogbe, A., Nugent, R., Spencer, G., Ralston, J., & Wilding, J. (2021). Economic impacts of overweight and obesity: current and future estimates for eight countries. *BMJ Global Health, 6*, e006351.

Onyia, A.F., Nana, T.A., Adewale, E.A., Adebesin, A.O., Adegboye, B.E., Paimo, O.K., De Campos, O.C., Bisi-Adeniyi, T.I., Rotimi, O.A., Oyelade, J.O. and Rotimi, S.O., 2023. Breast Cancer Phenotypes in Africa: A Scoping Review and Meta-Analysis. *JCO Global Oncology, 9*, p.e2300135

Osuchukwu, V. C., Anyanwu, P. E., Ling, J., & Hayes, C. (2021). A systematic review of the impact of sociocultural factors on West African Breast Cancer Diagnosis and Management. *Journal of Archives of Clinical Case Studies and Case Reports, 2*(10), 261–274.

Osuchukwu, V.C., 2022. *Treatment experiences of breast cancer patients in Nigeria: the impact of sociocultural factors as mediators of breast cancer treatment and outcomes* (Doctoral dissertation, University of Sunderland).

Osundolire, S., 2021. The prevalence of overweight and its association with heart disease in the US population. *Cogent Medicine, 8*(1), p.1923614.Pampel, F.C., Denney, J.T. and Krueger, P.M., 2012. Obesity, SES, and economic development: a test of the reversal hypothesis. *Social science & medicine, 74*(7), pp.1073–1081.

Pernar, C. H., Ebot, E. M., Wilson, K. M., & Mucci, L. A. (2018). The epidemiology of prostate cancer. *Cold Spring Harbor Perspectives in Medicine*. https://doi.org/ 10.1101/cshperspect.a030361

Powell-Wiley, T.M., Poirier, P., Burke, L.E., Després, J.P., Gordon-Larsen, P., Lavie, C.J., Lear, S.A., Ndumele, C.E., Neeland, I.J., Sanders, P. and St-Onge, M.P., 2021. Obesity and cardiovascular disease: a scientific statement from the American Heart Association. *Circulation, 143*(21), pp.e984–e1010.

Roth GA, Mensah GA, Johnson CO, Addolorato G, Ammirati E, Baddour LM, Barengo NC, Beaton AZ, Benjamin EJ, Benziger CP, Bonny A, Brauer M, Brodmann M, Cahill TJ, Carapetis J, Catapano AL, Chugh SS, Cooper LT, Coresh J, Criqui M, DeCleene N, Eagle KA, Emmons-Bell S, Feigin VL, Fernández-Solà J, Fowkes G, Gakidou E, Grundy SM, He FJ, Howard G, Hu F, Inker L, Karthikeyan G, Kassebaum N, Koroshetz W, Lavie C, Lloyd-Jones D, Lu HS, Mirijello A, Temesgen AM, Mokdad A, Moran AE, Muntner P, Narula J, Neal B, Ntsekhe M, Moraes de Oliveira G, Otto C, Owolabi M, Pratt M, Rajagopalan S, Reitsma M, Ribeiro ALP, Rigotti N, Rodgers A, Sable C, Shakil S, Sliwa-Hahnle K, Stark B, Sundström J, Timpel P, Tleyjeh IM, Valgimigli M, Vos T, Whelton PK, Yacoub M, Zuhlke L, Murray C, Fuster V; GBD-NHLBI-JACC

Global Burden of Cardiovascular Diseases Writing Group. Global Burden of Cardio-vascular Diseases and Risk Factors, 1990-2019: Update From the GBD 2019 Study. J Am Coll Cardiol. 2020 Dec 22;76(25):2982-3021. doi: 10.1016/j.jacc.2020.11.010. Erratum in: J Am Coll Cardiol. 2021 Apr 20;77(15):1958–1959.

Rudd, A.G., Hoffman, A., Grant, R., Campbell, J.T. and Lowe, D., 2011. Stroke throm-bolysis in England, Wales and Northern Ireland: how much do we do and how much do we need?. *Journal of Neurology, Neurosurgery & Psychiatry*, 82(1), pp.14–19.

Sacks, G., Kwon, J., & Backholer, K. (2021). Do taxes on unhealthy foods and bever-ages influence food purchases? *Current Nutrition Reports*, 10(3), 179–187. https://doi.org/10.1007/s13668-021-00358-0

Siegel, R. L., Miller, K. D., & Jemal, A. (2017). Cancer statistics 2017. *CA: Cancer Jour-nal for Clinicians*, 67(1), 7–30.

Singh, G.M., Danaei, G., Farzadfar, F., Stevens, G.A., Woodward, M., Wormser, D., Kaptoge, S., Whitlock, G., Qiao, Q., Lewington, S. and Di Angelantonio, E., 2013. The age-specific quantitative effects of metabolic risk factors on cardiovascular dis-eases and diabetes: a pooled analysis. *PloS one*, 8(7), p.e65174.

Sacco, R.L., Roth, G.A., Reddy, K.S., Arnett, D.K., Bonita, R., Gaziano, T.A., Heidenreich, P.A., Huffman, M.D., Mayosi, B.M., Mendis, S. and Murray, C.J., 2016. The heart of 25 by 25: achieving the goal of reducing global and regional premature deaths from cardiovascular diseases and stroke: a modeling study from the American Heart Association and World Heart Federation. *Circulation*, 133(23), pp.e674–e690.

Sushma, S.J. and Prasanna Kumar, S.C., 2017. Multi-stage Optimization Over Extracted Feature for Detection and Classification of Breast Cancer. In *Software Engineering Trends and Techniques in Intelligent Systems: Proceedings of the 6th Computer Sci-ence On-line Conference 2017 (CSOC2017), Vol 3 6* (pp. 276-283). Springer Interna-tional Publishing.

Temple, N. J., & Steyn, N. P. (2011). The cost of a healthy diet: A South African perspec-tive. *Nutrition*, 27(5), 505–508. https://doi.org/10.1016/j.nut.2010.09.005

Tremmel, M., Gerdtham, U.G., Nilsson, P.M. and Saha, S., 2017. Economic burden of obesity: a systematic literature review. *International journal of environmental research and public health*, 14(4), p.435.

Thomas, N. J., Lynam, A. L., Hill, A. V., Weedon, M. N., Shields, B. M., Oram, R. A., et al. (2019). Type 1 diabetes defined by severe insulin deficiency occurs after 30 years of age and is commonly treated as type 2 diabetes. *Diabetologia*, 62(7), 1167–1172. https://doi.org/10.1007/s00125-019-4863-8

Trayes, K. P., & Cokenakes, S. E. H. (2021). Breast cancer treatment. *American Family Physician*, 104(2), 171–178.

Tugendhaft, A., Manyema, M., Veerman, L. J., Chola, L., Labadarios, D., & Hofman, K. J. (2016). Cost of inaction on sugar-sweetened beverage consumption: implications for obesity in South Africa. *Public Health Nutrition*, 19(13), 2296–2304. https://doi.org/10.1017/S1368980015003006

Van de Poel, E., O'Donnell, O., & Van Doorslaer, E. (2009). Urbanization and the spread of diseases of affluence in China. *Economics & Human Biology*, 7(2), 200–216. https://doi.org/10.1016/j.ehb.2009.05.004

Vanderpuye, V., Grover, S., Hammad, N., Pooja, P., Simonds, H., Olopade, F., & Stefan, D. C. (2017). An update on the management of breast cancer in Africa. *Infectious Agent and Cancer*, 14, 12–13.

Vityala, Y., Tagaev, T., Zhumabekova, A., & Mamatov, S. (2022). Evaluation of metabolic syndrome, insulin secretion and insulin resistance in adolescents with overweight and obesity. *Metabolism: Clinical and Experimental*, 12.

Wahdan, M.H. (1996). The epidemiological transition. EMHJ - Eastern Mediterranean Health Journal, 2 (1), 8–2. 1996.

World Health Organisation (2019) World Health Statistics available at https://www.who.int/data/gho/publications/world-health-statistics accessed 01/07/2024

World Health Organization. (2020). https://apps.who.int/nha/database

World Obesity (2023). World Obesity Atlas available at https://www.worldobesity.org/resources/resource-library/world-obesity-atlas-2023 accessed 01/02/2023.World Health Organisation (2024). Breast Cancer. available at https://www.who.int/news-room/fact-sheets/detail/breast-cancer accessed 01/07/2024

WHO. (2014). Global status report on noncommunicable diseases. Geneva.

World Health Organisation (2021) Cardiovascular Diseases.avialabl at https://www.who.int/news-room/fact-sheets/detail/cardiovascular-diseases-(cvds),accessed 29/06/2024.

WHO. (2022a). New report shows progress and missed opportunities in the control of NCDs at the national level. In: World Health Organization. https://www.who.int/news/item/12-05-2022-new-report-shows-progress-and-missed-opportunities-in-the-control-of-ncds-at-the-national-level

WHO (2022b). Obesity rising in Africa, WHO analysis finds. Available at https://www.afro.who.int/news/obesity-rising-africa-who-analysis-finds accessed 01/07/2024

WHO (2023). World Health Organization. Breast Cancer fact-sheets. https://www.who.int/news-room/fact-sheets/detail/breast-cancer

Zeltner T, Riahi F, Huber J. Acute and Chronic Health Challenges in Sub-Saharan Africa: An Unfinished Agenda. Africa's Population: In Search of a Demographic Dividend. 2017 Jan 27:283–97. doi: 10.1007/978-3-319-46889-1

9

SICKLE CELL DISEASE IN AFRICA

Ade Ojelabi

Introduction

Sickle cell disease (SCD) is the most common type of monogenic disorder called haemoglobinopathies, which affects over 5% of the global population (1–5). It is a group of blood disorders inherited from both parents in an autosomal recessive fashion and is caused by an abnormality in the oxygen-carrying protein haemoglobin in the red blood cells, whereby the red blood cells become misshapen and break down. These disorders include more than 1,200 known structural haemoglobin variants, but the most common ones found in a substantial part of the global population are HbS, HbC and HbE, including almost 500 thalassemia mutations that affect the level of production of globin chains throughout prenatal and postnatal stages (5). The disease is associated with multisystem morbidity and high mortality (6,7), as well as premature death of the cells, resulting in a shortage of healthy red blood cells, obstruction of blood flow and unremitting pain. The blockage of blood flow to organs deprives affected organs of blood and oxygen, predisposing the affected individual to a weak immune system, infections, chronic pain and fatigue symptoms. The lack of oxygen-rich blood can fatally damage nerves and organs, including the kidneys, liver and spleen. Studies have shown that sickle cell anaemia (SCA) is a major cause of morbidity and mortality among those affected. SCA patients are burdened with aplastic crises, acute sequestration, hyper-haemolytic, and vaso-occlusive crises. Hyper-haemolytic crises are common in tropical Africa, with added complications due to recurrent episodes of malarial infection (8), but less commonly reported in temperate climates (9–11). Sickle cell patients also carry educational, psychological, financial, and socio-cultural burdens. The 63rd session of the

DOI: 10.4324/9781003467601-11

United Nations (UN) General Assembly in December 2008 passed a resolution to recognise SCA as a public health problem. The UN and its member states are thus to dedicate June 19 every year to create awareness about the condition. The severity of the disease varies and depends on several factors, including the level of foetal haemoglobin (HbF) produced or the coinheritance of α-thalassemia (5). In addition, phenotypic variability, environmental and socio-economic factors are also believed to represent important risk factors, although their specific influence is yet to be rigorously studied. SCD patients also have poor health-related quality of life along with their families when compared with the general population (12–14).

Definition and Aetiology

SCD belongs to a group of diseases caused by inherited disorders of haemoglobin. These disorders are generally referred to as haemoglobinopathies (genetic defects, i.e., abnormal haemoglobin in the blood). Approximately 5%–7% of the world population is affected with haemoglobinopathies (15). SCD is the most severe and common haemoglobinopathy, affecting over 5% of the world population (16,17). Haemoglobin is an iron-rich protein that transports oxygen in the blood and gives colour to the red cells. The haemoglobin molecule has two subunits, namely alpha globin and beta globin. The problem in sickle cell was brought about by a mutation in the beta (β) globin gene at position 6 of the beta subunit, where a replacement of the normal glutamic acid with the amino acid valine takes place (18). The disease damages and alters the shape of the red blood cells into a crescent (sickle) form. The sickle haemoglobin (HbS) is insoluble when deoxygenated. Due to low oxygen uptake of the cell, the shape of the cells is distorted from a healthy round disc to a crescent c-shape or sickle shape, a distortion referred to as sickling (19). Thus, the disease is known as SCD. The rigid sickle-shaped cells are hard (insoluble) and sticky compared with normal, healthy cells. The hardness may obstruct blood vessels, or they may stick together and obstruct blood vessels. These obstructions are responsible for harsh and painful complications (vaso-occlusive crises). The disease is also referred to as SCA as a result of the frequent breakdown of the red blood cells (haemolysis), resulting in anaemia. Due to haemolysis, survival of the blood cells may be reduced from the normal 110–120-day lifespan to around 20 days (20,21). The consequences of haemolysis also include jaundice, an aplastic crisis (red blood cells unable to mature, resulting in worsening anaemia) and retarded growth.

The Chromosomes

The chromosome structures of the SCD are referred to as haplotypes. There are four main African haplotypes and one Asian haplotype of the beta-globin chain genes. The African haplotypes are the Bantu, Benin, Cameroun and Senegal haplotypes. The Bantu (Central African Republic) haplotype is the most severe disease phenotype and is reputed to have twice the increased risk of complications and early mortality when compared with other haplotypes (22). The Asian or Arab-Indian haplotype has a mild disease phenotype associated with higher HbF. HbF has been shown to reduce the severity of the disease and thereby improve survival (23).

The homozygous (HbSS) chromosome is the most common form and is brought about by the individual affected inheriting HbS from both parents. This most severe form of SCD accounts for 70% of cases of the disease in the African population (24). The other common but milder form of SCD is HbSC, which is a co-inheritance of the βs and βc alleles to form HbSC. The HbSC is present in 25%–30% of the African population (15,24). This ratio is further supported by a longitudinal study of 230 African-American people with SCD, which reported that 71.7% had HbSS while 24.5% had HbSC (25). Other forms of sickle cell are HbS/β-thalassaemia found in people of Mediterranean origin, HbC and HbD common in Punjab and HbO among Arabs.

The History, Name and Description of SCD in Africa

Although Herrich was the first to publish a scientific article in 1910 to describe the shape of the cells responsible for the disease as "sickle shaped cell", Horton from Sierra Leone had earlier in 1874 given a written description of the clinical signs and symptoms of what is now referred to as SCD (26). Centuries before these, there had been cultural references in Africa to an illness referred to as "rainy season rheumatism" that appeared to be hereditary in families (27). The "rainy season" description was a result of observations that a colder temperature was associated with frequent pain crises in the affected. A multicentre study across Virginia in the US reported that adults with SCD experienced worsening disease conditions during colder seasons (28).

Epidemiology of Sickle Cell Disease or Trait

SCD occurs in 193 countries (15,29) and is regarded as the most predominant haemoglobinopathy in the world (15,17).

The prevalence in Africa is 2%, or 1 in 50 births, representing approximately 240,000 births annually (15,30). The sickle cell trait, or carrier status, is present in 5% of the world population (15,17). Globally, over 300 million people have the sickle cell trait (31) and are at risk of passing the gene to their children through the Mendelian inheritance principle. The prevalence of SCT ranges between 10% and 40% across Africa, but less than 2% in North and South Africa. In some West African countries, the carrier prevalence is between 15% and 30%

TABLE 9.1 Prevalence of SCD and Its Carrier Status

Country	SCD			SCT		Source
	Prevalence (%)	Population	Annual births	Prevalence (%)	Population	
Nigeria	2%–2.39	5m	90,000–150,000	24	40m	WHO, 2006, 2007; Nwogoh et al., 2012; Aliyu et al., 2008; Modell & Darlison, 2008; Piel et al., 2013; Brousse et al., 2014; Carey, 2014
DRC	2		40,000			Piel et al., 2013; Brousse et al., 2014; Ohene-Frempong, 2010
Ghana	2		15,000	23.9		Asare et al., 2018; Ohene-Frempong, 2010
Africa	2	12–15m	240,000			Makani et al., 2011; WHO, 2007; Modell & Darlison, 2008
India			40,000	3–7		Piel et al., 2013
Cuba				4		Granda et al., 1991
Brazil						Santos & Gomes Neto, 2013
World		20–25m	300,000	5	300m	Grant et al., 2011

and up to 45% among the Bantu people of Central Africa (see Table 9.1). This huge population of patients places a burden on the poor health care delivery system typical of African countries.

Spread of SCD

Malaria endemicity has been suggested as a factor responsible for the geographical spread and frequency of the occurrence of HbS. Alison (1954) suggested that the sickle cell trait offered protection against malaria infection. It has also been suggested that a significant correlation exists between the incidence of malaria and the prevalence of the HbS gene (24); carriers are found to exhibit resistance to all forms of plasmodium falciparum malaria (32); hence, those who survived malaria did pass on the gene to their children, acting like a selective factor that supported increased prevalence of the gene. The high prevalence of SCD in people from the malaria-endemic regions of Africa and the Mediterranean also seems to support this hypothesis (33). However, malaria has been found to be a risk factor for people with the double sickle gene HbSS (17) and contributes to mortality, anaemia and other crises in SCD (9,34).

Human migration, especially across continents, has been increasing since the 1960s (35). In 2015, 244 million people (3.3% of the world population) lived outside their country of origin due to the demand for their economic skills, escape from crises and better education (United Nations Population Fund, UNFPA, 2015). This, along with the slave trade, has been suggested to be responsible for the incidence of SCD in countries like the UK, the US and parts of Europe (36). SCD is found with varied incidence and prevalence in over 70% of the countries of the world (15), but it is traced to people from particular regions of the world, indicating that the spread may be due to migration. SCD is particularly common in Sub-Saharan Africa, Spanish-speaking regions in the Western Hemisphere, South and Central America, the Caribbean, India and Mediterranean countries (29) but there is current evidence of a rising population of people with SCD in countries like Ireland, Scandinavia, Australia and South Africa, which were previously free from the incidence of the disease (37). The disease has been described as the fastest-growing and most frequent inherited disorder in England (38) and is present in 193 countries around the world. Table 9.2 shows the prevalence of both SCD and the carrier status of SCT in selected countries.

Morbidity/Clinical Manifestations or Symptoms of SCD

The clinical manifestations of SCD range from mild symptoms to very severe symptoms across the ages. It has been suggested that genotype, the volume of HbF, and comorbidities could be responsible for the degree of severity (22,39–45). The clinical manifestations are both acute and chronic and include painful

TABLE 9.2 Prevalence of SCD and Its Carrier Status in High-Income Countries

	SCD		*SCT*		
Country	Prevalence	Population	Prevalence	Population	Source
UK	1 in 2,400	12,000–15,000		240,000	Brousse et al., 2014; NICE, 2016
USA	1 in 2,472	80,000–100,000		300,000	Centre for Disease Control and Prevention, 2016; Smith et al., 2006; Brousseau et al., 2010
France		12,000–15,000			Brousse et al., 2014; NICE, 2016

crises, vaso-occlusive episodes, stroke, anaemia, hand-foot syndrome, jaundice, frequent infections, delayed growth, vision problems, aplastic crises, acute chest syndrome, leg ulcers, priapism, pulmonary hypertension and organ damage (44,46–51). The disease also affects pregnancy; the sickling process may reduce the amount of oxygen going to the foetus. Morbidity and mortality are therefore high in pregnant women with SCD. Complications include increased risks of painful crises and preeclampsia, low birth weight, and heart enlargement. There is a 19% risk of spontaneous abortion, 21% of stillbirth, 32% risk of premature birth and 42% of intrauterine growth restriction (poor foetal growth) (52).

Mortality and Life Expectancy

SCD is a leading cause of the high infant mortality rate in Africa. The disease is responsible for above 5% of all under-five deaths in Africa, rising to 9% in West Africa and up to 16% in individual West African countries (2,15,32,37) and reducing life expectancy (53). Dacie described SCD as a "disease of childhood" (54) and the median age of survival was later estimated at 14.3 years (55). However, early childhood mortality has gradually reduced due to medical interventions, which include neonatal screening (NBS) for early detection (56), use of penicillin prophylaxis (57), pneumococcal immunisation (58,59), transcranial Doppler screening to detect patients at risk of stroke, blood transfusions (60,61) and other therapies like hydroxyurea (62) and bone marrow transplantation (63), along with parent education, better nutrition, hygiene and public health practices, have been responsible for the survival of 90%–95% of children with SCD into the first decade (64), especially in high-income countries. Quinn reported

TABLE 9.3 Median Survival of Individuals with Sickle Cell Disease

Genotype	US	UK	Jamaica	Nigeria
HbSS/HbSβ⁰	58	67	53–58.5	21
HBSC/HbSβ⁺				24
General Population		80–83		55–56

Sources: Elmariah et al., 2014; Gardner et al., 2016; Wirenga et al., 2001; Chijioke & Kolo, 2009; Yanni et al., 2009; Lanzkron et al., 2013.

that survival to age 5 increased from 96.8% in the period 1983–1987 to 99.2% in the period 2000–2007 (53). In high-resource countries like the UK and US, 95%–99% of children now survive into adulthood because of these interventions (37,53,65). In Africa, education and medical interventions such as screening, vaccines and antibiotics have contributed to the increase in the survival rate of children with SCD from less than 2% four decades earlier to nearly 50% (11,66). By 1994, life expectancy had significantly increased from a median of 14.3 years (55) to 42 years for males and 48 years for females (67). Recent estimates have also confirmed improvements in life expectancy, though short by about 20–30 years when compared with people with normal haemoglobin (NCBDDD, 2011) (See Table 9.3). The risk of premature and sudden death is, however, still high in SCD patients in spite of medical efforts (NCBDDD, 2011).

However, as patients with SCD grow older, they become susceptible to further disease complications such as chronic organ dysfunction or organ damage, renal failure, thromboembolism and iron overload (2,68,69), which predisposes them to high stress levels and negative emotions, as well as a life-long treatment regimen that in most cases is complex and multi-focused (70), a situation that negatively impacts their quality of life.

Impact of SCD

The impact of SCD on families is huge. The stress of taking care of a sickly child is always heavy on the mother, with attendant economic losses as the mother may not have to devote a larger portion of her time to caregiving. It is also attended with high levels of emotional distress, economic costs and physical exhaustion that could come through seemingly unending treatment seeking. Moreover, the entire family would be affected by the costs of caring for a child with a chronic lifelong disability while unavoidably neglecting the care of other children in the family. In a study of 225 caregivers of children with SCD in Nigeria, it was observed that caregivers carry significant financial, interpersonal and psychological burdens; they are unable to engage in gainful activities, lose financial benefits as a result of time spent on caring and have a presence of tension and hostility in the homes (71). On the other hand, SCD patients are predisposed to low esteem, feelings of hopelessness due to frequent pain, hospitalisations, loss of schooling (in children and adolescents) and loss of employment (in adults) and predisposed to depressive symptoms (5,72,73).

SCD patients and their families, especially, also carry stigma in society. Stigma is defined as "an attribute that is deeply discrediting" (74). It involves some type of labelling with negative consequences for the stigmatised individuals (75,76). Health-related stigma is the devaluation or social disqualification of individuals based on their health status (77). These may emanate from family members, the general public and health care providers (78) Parker describes a structural concept of stigma as one that "feeds upon, strengthens and reproduces existing inequalities of class, race, gender and sexuality" (79). People with SCD do experience stigmatisation due to race, disease status, socioeconomic status, delayed growth and puberty and having chronic and acute pain that needs to be managed with opioids (80). Individuals with SCD reported being stigmatised as drug seekers or drug addicts and having their experiences of pain discredited by healthcare providers. In the African set up, mothers of SCD children could experience "discrediting attributes" including blaming for the illness of the child and accusation of unfaithfulness, as fathers often refuse to admit to having any role to play in the disease condition of the child.

Public Health Implications

SCD presents a significant challenge to public health due to under-five mortality, which was estimated to be 5%–16% in individual West African countries (SCAF, 2016, 58; WHO, 2006). Added to this is the high rate of deaths due to SCD-related complications in adolescents and pregnant women in Africa (81). Globally, the chronicity of the disease and high rate of hospital utilisation increase the burden on health facilities. Moreover, the disability-adjusted life years (DALY) from SCD have been found to be comparable to the DALY from cervical cancer and greater than the DALYs of chronic kidney disease related to diabetes mellitus or hypertension (37). SCD, though less common, has a higher rate of health care service utilisation than diabetes, cardiovascular disease and cancer (82,83).

SCD and the Healthcare System

The health-seeking behaviour of SCD patients due to disease-related complications raises health costs and puts significant pressure on the utilisation of healthcare facilities. In the US, the health cost associated with SCD has been estimated at $2 billion annually (84); an average of $8.7 million was required to care for an SCD patient from 0–50 years, apart from other costs associated with social workers time and efforts (85). In 2010–2011, England spent over £18–20 million on SCD-related cases (38). In the Democratic Republic of Congo (DRC), the cost of care in a paediatric ward was estimated at $1,000 per patient (86), and in Nigeria, a study suggested that the average cost of blood transfusion among paediatrics with SCD was above $3,000 (87). Another study put the cost of care per hospitalisation for children at $132.67, with an average of 2.5 hospitalisation per child (88). The implication of this is that a minimum-wage earner who has a child with SCD may spend about half of his annual salary on hospitalisation. Seventy percent of Nigerians earn less than 1 USD per day, according to the 2011 World Bank report. On the other hand, adults with SCD spend twice the cost for children with SCD on care (89). However, despite the high burden of SCD in Africa, especially Nigeria (2,90), many of the standard management practices are lacking (33) due to a shortage of requisite personnel and equipment, resulting in suboptimal care. A survey conducted by the Nigerian SCD network (NSCDN) in 2011 reported that while all clinics administered folic acid and malaria prophylaxis, only 8 of the 18 clinics surveyed prescribed penicillin prophylaxis (33) while none of the centres offered pneumococcal vaccine routinely. Moreover, despite the disease being among the priority of top ten non-communicable diseases, many African countries are yet to have or implement a national policy on SCD.

African Healthcare Systems

The African healthcare system is a main factor in the suboptimal management of the disease. Healthcare delivery is structured along the widely used three levels of care. Primary, secondary and tertiary (91). However, government commitment to improved and affordable healthcare delivery is low (WHO, 2004). For example, the 2,000 World Health Report ranked Nigeria as 187 of the 191-member nations for its health systems performance (91). There is inadequate government allocation to health, high out-of-pocket expenditure, a lack of an integrated system for disease prevention, surveillance and treatment and low supervision of healthcare providers (92).

Table 9.4 shows the wide gap in percentage of government contributions to health in selected African countries with a high prevalence of SCD compared with the UK, the US and France. Government contribution ranges from 4% to 16% in the DRC, 18% to 49% in Nigeria and 27% to 49% in Ghana, whereas it is 76% to 82% in the UK, 70% to 75% in France and 44% to 51% in the US.

Delivery of healthcare is regarded more as a personal affair, which means assessing healthcare depends on patients' ability to pay for basic laboratory and physician services, which have worsened the disease burden (FMOH, 2004). African countries operate out-of-pocket expenses (OOPS) to pay for medical services. While OOPS ranges from 4% to 16% in France, 13% to 18% in the UK and 11% to 15% in the US, the reverse is the case in Africa. The OOPS accounts for

TABLE 9.4 Gap in Percentage of Government Contributions to Health in Selected African Countries

Country	Means	2000	2006	2012	2019
DRC	Govt	4.0	5.2	16.1	15.8
	OOPS	51.1	67.9	40.3	38.3
Ghana	Govt	27.8	40	49.2	40.2
	OOPS	52.6	38.8	38.3	36.2
Nigeria	Govt	18.3	21.2	16.2	13,9
	OOPS	60.2	70.5	72.8	70.5
France	Govt	72.7	71.3	70.3	75.3
	OOPS	4.0	5.2	16.1	15.8
UK	Govt	76.7	82.1	81.2	79.5
	OOPS	17.7	13.3	14.6	17.1
USA	Govt	44.4	46.3	48.8	50.8
	OOPS	15.1	13.7	12.3	11.3

Note: OOPS – Out-of-pocket expenses.

38% to 68% in the DRC, 36% to 53% in Ghana and 70% to 75% in Nigeria (see Table 9.1). Out-of-pocket health expenditures present a large and sometimes catastrophic burden on a household; 100 million people are pushed into poverty every year because they have to pay directly for their health care (93). Also, the OOPS health financing system makes good healthcare inaccessible and unaffordable to the majority (33,91,92,94). Moreover, patients often find consultations and medications costly relative to other health-related expenses (94). According to the Ghana Ministry of Health, the 2003 National Health Insurance Scheme (NHIS) had enrolled two-thirds of the population by mid-2009, but the poorest remained outside the scheme. In Nigeria, the NHIS currently applies only to employees of the federal government (92). The African system is also characterised by the absence of an integrated system for disease prevention, surveillance and treatment, which reflects the lack of targeted efforts at outreach, health promotion and disease prevention activities designed to reach the people where they are (92).

Lay Perspectives/Cultural Views of SCD in Some African Countries

There are various cultural views and concepts of SCD in various African communities. Understanding these is necessary because how they perceive the cause and trend of the disease may be useful in orientating their social behaviour and is likely to be a product of their specific social and cultural circumstances (95). Moreover, while science has shown that SCD is inherited, most lay people still attribute the cause of illness to lie with the patient, the natural world, the social world or the supernatural world (96).

SCD is thought of as a mysterious ailment with no cure. A child with SCD in a family is believed to be a curse. In Nigeria, the Yorubas tag them as "Abiku" meaning "born to die", to describe their short life and premature death, mostly before age 5, and to express hopelessness on the possibility of the child surviving to adulthood. A variant of this from Ghana is "*Ene mewu: Okyena me wu*", meaning "I can die today, I can die tomorrow". The Igbos will refer to them as "*Ogbanje*", evil child' (97), which is seen as supernatural revenge against the family.

Ghanaians often refer to SCD as "*Nto, yare*", meaning "a bought disease", reflecting the belief that SCD was purchased by one's enemy or spirit mediums to afflict and bring hardships upon such families through the birth of a child with the sickness. In other words, they do not see it as an inherited disease but as the handiwork of an imaginary enemy or spiritual forces. Children with SCD are also regarded as "agbana", financial drain pipes to the family or "*sika be sa*", "money will finish" reiterating the belief that the enemy uses the illness to drain the family finances.

The severe nature of SCD, with its features of unremitting pain and long-term symptoms, makes its cause adduced to supernatural phenomena such as ancestral curses or affliction by witches or evil spirits. Hence, families of affected individuals are more likely to seek spiritual rather than medical "solutions" to the problem. Actually, supernatural explanations for misfortunes are a common phenomenon in Africa (98). Aside from supernatural explanations, whatever disease is found in a child is often attributed to the mother, such that the father is absolved of any responsibility as a cause of the child's illness. Invariably, fathers are resistant to accepting roles in the child's SCD condition. This gender blaming is common in African community settings (99,100).

Traditional "Solutions" to Sickle Cell Disease

Africans, in most cases, attribute their problems with spiritual forces (101). A slight perceived deviation from the expected norms in finances or health will be blamed on an external force, namely someone using sorcery or witchcraft against them (102). Hence, they look for solutions by consulting oracles, sacrificing to the gods or visiting prayer houses. For those who have converted to Christianity, they seek help through prayer and fasting to find solutions. A Nigerian newspaper, the *Guardian*, in its editorial review of April 4, 2019, opined that spiritual cleaning is being practiced for SCD persons in order to determine how long such a child would live and whether or not the child would survive, so as to know if further rituals and sacrifices are imperative.

Discussion and Policy Measures

SCD is a public health concern with the growing population of people with SCD. Annual births in Africa are projected to increase from 240,000 (11) to

400,000 by 2050 (4,15). The need to evolve effective policies for managing the disease in African countries becomes imperative. Counselling is commonly acknowledged as an important means of managing genetic disorders in some parts of Africa (90,100) and developed countries (103). Moreover, effective treatment is limited due to challenges associated with communicating complex health-related concepts, resource limitations and emotional concerns. Scholars, however, believe that understanding the concept of "healthy carrier status" and both parents accepting their roles could be helpful to the patients and the caregivers, especially to eliminate the risk of blame and stigmatisation of mothers (104). Although there is a potential concern that providing genetic information can generate or increase stigma (105), there is evidence that "blaming" within families often occurs in the absence of any biomedical explanations based on lay understandings of inheritance and cause (104). Therefore, generating more understanding of the origins of SCD, including the roles of parents and their extended families, can provide an important means of reducing or countering the negative attitudes of stigmatising mothers. And also provide a useful way of initiating discussions about SCD in counselling. These could be further enhanced by sharing information on inheritance. Efforts must be made to ensure access to health facilities and effective care and counselling. Other potentially effective interventions may include continuous education, advocacy and forming self-help groups or associations with deliberate efforts to address gender inequities and strengthen the rights of mothers.

Conclusion

Africa, especially Sub-Saharan Africa, carries a huge burden of SCD, representing over 70% of SCD cases in the world. The continent lacks adequate policies and an effective healthcare system to cater to people living with SCD. Also, the OOPS of these countries and the poverty low-income status of most countries in Africa do not provide help in addressing the burden. In most African countries, newborn screening is non-existent or in its infant stage. Stigmatisation also contributes to the psychological burden of people living with SCD and their caregivers, most especially the mothers, who are often accused of the cause of the disease, as well as the tendency to attribute the problem to spiritual or supernatural origin rather than biomedical explanations that could help parents accept responsibilities. Deliberate policies, effective counselling and health financing could go a long way towards helping in the management of the disease, reducing the physical burden of the disorder, and improving their health-related quality of life (5,106).

References

1. WHO. Report by the Secretariat of the Fifty-Ninth World Health Assembly A59/9. 2006.

2. Aliyu ZY, Gordeuk V, Sachdev V, Babadoko A, Mamman AI, Akpanpe P, et al. Prevalence and risk factors for pulmonary artery systolic hypertension among sickle cell disease patients in Nigeria. *Am J Hematol*. 2008;83(6):485–490.

3. Piel FB, Patil AP, Howes RE, Nyangiri OA, Gething PW, Williams TN, et al. Global distribution of the sickle cell gene and geographical confirmation of the malaria hypothesis. *Nat Commun*. 2010;1(1), 1-7.

4. Piel FB, Hay SI, Gupta S, Weatherall DJ, Williams TN. Global burden of sickle cell anaemia in children under five, 2010–2050: modelling based on demographics, excess mortality, and interventions. *PLoS Med*. 2013;10(7):e1001484.

5. Ojelabi AO. *Quality of life and its predictor markers in sickle cell disease in Ibadan South West Nigeria*. University of Sunderland; 2018.

6. Juwah AI, Nlemadim A, Kaine W. Clinical presentation of severe anemia in pediatric patients with sickle cell anemia seen in Enugu, Nigeria. *Am J Hematol* [Internet]. 2003;72(3):185–191. Available from: http://doi.wiley.com/10.1002/ajh.10285

7. Lucchesi F, Figueiredo MS, Mastandrea EB, Levenson JL, Smith WR, Jacinto AF, et al. Physicians' perception of sickle-cell disease pain. *J Natl Med Assoc* [Internet]. 2016;108(2):113–118. Available from: http://doi.org/10.1016/j.jnma.2016.04.004

8. Fleming AF, Storey J, Molineaux L, Iroko EA, Attai EDE. Abnormal haemoglobins in the Sudan savanna of Nigeria: I. Prevalence of haemoglobins and relationships between sickle cell trait, malaria and survival. *Ann Trop Med Parasitol*. 1979;73(2):161–172.

9. Williams TN, Obaro SK. Sickle cell disease and malaria morbidity: a tale with two tails. *Trends Parasitol* [Internet]. 2011;27(7):315–320. Available from: http://doi.org/10.1016/j.pt.2011.02.004

10. Booth C, Inusa B, Obaro SK. Infection in sickle cell disease: a review. *Int J Infect Dis*. 2010;14(1):e2–e12.

11. Makani J, Cox SE, Soka D, Komba AN, Oruo J, Mwamtemi H, et al. Mortality in sickle cell anemia in Africa: a prospective cohort study in Tanzania. *PLoS One*. 2011;6(2):e14699.

12. Tunde-Ayinmode MF. Psychosocial impact of sicke cell disease on moethers of affected children seen at University of Ilorin Teaching Hospital, Ilorin, Nigeria. *East Afr Med J*. 2007;84(9):410–419.

13. Brandow AM, Brousseau DC, Pajewski NM, Panepinto JA. Vaso-occlusive painful events in sickle cell disease: impact on child well-being. *Pediatr Blood Cancer*. 2010;54(1):92–97.

14. McClish DK, Penberthy LT, Bovbjerg VE, Roberts JD, Aisiku IP, Levenson JL, et al. 2005. Health related quality of life in sickle cell patients: the PiSCES project. *Health Qual Life Outcomes* [Internet]. 2016;3(1):50. Available from: https://www.scopus.com/inward/record.uri?eid=2-s2.0-84922229233&partnerID=40&md5=97db00cab6609d53b6b7af5de3613d61

15. Modell B, Darlison M. Global epidemiology of haemoglobin disorders and derived service indicators. *Bull World Health Organ*. 2008;86(6):480–487.

16. WHOQOL group, others. The World Health Organization quality of life assessment (WHOQOL): position paper from the World Health Organization. *Soc Sci Med* [Internet]. 1995;41(10):1403–1409. Available from: http://www.sciencedirect.com/science/article/pii/027795369500112K

17. World Health Organization. The Global Burden of Disease: 2004 update [Internet]. 2008;146. Available from: https://www.who.int/publications/i/item/9789241563710

18. Sant'Ana PG dos S, Araujo AM, Pimenta CT, Bezerra MLPK, Junior SPB, Neto VM, et al. Clinical and laboratory profile of patients with sickle cell anemia. *Rev Bras Hematol Hemoter* [Internet]. 2017;39(1):40–45. Available from: http://doi.org/10.1016/j.bjhh.2016.09.007

19. Pauling L, Itano HA, Singer SJ, Wells IC. Sickle cell anemia, a molecular disease. *Science*. 1949;110(2865):543–548.

20. Wilson RE, Krishnamurti L, Kamat D. Management of sickle cell disease in primary care. *Clin Pediatr (Phila)*. 2003;42(9):753–761.

21. Allison AC. Turnovers of erythrocytes and plasma proteins in mammals. *Nature*. 1960;188(4744):37.

22. Powars D, Hiti A. Sickle cell anemia: βS gene cluster haplotypes as genetic markers for severe disease expression. *Am J Dis Child*. 1993;147(11):1197–1202.

23. Tewari S, Rees D. Morbidity pattern of sickle cell disease in India: a single centre perspective. *Indian J Med Res*. 2013;138(3):288.

24. Rees DC, Williams TN, Gladwin MT. Sickle-cell disease. *Lancet*. 2010;376(9757): 2018–2031.

25. Sogutlu A, Levenson JL, McClish DK, Rosef SD, Smith WR. Somatic symptom burden in adults with sickle cell disease predicts pain, depression, anxiety, health care utilization, and quality of life: the PiSCES project. *Psychosomatics*. 2011;52(3):272–279.

26. Adewoyin AS. Management of sickle cell disease: a rview for physician education in Nigeria (sub-saharan Africa). *Anemia*. 2015 (1) p 791498

27. Konotey-Ahulu FID. (1996) The sickle cell disease patient: natural history from a clinico-epidemiological study of the first 1550 patients of Korle Bu Hospital Sickle Cell Clinic.Tetteh-A'Domeno, Watford.

28. Smith WR, Penberthy LT, Bovbjerg VE, McClish DK, Roberts JD, Dahman B, et al. Daily assessment of pain in adults with sickle cell disease. *Ann Intern Med*. 2008;148(2):94–101.

29. Center for Disease Control and Prevention. Sickle Cell Disease (SCD). 2011. Available from: http//www cdc gov/NCBDDD/sicklecell/data html.

30. WHO. Management of haemoglobin disorders. In: Report of Joint WHO-TIF meeting on the management of haemoglobin disorders Nicosia, Cyprus. 2007, pp. 16–18.

31. Grant AM, Parker CS, Jordan LB, Hulihan MM, Creary MS, Lloyd-Puryear MA, et al. Public health implications of sickle cell trait: a report of the CDC meeting. *Am J Prev Med* [Internet]. 2011;41(6 SUPPL.4):S435–S439. Available from: http://doi.org/10.1016/j.amepre.2011.09.012

32. Serjeant GR, Serjeant BE. *Sickle cell disease*. Vol. 3. New York: Oxford University Press; 1992.

33. Galadanci N, Wudil BJ, Balogun TM, Ogunrinde GO, Akinsulie A, Hasan-Hanga F, et al. Current sickle cell disease management practices in Nigeria. *Int Health*. 2013;6(1):23–28.

34. McAuley CF, Webb C, Makani J, Macharia A, Uyoga S, Opi DH, et al. High mortality from P. falciparum malaria in children living with sickle cell anemia on the coast of Kenya. *Blood*. 2010;116(10):1663–1668.

35. OECD. Iii. quality of life ©. 2011;19–35.

36. Modell B, Darlison M, Birgens H, Cario H, Faustino P, Giordano PC, et al. Epidemiology of haemoglobin disorders in Europe: an overview. *Scand J Clin Lab Invest*. 2007;67(1):39–70.

37. Ware RE. Is sickle cell anemia a neglected tropical disease? *PLoS Negl Trop Dis.* 2013;7(5):e2120.
38. Pizzo E, Laverty AA, Phekoo KJ, AlJuburi G, Green SA, Bell D, et al. A retrospective analysis of the cost of hospitalizations for sickle cell disease with crisis in England, 2010/11. *J Public Health (Oxf).* 2015;37(3):529–539.
39. Ballas SK, Lewis CN, Noone AM, Krasnow SH, Kamarulzaman E, Burka ER. Clinical, hematological, and biochemical features of Hb SC disease. *Am J Hematol.* 1982;13(1):37–51.
40. Nagel RL, Ranney HM. Genetic epidemiology of structural mutations of the beta-globin gene. *Semin Hematol.* 1990;27(4):342.
41. Gill FM, Sleeper LA, Weiner SJ, Brown AK, Bellevue R, Grover R, et al. Clinical events in the first decade in a cohort of infants with sickle cell disease. Cooperative Study of Sickle Cell Disease [see comments]. *Blood.* 1995;86(2):776–783.
42. Chang Y-PC, Maier-Redelsperger MI, Smith KD, Contu L, Ducrocq R, De Montalembert M, et al. The relative importance of the X-linked FCP locus and β-globin haplotypes in determining haemoglobin F levels: a study of SS patients homozygous for βS haplotypes. *Br J Haematol.* 1997;96(4):806–814.
43. Thomas PW, Higgs DR, Serjeant GR. Benign clinical course in homozygous sickle cell disease: a search for predictors. *J Clin Epidemiol.* 1997;50(2):121–126.
44. Ohene-Frempong K, Weiner SJ, Sleeper LA, Miller ST, Embury S, Moohr JW, et al. Cerebrovascular accidents in sickle cell disease: rates and risk factors. *Blood.* 1998;91(1):288–294.
45. Ashley-Koch A, Yang Q, Olney RS. Sickle Hemoglobin (Hb S) allele and sickle cell disease: a HuGE review. *Am J Epidemiol Huge Genome Epidemiol Rev.* 2000;151(9):839–845.
46. Powars DR. Sickle cell anemia and major organ failure. *Hemoglobin.* 1990;14(6):573–598.
47. Hernigou P, Galacteros F, Bachir D, Goutallier D. Deformities of the hip in adults who have sickle-cell disease and had avascular necrosis in childhood. A natural history of fifty-two patients. *J Bone Joint Surg Am.* 1991;73(1):81–92.
48. Castro O, Brambilla DJ, Thorington B, Reindorf CA, Scott RB, Gillette P, et al. The acute chest syndrome in sickle cell disease: incidence and risk factors. *Blood.* 1994;84(2):643–649.
49. Oliveira CC de, Ciasca SM, Moura-Ribeiro M. Stroke in patients with sickle cell disease: clinical and neurological aspects. *Arq Neuropsiquiatr.* 2008;66(1):30–33.
50. Scheinman JI. Sickle cell disease and the kidney. *Nat Rev Nephrol.* 2009;5(2):78.
51. Ladizinski B, Bazakas A, Mistry N, Alavi A, Sibbald RG, Salcido R. Sickle cell disease and leg ulcers. *Adv Skin Wound Care.* 2012;25(9):420–428.
52. Oteng-Ntim E, Chase AR, Howard J, Khazaezadeh N, Anionwu EN. Sickle cell disease in pregnancy. *Obstet Gynaecol Reprod Med.* 2008;18(10):272–278.
53. Quinn CT, Rogers ZR, Mccavit TL, Buchanan GR. Improved survival of children and adolescents with sickle cell disease. *Blood J.* 2010;115(17):3447–3452.
54. Dacie JV. *The haemolytic anaemias: congenital and acquired.* Vol. 2. London: J & A Churchill1960.
55. Diggs LM. Anatomic lesions in sickle cell disease. In: Abramson H, Bertles JF, Wethers DL, editors. *Sickle cell disease: diagnosis, management, education, and research.* St Louis: C. V. Mosby; 1973, pp. 189–229.

56. Wang CJ, Kavanagh PL, Little AA, Holliman JB, Sprinz PG. Quality-of-care indicators for children with sickle cell disease. *Pediatrics*. 2011;128(3):484–493.

57. Cober MP, Phelps SJ. Penicillin prophylaxis in children with sickle cell disease. *J Pediatr Pharmacol Ther*. 2010;15(3):152–159.

58. Hardie R, King L, Fraser R, Reid M. Prevalence of pneumococcal polysaccharide vaccine administration and incidence of invasive pneumococcal disease in children in Jamaica aged over 4 years with sickle cell disease diagnosed by newborn screening. *Ann Trop Paediatr*. 2009;29(3):197–202.

59. Ellison AM, Ota KV, McGowan KL, Smith-Whitley K. Pneumococcal bacteremia in a vaccinated pediatric sickle cell disease population. *Pediatr Infect Dis J*. 2012;31(5):534–536.

60. Malouf Jr AJ, Hamrick-Turner JE, Doherty MC, Dhillon GS, Iyer RV, Smith MG. Implementation of the STOP protocol for stroke prevention in sickle cell anemia by using duplex power Doppler imaging. *Radiology*. 2001;219(2):359–365.

61. Lee MT, Piomelli S, Granger S, Miller ST, Harkness S, Brambilla DJ, et al. Stroke Prevention Trial in Sickle Cell Anemia (STOP): extended follow-up and final results. *Blood*. 2006;108(3):847–852.

62. Charache S. Hydroxyurea as treatment for sickle cell anemia. *Hematol Clin*. 1991;5(3):571–583.

63. Bhatia M, Kolva E, Cimini L, Jin Z, Satwani P, Savone M, et al. Health-related quality of life after allogeneic hematopoietic stem cell transplantation for sickle cell disease. *Biol Blood Marrow Transplant*. 2015;21(4):666–672.

64. Quinn CT, Rogers ZR, Buchanan GR. Survival of children with sickle cell disease. *Blood*. 2004;103(11):4023–4027.

65. Telfer P, Coen P, Chakravorty S, Wilkey O, Evans J, Newell H, et al. Clinical outcomes in children with sickle cell disease living in England: a neonatal cohort in East London. *Haematologica*. 2007;92(7):905–912.

66. Brousse V, Makani J, Rees DC. Management of sickle cell disease in the community. *BMJ*. 2014;348:g1765.

67. Platt OS, Brambilla DJ, Rosse WF, Milner PF, Castro O, Steinberg MH, et al. Mortality in sickle cell disease--life expectancy and risk factors for early death. *N Engl J Med*. 1994;330(23):1639–1644.

68. Powars DR, Chan LS, Hiti A, Ramicone E, Johnson C. Outcome of sickle cell anemia: a 4-decade observational study of 1056 patients. *Medicine (Baltimore)*. 2005;84(6):363–376.

69. Ogun GO, Ebili H, Kotila TR. Autopsy findings and pattern of mortality in Nigerian sickle cell disease patients. *Pan Afr Med J*. 2014;18:1–4.

70. Thomas JA, Lipps GE. Subjective well-being of adults with homozygous sickle cell disease in Jamaica. *West Indian Med J*. 2011;60(2):181–187.

71. Adegoke SA, Kuteyi EA, Ohaeri JU, Shokunbi WA, Olaniyi JA, Alagbe AE, et al. Psychosocial burden of sickle cell disease on caregivers in a Nigerian setting. *Ann Intern Med*. 2012;4(1):94–101.

72. Anie KA. Psychological complications in sickle cell disease. *Br J Haematol*. 2005;129(6):723–729.

73. Ojelabi AO, Bamgboye AE, Ling J. Preference-based measure of health-related quality of life and its determinants in sickle cell disease in Nigeria. *PLoS One*. 2019;14(11):e0223043.

74. Goffman, E. (1963). Embarrassment and Social Organization. In N. J. Smelser & W. T. Smelser (Eds.), *Personality and social systems* (pp. 541–548). Toronto: John Wiley & Sons, Inc. https://doi.org/10.1037/11302-050

75. Link BG, Phelan JC. Labeling and stigma. In: *Handbook of the sociology of mental health*. Springer; 2013, Available via https://link.springer.com/chapter/10.1007/978-94-007-4276-5_25 accessed 29/06/2024

76. Adeyemo TA, Ojewunmi OO, Diaku-Akinwumi IN, Ayinde OC, Akanmu AS. Health related quality of life and perception of stigmatisation in adolescents living with sickle cell disease in Nigeria: a cross sectional study. *Pediatr Blood Cancer*. 2015;62(7):1245–1251.

77. Weiss MG, Ramakrishna J, Somma D. Health-related stigma: rethinking concepts and interventions 1. *Psychol Health Med*. 2006;11(3):277–287.

78. Scambler G. Health-related stigma. *Sociol Health Illn*. 2009;31(3):441–455.

79. Parker R, Aggleton P. HIV and AIDS-related stigma and discrimination: a conceptual framework and implications for action. *Soc Sci Med*. 2003;57(1):13–24.

80. Haywood Jr C. Disrespectful care in the treatment of sickle cell disease requires more than ethics consultation. *Am J Bioeth*. 2013;13(4):12–14.

81. Dennis-Antwi JA, Dyson S, Frempong KO. Healthcare provision for sickle cell disease in Ghana: challenges for the African context. *Divers Equal Heal Care*. 2008;5(4), 241–254.

82. Davis H, Moore Jr RM, Gergen PJ. Cost of hospitalizations associated with sickle cell disease in the United States. *Public Health Rep*. 1997;112(1):40.

83. AlJuburi G, Laverty AA, Green SA, Phekoo KJ, Banarsee R, Okoye NVO, et al. Trends in hospital admissions for sickle cell disease in England, 2001/02–2009/10. *J Public Health (Bangkok)* [Internet]. 2012;34(4):570–576. Available from: https://academic.oup.com/jpubhealth/article-lookup/doi/10.1093/pubmed/fds035

84. Kauf TL, Coates TD, Huazhi L, Mody-Patel N, Hartzema AG. The cost of health care for children and adults with sickle cell disease. *Am J Hematol*. 2009;84(6):323–327.

85. Ballas SK. The cost of health care for patients with sickle cell disease. *Am J Hematol*. 2009;84(6):320–322.

86. World Health Organization. Preventing suicide. *CMAJ*. 2014;143(7):609–610.

87. Lagunju IA, Brown BJ, Sodeinde OO. Chronic blood transfusion for primary and secondary stroke prevention in Nigerian children with sickle cell disease: a 5-year appraisal. *Pediatr Blood Cancer*. 2013;60(12):1940–1945.

88. Adegoke SA, Abioye-Kuteyi EA, Orji EO. The rate and cost of hospitalisation in children with sickle cell anaemia and its implications in a developing economy. *Afr Health Sci*. 2014;14(2):475–480.

89. Pizzo E, Laverty AA, Phekoo KJ, AlJuburi G, Green SA, Bell D, et al. A retrospective analysis of the cost of hospitalizations for sickle cell disease with crisis in England, 2010/11. *J Public Health (Bangkok)*. 2014;37(3):529–539.

90. Akinyanju OO. A profile of sickle cell disease in Nigeria. *Ann N Y Acad Sci*. 1989;565:126–136.

91. Asuzu MC. Commentary: The necessity for a health systems reform in Nigeria. *J community Med Prim Heal Care*. 2004;16(1):1–3.

92. Obansa SAJ, Orimisan A. Health care financing in Nigeria: prospects and challenges. *Mediterr J Soc Sci*. 2013;4(1):221–236.

93. Elmariah H, Garrett ME, De Castro LM, Jonassaint J, Ataga KI, Eckman J, et al. Factors associated with survival in a contemporary adult sickle cell disease cohort. *Am J Hematol*. 2014;89(5):530–535.

94. Ogunbekun I, Ogunbekun A, Orobaton N. Private health care in Nigeria: walking the tightrope. *Health Policy Plan.* 1999;14(2):174–181.

95. Blaxter M, Cox BD, Buckle ALJ, Fenner NP, Golding JF, Gore M, et al. *The health and lifestyle survey.* London: Tavistock/Routledge; 1990.

96. Helman CG. *Culture, health and illness. Gender and reproduction.* Oxford: Planta Tree; 2000.

97. Nzewi E. Malevolent ogbanje: recurrent reincarnation or sickle cell disease? *Soc Sci Med.* 2001;52(9):1403–1416.

98. Parkin DJ. *Sacred void: spatial images of work and ritual among the Giriama of Kenya.* Cambridge University Press; 1991.

99. Bamisaiye A, Bakare CGM, Olatawura MO. Some social-psychologic dimensions of sickle cell anemia among nigerians: the implications for genetic counseling. *Clin Pediatr (Phila).* 1974;13(1):56–59.

100. Naveed M, Phadke SR, Sharma A, Agarwal SS. Sociocultural problems in genetic counselling. *J Med Genet.* 1992;29(2):140.

101. Anthony A. Factors influencing health beliefs among people in South West, Nigeria. *Afr Res Rev.* 2008;2(1):177–197.

102. Ameh SJ, Tarfa FD, Ebeshi BU. Traditional herbal management of sickle cell anemia: lessons from Nigeria. *Anemia.* 2012;2012:607436.

103. Atkin K, Ahmad WIU, Anionwu EN. Screening and counselling for sickle cell disorders and thalassaemia: the experience of parents and health professionals. *Soc Sci Med.* 1998;47(11):1639–1651.

104. Marsh VM, Kamuya DM, Molyneux SS. 'All her children are born that way': gendered experiences of stigma in families affected by sickle cell disorder in rural Kenya. *Ethn Health.* 2011;16(4–5):343–359.

105. Tekola F, Bull S, Farsides B, Newport MJ, Adeyemo A, Rotimi CN, et al. Impact of social stigma on the process of obtaining informed consent for genetic research on podoconiosis: a qualitative study. *BMC Med Ethics.* 2009;10(1):1–10.

106. Ojelabi A, Graham Y, Ling J. Health-related quality of life predictors in children and adolescents with sickle cell disease: a systematic review. *Int J Trop Dis Heal.* 2017;22(2):1–14.

10

SOCIAL INEQUALITIES AND HEALTH SECURITY IN GHANA AND NIGERIA

Cynthia Okpokiri and Vincent Adzahlie-Mensah

Introduction

The Context of Social Inequalities and Health Security in Ghana and Nigeria

Sub-Saharan Africa (SSA) remains afflicted by entrenched poverty and alarmingly high and rising inequality (see Seery et al., 2019). As the gap between rich and poor continues to grow in many African countries, health security threats, especially those emanating from infectious diseases, accentuate the importance of reducing the vulnerability of societies and the need for individual states to act effectively to contribute to public health security (Heymann et al., 2015; Moon et al., 2015). The emergence of COVID-19 and the experience of Ebola in SSA indicate that the most vulnerable and disadvantaged members of society bear the largest toll of infectious diseases (Moodie et al., 2021; Moon et al., 2015). As the COVID-19 pandemic raged through the world, health experts warned that African countries faced an existential threat in which strained public health systems could become quickly overwhelmed if the virus took hold, although SSA countries were largely spared. People in SSA rate their health and healthcare among the lowest in the world (Deaton and Tortora, 2015; Moon et al., 2015), and this is borne out in real terms (Makinde, 2015). Concerns about the quality of healthcare are founded in an awareness of social inequalities and health security risks that are overtly present in SSA countries. Health security risks are heightened for socially excluded and marginalised groups and exacerbated by policy-level gaps in health service provision and disparities in the availability and quality of health facilities as well as personnel (Deaton and Tortora, 2015;

DOI: 10.4324/9781003467601-12

Fasomuni et al., 2022; Seery et al., 2019). In this chapter, we explore the health security risks faced by socially excluded and marginalised groups in inner cities and poor rural communities in the countryside. We also explain why we chose to discuss inequalities and health security in Ghana and Nigeria.

Ghana maintains a key position in a rising Africa because of its political stability and its friendly relations with other nations (Killick, 2010). Ghana is positioned to perform a frontline role in the public health security of the region, although that might require considerable amounts of resources from the government (Assan et al., 2020). Despite being the first country in SSA to become independent with a promise to lead the economic prosperity of Africa, Ghana ranks 22 in the African inequality ranking and 144 in the global ranking. Academic discussions trace the history of social inequalities in Ghana to the country's colonial legacy and how that has been further accentuated by post-colonial development policies and strategies (Aryeetey et al., 2009). Research highlights that Ghana needs a realistic national hospital and medical emergency response programme designed on the principle of equitable distribution of appropriate equipment and supplies and well-trained emergency medical personnel (Drislane et al., 2014; Mensah et al., 2010; Norman et al., 2012). Studies show a wider income distribution gap between the poorest and richest households, marked disparities between the affluent urban areas and the impoverished rural areas, and a gendered bias in the distribution of wealth assets despite a general reduction in the incidence of income poverty (Osei-Assibey, 2014). Social inequalities persist despite many policy interventions, including the National Health Insurance Scheme and the introduction of the Ministry of Gender, Children, and Social Protection, and funding and implementation challenges remain. Like in Nigeria, many of the social interventions in Ghana suffer because of resource constraints, poor implementation or a lack of operational effectiveness, and corrupt practices. Assan et al. (2020) note that Ghana needs to first reinvigorate its national health system through building a research culture, improving the capacity of national policymakers regarding health governance, addressing international influence in matters of public health security and how that can impact the region, coordinating the capacity with international partners to mobilise resources to pursue a collective fight for the global health agenda.

Health indicators in Nigeria are some of the worst in Africa in terms of the distribution of health facilities (USAID, 2021), and these have implications and options for universal health coverage (Makinde et al., 2018). Most people in Nigeria have developed out-of-pocket spending and strategies for coping with payments for healthcare (Onah and Govender, 2014; Onwujekwe et al., 2010). The country has one of the fastest-growing populations globally, remains Africa's most populous nation, and its economic potential is unparalleled on the continent. In spite of its petroleum oil and natural gas wealth, Nigeria is a highly unequal society, where inequalities lie along several different dimensions interacting in complex ways, including retrogressive taxation of the poor, elite capture, multifarious ethnic divisions, wealth concentrated in the Christian South, and the domination of political power by the Hausa-Fulani in the North, a legacy of British colonial machinations in the country (Archibong, 2018). Nigeria has the unenviable distinction of languishing at the bottom of the global inequality ranking. There is stagnation in social spending as well as underinvestment in health and education. As of 2019, one in ten children in Nigeria dies before they reach their fifth birthday. Despite its highly educated elite, more than 10 million children, particularly in the North (with girls constituting 60%), do not go to school (Fasominu et al., 2022). In 2018, Nigeria was ranked 157th on the United Nations Development Programme's Human Development Index (HDI) among countries fighting inequalities.

This chapter draws on available data from both Ghana and Nigeria to explore the implications of social inequalities on the health security threats in SSA. We used some evidence from national-level Joint External Evaluation (JEE) data in Ghana and Nigeria to explore the intersections that exist between social inequalities and health security. Our focus is mainly on how national capacity deficits exacerbate risks for people who are socially marginalised. We analysed the core capacity to prevent, to detect, and to manage health security threat issues and the countermeasures that exist for responding to health security threats to protect poor and vulnerable people, especially in rural areas and inner cities in Ghana and Nigeria.

A Note on Health Security – Theoretical Perspective

For the purposes of this chapter, we take health security to mean the capacity to prevent, detect, and respond to public health risks. Health security rose to prominence as a means of capturing "the complex interplay between the spread of infectious diseases beyond territorial borders" with attendant impacts on state stability (Moodie et al., 2021: 8). The world was ushered into a new era of novel risks, including the COVID-19 pandemic, which has tested the international community's pandemic preparedness and the potential for building a cohesive, multilateral response. For SSA, the recent stories of HIV and Ebola brought health security to the fore (Heymann et al., 2015; Moodie et al., 2021; Moon et al., 2015). The spread of infectious diseases has made the field active in various dimensions (Aldis, 2008; Michaud et al., 2019; Morrison, 2014; Yuk-ping and Thomas, 2010). Traditional conceptions of health security have been challenged, and thinking has shifted dramatically (Moodie et al., 2021). However, the rapid expansion of discussions around health security has not succeeded in setting the parameters and defining the conceptual and policy contours of health security (Moodie et al., 2021; Rushton, 2011).

Many Western countries have developed national security responses in line with "awareness of the threat that infectious disease outbreaks could pose to their citizens" and their countries' economic and political stability (Davies, 2008: 298). They consider such responses as protection for their populations, especially against external threats that undermine usual public health functions such as routine immunisation, screening, and health promotion (Yuk-ping and Thomas, 2010). Health challenges now feature prominently within Ghana's National Security Strategy (2020), highlighting them as a central theme even when some (e.g., Aldis, 2008; Heymann et al., 2015) continue to view health security as a public health concept. Caballero-Anthony (2006) and Enemark (2007) discussed how reframing public health as a health security issue can improve capacity both within and across countries to deal with outbreaks of infectious diseases – specifically those that inspire a level of dread disproportionate to their ability to cause illness and death – whether as a result of a natural process or human agency. Health workers and policymakers in developing countries and within the United Nations understand the term in a broader public health context (Aldis, 2008). Within the United Nations Development Programme (UNDP), health security is listed as number three (after economic and food security) in the threat domains of human security (UNDP, 1994). Health security includes ensuring a minimum level of protection from both communicable and non-communicable diseases and unhealthy lifestyles. The Office of the Assistant Secretary for Preparedness and Response (2015) explained that the relevance of national health security is twofold: (1) build community resilience; and (2) strengthen and sustain health and emergency response systems. These conceptualisations frame health security as a human security issue, with the dominant criteria for identifying a health security concern being: (a) the scale of the disease burden; (b) the urgency for action; (c) the scale of the impact on society; and (d) the interdependencies or externalitiewith the potential to cause ripple effects.

Adopting a social epidemiology approach, this chapter follows axiomatic understandings of human security, which holds that a people-centred, multi-disciplinary model is required for a holistic understanding of security threats and responses (Commission on Human Security, 2003: 4). We take the question beyond vulnerability studies by not concerning ourselves with the literature on traditional security threat analysis, which focuses on how potential adversaries exploit system weaknesses to achieve their goals (Myagmar et al., 2005; Oladimeji et al., 2006; Swiderski and Snyder, 2004). Meanwhile, we acknowledge the importance of risk mitigation policy in terms of architecture, functionality, and configuration, as well as minimising exposure to considerable threats and vulnerabilities (Steven and Peterson, 2008). We examined health security in terms of capacity to prevent, detect, and respond within the context of deep and persistent social inequalities in SSA countries. We operationalise the view of International Health Regulation (IHR) (2005) and propositions by WHO (2013) to define a health security threat as a condition that presents or could present significant and sustained harm to a broad range of humans, irrespective of origin or source. These threats include public health risks (IHR, 2005) identified based on the scale of the event in terms of populations at risk (with attention to vulnerable and marginalised groups) and the urgency of mounting the response (WHO, 2013).

Health security encompasses counter measures such as the assemblage of a well-trained critical group of infectious disease professionals, the availability of training institutions, and properly resourced research centres funded by business, civil society, and. Such bodies should have the capacity to develop vaccines and stockpile medications government to combat infectious disease outbreaks, establish mechanisms to support continuous surveillance of events to determine their potential impact on public health, and determine whether an emergency response is required (WHO, 2013). However, poor leadership by many SSA governments and the incessant concerns around political instability, coupled with planning processes where a multitude of domestic agendas compete with international influences, mean that considerations of public health issues will continue to receive less attention, thereby posing threats to the continental and global health order. It is unclear how SSA countries have arrived at this juncture. It is also unclear what their citizens' perspectives are concerning levels of national preparedness or capacity to detect, prevent, and respond to threats. This is a task we take up in this chapter in terms of the implications in the context of the geospatial social inequalities in Ghana and Nigeria.

Methodology

We used secondary data from the World Health Organisation's (WHO) JEE of Ghana and Nigeria's progress on the International Health Regulations (2005). The Ghana case study relied on data from the WHO's (2017) country-led JEE. The Nigeria case relied on secondary data drawn from the country's mid-term country-led JEE results (Nigeria Centre for Disease Control, 2020). These were the latest results from each country at the time of our review. The JEE process, which is a critical component of the IHR (2005) Monitoring and Evaluation Framework, shows the extent to which a country is progressing on health security indicators. JEE and its approach help to spotlight the need for better preparedness and ensure compliance with IHR by countries signatory to it. With the COVID-19 pandemic, there was more focus on the JEE's utility to better understand response indicators, such as time-to-first case detection (Fasominu et al., 2022). The JEE was designed for epidemic-prone diseases, not necessarily pandemics. A major distinction between both public health events is that epidemics are expected to be primarily managed by the health sector, whereas pandemics require a whole-of-society approach including cutting through bureaucracy across different levels of society.

Furthermore, the JEE does not measure critical indicators of pandemic preparedness, such as health system resilience. However, recognising this limitation has helped guide and support advocacy efforts for strengthening health security. The JEE highlights that health security capacity may not necessarily translate to having the capability to respond to public health events. Although capabilities can only be observed during real-world events, the JEE remains critical to help structure national action planning for health security, providing a common language and framework for countries to work towards (Fasominu et al., 2022). Nonetheless, using the JEE as a tool for IHR monitoring and evaluation framework remains the most viable assessment of health security capabilities. The JEE is conducted every five years to measure core capabilities to prevent, detect, and respond to health security issues. It has been helpful in assessing the health security preparedness of developing countries that have weak security systems. Ghana and Nigeria, like other SSA countries, are known to have weak, inadequate, and fragile health systems and facilities. The scores speak to the risks posed by the unequal distribution of health facilities, geographic distribution disparities in health service provision, the surge capacity of facilities, and gaps in national policies aimed at addressing health security issues. We examined the scores in terms of how they relate to social inequalities in health service provision and delivery in Ghana and Nigeria.

Social Inequality and Health Security in Ghana

COVID-19 exposed lapses in Ghana's health delivery system. At the height of the pandemic, Ghana's president announced his intention to build 88 district hospitals. As of February 2022, the hospitals were yet to be built. However, urban centres in Ghana are well-served with health facilities, including clinics, hospitals, and pharmacies. The story in rural areas is different. Rural areas usually have no modern healthcare services meaning patients are forced to either rely on traditional African medicine or travel great distances for healthcare. The healthcare system in rural areas mainly consists of health posts, health centres, and clinics, whereas urban areas boast of polyclinics, district hospitals, regional hospitals, general hospitals, tertiary hospitals, and national hospitals.

Our analysis of Ghana's WHO JEE (2017) results showed there are several deficits in the country's health security preparedness based on the principles of the International Health Regulations (2005) (Table 10.1).

The scores show that Ghana's health security risk preparedness lags behind in all the capacity areas – prevention, detection, and response. The problem is more pronounced in the response area, where the country's scores were less than half of the expected total score of five points in all capacity areas. The capacity

TABLE 10.1 Health Security Risk Preparedness

Technical Area	Capacities	Scores	100
Prevent	National legislation, policy, and financing	2	40%
	IHR coordination, communication, and advocacy	3	60%
	Antimicrobial resistance	1.3	26%
	Zoonotic disease	3	60%
	Food safety	2	40%
	Biosafety and biosecurity	2	40%
	Immunisation	3.5	70%
Detect	National laboratory system	2.3	46%
	Real-time Surveillance	2.75	55%
	Reporting	2.5	50%
	Human resources	2.6	53%
Response	Emergency preparedness	2	40%
	Emergency response operations	1.5	30%
	Linking public health and security authorities	2	40%
	Medical countermeasures and personnel deployment	1	20%
	Risk communications	2.4	48%

area where the country was least prepared is medical countermeasures and personnel deployment, where the country scored only 1 (20%) out of the maximum score of 5. This was followed by emergency response operations (30%) and emergency preparedness (40%). Regarding linking public health and security authorities, the country scored 2 (40%) out of 5. In the prevent area, the best performing capacity areas were: (a) immunization, where the country scored 3.5 (70%) out of the total score of 5; (b) IHR coordination, communication, and advocacy, where the country scored 3 (60%) out of 5; (c) and zoonotic disease, where the country scored 3 (60%). The capacity areas in the prevent dimension where the country appears least prepared were antimicrobial resistance (26%), food safety (40%), and national legislation, policy, and financing (40%). Ghana's preparedness in the detect dimension was average across all capacity areas of the national laboratory system (46%), real-time surveillance (55%), reporting (50%), and human resources (53%).

The Government of Ghana has a satisfactory legal framework, including the laws and regulations that require new or modified legislation and regulations to support and enable the implementation of IHR (2005). The main legal frameworks include the Economic Community of West African States (ECOWAS) protocols on health (1975), the Public Health Act, 2012 (Act 851), and the Ordinance (Laws of Gold Coast, 1951). However, the results showed that active national oversight and enforcement mechanisms are needed for both biosafety and biosecurity, in addition to adequate funding. The recommendations from the 2017 JEE included the development of a consolidation plan that outlines the transfer of dangerous pathogens and toxins into a minimum number of facilities; routine external quality assessments at all laboratories; and staff training programmes on dangerous pathogens and toxins needed for public health and clinical laboratories. Among the key challenges identified are a lack of national regulations for the transport of infectious substances, a "train-the-trainer" programme for biosafety and biosecurity, and a lack of capacity to ensure proper and timely maintenance of facilities and equipment.

Although immunisation is the area where Ghana scored the highest (70%), the JEE (2017) analysis highlights that there is limited access to immunisation services in many hard-to-reach areas, especially the Volta Basin area, also known as the Afram Plains. Ghana uses routine immunisation, outreach activities, and supplementary immunisation activities to reach those living in hard-to-reach areas.

Disease monitoring systems exist across the country to identify unknown diseases and report at early stages to avoid surges. However, there are many problems. The Integrated Disease Surveillance and Response (IDSR) works well in well-populated areas but relies on community-based surveillance in hard-to-reach areas. Outside the capital, the system relies heavily on community volunteers who are largely unskilled and not dedicated to disease surveillance. Their training is flawed in the sense that it is limited to the identification of conditions that are prevalent in their communities. They do not receive generic training to identify conditions that are *alien* to their communities, and the manual reporting system used by the untrained community volunteers means that reports take time to get to central management systems. There is currently no national quality standard for laboratory testing, and the Food and Drugs Authority (FDA) has challenges with appropriate testing as required under the Public Health Act, 2012 (851). While the FDA has some capacity to test for both chemical and biological threats in foods and water, this system is ad hoc and not routinely implemented. There is minimal oversight in the largest slaughterhouses in the capital area, while facilities outside the capital area are not typically inspected. Furthermore, the JEE report (p. 29) notes that there is "a lack of interest among staff in health facilities (management level) to conduct data analysis … [and] the majority of health facilities are not analysing data." No information is gathered on a regular basis from nuclear plants, the radiation protection office, or the nuclear regulatory body. No data are collected from the birth and death registries for surveillance purposes. There is an irregular and weak capacity for the analysis of epidemiological data at all levels.

The JEE report also explains that people in rural areas are prone to health challenges, as Ghana is yet to develop a specimen referral network and transportation system, implement a plan to standardise and harmonise testing methods, or establish a sustainable supply of laboratory reagents and methods to procure modern equipment. There are huge risks, as the nation is yet to establish a mechanism for the regulation of laboratory practice and to complete the Strengthening Laboratory Management Toward Accreditation (SLMTA) process as part of an overall quality improvement system. Most laboratories outside the regional capitals lack the equipment for the required tests, and frequent shortages of laboratory supplies are experienced. Ghana is heavily dependent on donors, and there is no in-country production of media, kits, or reagents for the performance of core laboratory tests. Frequent stock disruption of media, reagents, and test kits for processing core laboratory tests is a challenge for laboratories outside the capital.

Although some infectious diseases such as AIDS, COVID-19, and Ebola have been traced to human–animal interactions (Moodie et al., 2021; Moon et al., 2015), the JEE report (p. 27) notes that there are inadequate veterinary staff in Ghana (at both professional and technical levels) and no "linkages exist between colleagues in human health and animal health for reporting at any level." While there is legislation in place that allows the government to detain/quarantine any individual who presents a public health risk (Public Health Act, 2012 Act 851), there are no formal protocols between public health, animal health, and security authorities on collaboration to respond to a public health emergency.

In terms of human resources, there are many issues. First, the health workforce is focused at the central level. There are fundamental disparities as multidisciplinary health regulation capacity (epidemiologists, veterinarians, clinicians, and laboratory specialists or technicians) is available at the national level and not in some of the regions. Nationwide, there is a general lack of epidemiologists, skilled animal health personnel, and experts for chemical and radiological threats. Thus, human workforce resources to implement IHR core capacity requirements in Ghana are geographically unevenly distributed and skewed towards the southern parts of the country, particularly in the areas around the capital. Highly skilled health workers, including medical doctors, nurses, pharmacists, and allied health professionals, are concentrated in the Greater Accra and Ashanti regions. In areas outside the regional capitals, disease control officers serve as epidemiologists in the districts. Second, there is no workforce strategy specifically for the public health sector. There is no formal plan in place for sending and receiving health personnel during public health emergencies. A plan for training and maintaining the medical personnel who would respond via a formal readiness roster is also lacking. No incentives are in place to maintain the existing public health workforce within the country, especially in rural areas where living conditions do not support the quality of life attainable in urban areas. Third, there are inadequate numbers of personnel to secure IHR implementation, especially in the areas of animal health, chemical events, radiation emergencies, and skilled personnel in other sectors. Fourth, there is a lack of emphasis on enhancing capacity for nuclear, biological, and chemical countermeasures across the security agencies, as a result of which there is a need for specialised units within the various security agencies to deal with public health interactions.

Regarding emergency operations, Ghana does not have someone in the role of Emergency Operations Centre coordinator. Therefore, no system is in place to activate a coordinated emergency response rapidly (within 120 minutes). Also, case management guidelines are not available for all priority diseases. Communication teams have, however, been established and trained for each of the ten original regions. It has not been established that the six newly created regions have such teams. Also, all the newly created regions do not have regional hospitals. Similar structures do not yet exist at the district, subdistrict, or community levels. Some of the regions have health promotion officers, while others do not.

Overall, there are geographic disparities in terms of the distribution of facilities. Regional hospitals exist in 10 out of the 16 regions. This implies that, in some regions, the surge capacity is not available to respond to public health emergencies of national or international concern. Access to quality healthcare is therefore easier in the traditional regions. Some districts have polyclinics, while others have district hospitals. While it can be argued that no nation has the same quality of facilities across the length and breadth of its territories, the problem is more pronounced for Ghana because of poor road networks connecting rural areas to the urban areas where the tertiary facilities are localised. The effects include preventable mortality rates, congestion at referral hospitals, and long hours of waiting for laboratory results prior to treatment.

Ghana's health security capacity at the points of entry (PoEs) appears to be underdeveloped. Performance in terms of routine capacities established at points of entry is 3 (60%) out of 5, whereas the score for effective public health response at points of entry is 2 (40%) out of 5, as seen in the following table. This means that disease surveillance capacity at points of entry is weak (Table 10.2).

The challenge is more pronounced with the existence of many unapproved entry points that allow nationals from other countries to enter the country at will. Given the artificial colonial boundaries, many border towns in Ghana have fluid situations that allow people to live in two different countries at the same time. In some communities, one family may have their bedroom in Togo or the Ivory Coast while their kitchen and farmlands are in Ghana. This makes border regulation difficult. However, the localisation of health facilities and personnel in urban areas has affected the effectiveness of public health response at points of entry, as most points of entry are outside the capital. Basic things such as the availability of ambulances, basic facilities for the convenience of travellers, and routine inspection programmes at PoEs are limited. There are inadequate resources (personnel, offices, and equipment) for port health services. As a result, conducting routine vector and reservoir control activities is a challenge. Ghana does not have a specific public health emergency contingency plan, for example, to support the transfer of ill travellers from the points of entry to appropriate medical

TABLE 10.2 IHR-Related Hazards and Points of Entry in Ghana

IHR-related Hazard	Thematic	Score	%
Points of entry	Routine capacities established at points of entry	3	60
	Effective public health response at points of entry	2	40
Chemical events	Mechanisms established and functioning for detecting and responding to chemical events or emergencies	2	40
	Enabling environment in place for the management of chemical events	2	40
Radiation emergencies	Mechanisms established and functioning for detecting and responding to radiological and nuclear emergencies	2	40
	Enabling environment in place for the management of radiological and nuclear emergencies	3	60

facilities. Ground crossing points have no ambulances readily available to take care of emergency situations at the points of entry.

In terms of the capacity of chemical events, the score for mechanisms established and functioning for detecting and responding to chemical events or emergencies is 2 (40%). The score for the enabling environment in place for the management of chemical events is also 2 (40%). In terms of radiation emergencies, Ghana scored 2 (40%) out of 5 for capacity to deal with mechanisms established and functioning for detecting and responding to radiological and nuclear emergencies. Ghana performed better in terms of the enabling environment in place for the management of radiological and nuclear emergencies, where the score was 3 (60%). However, the JEE report recommends that information sharing and collaboration between involved sectors on chemical safety need to be strengthened concerning awareness of surveillance and reporting of human cases of chemical events (World Health Organisation, 2017).

Overall, Ghana obtained pass scores on only 8 out of the 22 indicators. Out of the eight areas where the country obtained pass scores, only five were above average (60% or more). This means that Ghana's health security preparedness is weak, especially when the highest score the nation obtained on any capacity indicator was 70% for immunisation.

Ghana's National Security Strategy (2020) states that the government intends to develop a five-year National Health Security Policy that outlines the efforts required to pursue a cost-effective and efficient healthcare delivery system. The probability-impact matrix in Ghana's first ever National Security Strategy (2020) identifies pandemics as a high-probability threat. The National Security Strategy (2020: 40) identifies what it calls two "fundamental strategies" that are possible during times of outbreaks of major health hazards or pandemics. These are (a) mitigation measures to slow down the rate and spread of infection to reduce peak health demand while protecting those most at risk of severe disease from infection, and (b) suppression measures, which aim to reverse the epidemic by reducing case numbers to low levels and maintaining that situation indefinitely. While this is being developed, the health security system remains fragile, to the consistent disadvantage of poor, marginalized, and vulnerable people in society. The National Health Insurance Scheme, which aims to provide access to health care delivery, continues to be ineffective and underaccessed, and many have lost confidence in the viability of their insurance cards (Jehu-Appiah et al., 2011; Mensah et al., 2010).

Social Inequalities and Health Security in Nigeria

Existing evidence from the literature shows Nigeria's health security preparedness is not in good shape as there are large inequalities in health care provision across states (Okoli et al., 2020). The evidence from the JEE process shows the nation lacking on several health security indicators (Table 10.3).

As in the case of Ghana, the JEE scores show that Nigeria's health security risk preparedness lags behind in all the capacity areas: prevention, detection,

TABLE 10.3 IHR-Related Hazards and Points of Entry in Nigeria

Technical Area	Thematic Areas	Scores	100
Prevent	National legislation, policy, and financing	2	40%
	HR coordination, communication, and advocacy	2	40%
	Antimicrobial resistance	2	40%
	Zoonotic disease	3	60%
	Food safety	1	20%
	Biosafety and biosecurity	1.5	30%
	Immunisation	3	60%
Detect	National laboratory system	2.8	56%
	Surveillance	2.7	54%
	Reporting	3.5	70%
	Human resources	2.8	56%
Response	Emergency preparedness	1.5	30%
	Emergency response operations	3.3	66%
	Linking public health and security authorities	2	40%
	Medical countermeasures and personnel deployment	1.7	34%
	Risk communications	3	60%

TABLE 10.4 IHR-Related Hazards and Points of Entry

IHR-related Hazard	Thematic	Score	%
Points of entry	Routine capacities established at points of entry	3	60
	Effective public health response at points of entry	1	20
Chemical events	Mechanisms established and functioning for detecting and responding to chemical events or emergencies	1	20
	Enabling environment in place for the management of chemical events	2	40
Radiation emergencies	Mechanisms established and functioning for detecting and responding to radiological and nuclear emergencies	3	60
	Enabling environment in place for the management of radiological and nuclear emergencies	3	60

and response. The problem is more pronounced in the preventive and response domains, where the country's scores were below average in most capacity areas. The capacity areas where the country was least prepared were food safety (20%), biosafety and biosecurity (30%), emergency preparedness (30%), and medical countermeasures and personnel deployment (34%). In the prevent area, the best-performing capacity areas were a) immunisation, where the country scored 3 (60%) out of the total score of 5, and for zoonotic disease, where the country scored 3 (60%). In addition, Nigeria failed in all capacity areas in the prevent domain, including antimicrobial resistance (40%), national legislation, policy, and financing (40%), IHR coordination, communication, and advocacy, where the country scored 2 (40%) out of 5. In the response domain, Nigeria is faring better in the areas of emergency response operations (66%) and risk communication (60%). Aside from that, the country failed in all capacity areas in the detect domain. Regarding linking public health and security authorities, the country scored 2 (40%) out of 5. Nigeria passed satisfactorily in all capacity areas in the detect domain. The score for reporting (70%) was the best, followed by the national laboratory system (56%), real-time surveillance (54%), and human resources (56%). However, the performance ratings should be read with caution, as the scores for Nigeria were obtained in 2019 and those for Ghana in 2017 (Table 10.4).

With reference to health security capacity at the points of entry (PoEs), routine capacities established at points of entry are 3 (60%) out of 5, whereas the score for effective public health response at points of entry was 20%. This means that response capacity at PoEs is weak. This is worse than the situation in Ghana.

Aside from that, the challenge is more pronounced in Nigeria given the size of its land mass, the number of landlocked countries it shares boundaries with, political conflicts, and the existence of many unapproved entry points that allow nationals from other countries to enter the country at will. Nigeria does not have formal data on the number of people from neighbouring Niger who have immigrated into Nigeria, but there is sufficient anecdotal evidence to suggest that hundreds of thousands of citizens from Niger are living in Nigeria without formal emigration processing. Most of these migrants tend to flee from the impact of climate change, which is rapidly increasing desertification in Niger, Islamic religious conflict and political instability, and limited economic opportunities, to seek refuge within their wealthier neighbour, Nigeria.

On the performance scales, the chemical event capacity is the least developed in the Nigerian context. The score for mechanisms established and functioning for detecting and responding to chemical events or emergencies was 1 (20%) out of 5. The score for the enabling environment in place for the management of chemical events was 2 (40%) out of 5. Given the size of Nigeria, this is problematic for understandable reasons. Meanwhile, Nigeria's capacity for radiation emergencies was rated as better developed than its capacity for chemical events. In respect of mechanisms established and functioning for detecting and responding to radiological and nuclear emergencies, the country's capacity scored 3 (60%) out of 5. Nigeria also obtained a score of 3 (60%) on the indicator of an enabling environment in place for the management of radiological and nuclear emergencies. Overall, Nigeria obtained pass scores on 11 out of the 22 indicators. Out of the 11 areas where the country passed, only 8 were above average (60% or more). This meant that Nigeria's health security preparedness is questionable, especially when the highest score obtained on any capacity indicator was 70%.

The main enabler of access to health services in Nigeria is the National Health Insurance Scheme. However, there are many inequalities that affect the viability of the scheme (Otu, 2018). Many people who subscribed to the National Health Insurance Scheme are unable to use it because of distance, as the majority of the facilities are in urban areas, in the industrial and commercial parts of the country. The distribution of the state general hospitals and local community dispensaries is therefore structurally and geographically imbalanced (Fasominu et al., 2022). The private sector, whose primary motive is profit maximization, operates mainly in urban centres. This results in unequitable distribution in the provisioning of services, with rural dwellers affected more in this regard (Nwakeze and Kandala, 2011).

Fasominu et al. (2022) note that access to the facilities, particularly in the case of emergencies, is likely to be poor due to the long distance of the referral centre for wards with limited primary healthcare facilities, coupled with a poor road network and a lack of operational ambulance services. Adano (2008) argues that factors capable of influencing the supply of healthcare services revolve around available manpower, determined largely by the hiring process of the health system, deployment procedures, and compensation packages. There are long-standing issues with rural-to-urban migration of health care professionals, with adverse consequences for the supply of health services. The outflow of healthcare professionals affects the supply of healthcare services in remote areas, to the consistent advantage of the urban and city centres; this disparity is reflected in the national scores.

As Nwakeze and Kandala (2011) explain, the determinants of health-seeking behaviour of poor people in Nigeria are influenced by a number of factors, including the lack of physical access and inconvenient opening/closing hours. For some populations, distance also implies hidden costs of seeking "free" treatment, while for others, it implies paying more to access quality service that is closer. The hidden cost includes the opportunity costs of time spent in travel, waiting for treatment, and buying drugs, as well as the costs of transport, and informal payments demanded by health workers and other staff (Otu, 2022). Sometimes, neglect of health facilities creates unacceptable conditions such as inadequate/broken equipment and dirty facilities, which mean denial of or reduced access to health services. Staff in remote areas are engaged in absenteeism because they are demotivated. The opposite happens in urban centres, where staff shortages mean that skilled staff may be concurrently employed at different facilities. In addition, the behaviour of some health staff can be unprofessional, influencing the quality of services and people's access to the limited available drugs. Other factors identified include consumer/patient characteristics, such as income, social class, household or cultural (religious and ethnic) characteristics, knowledge of available healthcare, and education. Lack of education and general understanding of health problems, as well as lower priority being given to the health needs of poor people and women in particular, are important pressure points.

Risk Mitigation

The scores from the JEE of the International Health Regulation for both Ghana and Nigeria show the countries are largely unprepared for health security issues. The absence of emergency preparedness programmes with surge capacity planning can lead to poor outcomes. The low scores for emergency response operations, linking public health and security authorities, and medical countermeasures and personnel deployment mean that Ghana and Nigeria have acute problems with health security that can severely affect the poor and vulnerable people, especially women and children in rural communities. When linked with inadequate infrastructure, geographic distribution disparities, low surge capacity of facilities in rural areas, and the ways in which socially excluded groups rely on traditional cultural practices for disease prevention, health security risks are likely to be pervasive. The lack of standard operating procedures (SOPs) for case management and response and problems with data collection and processing create grounds for serious health security breaches. The distribution of health services tends to favour urban areas with high population density more than rural dwellers, hence deprivation. This affects access to facilities, satisfaction with quality, especially in terms of gender inequalities, and the attitudes of health professionals (Otu, 2018).

Poor capabilities at the points of entry mean that disease surveillance is weak in those areas. Porous entry points also increase the avenues for smuggling fake drugs and other chemicals into the country, especially to rural areas. The fake drugs are sold to both the rural and urban poor. It also means that there are high risks of cross-border transmission of infectious diseases that can spread quickly, with few systems in place to prevent, detect, and respond to the spread.

Gaps in policy, practices, and localisation of health facilities in urban areas reinforce social inequalities. Localisation of health facilities in urban areas presents health security risks to socially excluded and marginalised groups in the inner cities and in poor rural communities in the countryside. The risk factors associated with unequal distribution of health facilities range from poor quality of care for those away from urban centres to higher child and maternal mortality and morbidity rates in hard-to-reach areas. At the same time, status and cultural norms that are pervasive in rural areas tend to reduce the utilisation of health services significantly. The localisation of health facilities in urban areas exists concomitantly with personnel deployment gaps that further erode effectiveness and equity in health service provision. Geographic disparities between urban areas and the countryside make it difficult for health professionals to accept postings to rural areas where poor and marginalised groups are located. Health professionals do not accept posting to rural areas due to the lack of basic facilities, poor road networks, and decent accommodation. Inadequate facilities and personnel gaps in rural areas leave the population vulnerable to fake drugs, poor quality care, and the burden of travelling long distances to access facilities.

Political expediency may undermine professional choices in both countries, where the locations of new health facilities are sometimes selected based on party commitment or used as a reward to faithful voters (Aliyu et al., 2020). This does not only affect distribution capacity but also the utilisation of public health facilities. Setting aside political sentiments and embracing the locational viability of healthcare interventions will enable health planners to target locations with genuine health needs and to improve capacities across a broader spectrum of the population (Otu, 2018). Location-Allocation Models that allow planners to site health facilities at optimised locations using simple parameters about the users and the proposed facilitiesare not used to site health facilities in either Ghana or Nigeria.

Otu (2018) explains the effects of geographic disparities, noting that the influence of traditional health care practitioners tends to be stronger in suburban and rural areas where geographical access to modern healthcare is limited. There are consequences for acceptability. Lack of acceptability is one of the leading causes of low utilisation of government-managed health facilities in developing countries (Akin and Hutchinson, 1999). Acceptability is influenced by perceptions of quality, social status, faith, and other attributes of the health service (Penchansky and Thomas, 1981). Although the declaration of Alma-Ata emphasised the provision of primary health services that are culturally acceptable (Peters et al., 2008), the assessment of core capacities shows that policy does not exist to regulate the distribution of facilities, personnel, or reagents for laboratory activities and surveillance across the nation. This limited capacity leaves many aspects and issues unaddressed in ways that further deepen social inequalities related to location, gender, and age. Elderly people are usually also more likely to have difficulty accessing health in a society where inequalities persist.

The capacity for management of chemical events, such as laboratory capacity for performing rapid risk assessments and training health workers in the management of cases, needs to be strengthened. Policies and guidelines for surveillance and response need to be developed and integrated into the health system. The low capacity emergency response plan emphasises the need to clearly define the roles and responsibilities of the relevant parties in detection, surveillance, and response using comprehensive policy statements. Such policies should incorporate harmonised surveillance protocols and SOPs, including timeliness of reporting and information sharing across sectors and agencies, and institutionalised coordination. Poor network connectivity and internet coverage affect data entry on electronic health platforms at the district level and should be addressed. The limited capacity to conduct tests and analysis at facilities and within some districts creates risks, especially for people who are socially excluded, have limited education, or are unable to read, and those living in the countryside with little access to information.

Conclusion

To assess social inequalities in health, interrogating health security threats with reference to the core capacities – prevention, detection, and response – is crucial. We used the core capacity scores to explore how gaps in policy practices and the localisation of health facilities reinforce social inequalities. We analysed the implications for the quality of care, personnel deployment gaps, and health security threats for poor and marginalised groups. In our view, Ghana and Nigeria are not prepared for health security threats, and social inequalities deepen the threats faced by the majority of the populations. Considering that dealing with new global health emergencies requires multi-stakeholder involvement and mobilisation, institutional and regulatory measures, systems of preparedness, early identification, and effective response (Aldis, 2008; Calain, 2007).

This chapter makes significant contributions in several ways relating to policy and practice. Concerning policy, it provides knowledge on how Ghana and Nigeria are prepared to deal with health security, the systems that exist to deal with health security challenges, and the gaps that exist in policy and regulatory frameworks. For practice, it provides useful knowledge on the gaps in health security preparedness by questioning the practical measures relating to social inequalities linked with geographic disparities and the implications for health security threats. Our discussions point to some core issues: social inequalities affect health service provision, and health seeking behaviour, thus prompting the discussion towards considerations of health as a national security concern. The cases of Ghana and Nigeria show that both countries have not developed the capacities needed to prepare for health security risks. Given the declining global cohesion, regional African bodies, including the ECOWAS and the African Union, should develop the capacity to use their platforms to advance sustainable mechanisms to reduce social inequalities and improve health security. For both countries, it would be helpful to strengthen the link between public health and security agencies with a special department within the security services responsible for public health emergencies. To reduce health security risks for poor and marginalised groups, there is a need to address inequalities in service delivery, health workforce distribution, strategic information dissemination, and health financing.

References

Adano, U., 2008. The health worker recruitment and deployment process in Kenya: an emergency hiring program. *Human Resources for Health*, 6, pp.1-3.

Akin, J.S. and Hutchinson, P., 1999. Health-care facility choice and the phenomenon of bypassing. *Health Policy and Planning*, 14(2), pp.135-151.

Aldis, W. (2008). Health security as a public health concept: A critical analysis. *Health Policy*, 23(6), 369–375.

Aliyu, U. A., Kolo, M. A. & Chutiyami, M. (2020). Analysis of distribution, capacity and utilization of public health facilities in Borno, North-Eastern Nigeria. Pan African Medical Journal, 35(39), 1–10.

Archibong, B., 2018. Historical origins of persistent inequality in Nigeria. Oxford Development Studies, 46(3), pp.325-347.

Aryeetey, E., Owusu, G. & Mensah, E.J. 2009. An Analysis of Poverty and Regional Inequalities in Ghana. Working Paper Series 27, GDN, Washington/New Delhi

Assan, A., Akbari Sari, A. & Takian, A. (2020). Ensuring sustainable development in Ghana: Public health security and policy concerns. Iran Journal of Public Health, 49(8), 1580–1581.

Caballero-Anthony, M., 2006. Bridging development gaps in Southeast Asia: Towards an ASEAN community. Revista UNISCI, (11), pp.37-48.

Calain, P., 2007. From the field side of the binoculars: a different view on global public health surveillance. *Health Policy and Planning*, *22*(1), pp.13-20.

Davies, S. E. (2008). Securitizing infectious disease. *International Affairs*, 84(2), 295–313.

Deaton, A. S. & Tortora, R. (2015). People in sub-Saharan Africa rate their health and health care among the lowest in the world. *Health Affairs*, 34(3), 519–527. https://www.healthaffairs.org/doi/10.1377/hlthaff.2014.0798

Drislane FW, Akpalu A, Wegdam HH. The medical system in Ghana. Yale J Biol Med. 2014 Sep 3;87(3):321-6.

Enemark, C., 2007. Disease and security: natural plagues and biological weapons in East Asia. Routledge.

Fasominu, O., Okunromade, O., Oyebanji, O., Lee, C. T., Atanda, A., Mamadu, I., Okudo, I., Okereke, E., Ilori, E. & Ihekweazu, C. (2022). Reviewing health security capacities in Nigeria using the updated WHO joint external evaluation and WHO benchmarks tool: Experience from a country-led self-assessment exercise. Health Security, 20(1), 74–86.

Ghana Government (2012). Public Health Act. Available at https://www.moh.gov.gh/wp-content/uploads/2016/02/Public-Health-Act-851.pdf. Acessed 30/06/2024.

Heymann, D. L., Chen, L., Takemi, K., Fidler, D. P., Tappero, J. W., Thomas. M. J., Kenyon, T. A., Frieden, T. R., Yach, D., Nishtar, S., Kalache, A., Olliaro, P. L., Horby, P., Torreele, E., Gostin, L. O., Ndomondo-Sigonda, M., Carpenter, D., Rushton, S., Lillywhite, L., Devkota, B., Koser, K., Yates, R., Dhillon, R. S. & Rannan-Eliya, R. P. (2015). Global health security: The wider lessons from the West African Ebola virus disease epidemic. *Public Policy*, 385, 1884–1901.

Jehu-Appiah, C., Aryeetey, G., Spaan, E., de Hoop, T., Agyepong, I. & Baltussen, R. (2011). Equity aspects of the National Health Insurance Scheme in Ghana: Who is enrolling, who is not and why? *Social Science & Medicine*, 72, 157–165.

Killick, T. (2010). *Development economics in action second edition: A study of economic policies in Ghana*: Routledge.

Makinde, O. A. (2015). Health care in sub-Saharan Africa. *Health Affairs*, 34(7), 1254– https://www.healthaffairs.org/doi/10.1377/hlthaff.2015.0459 Laws of Gold Coast (1951) available at https://lawcat.berkeley.edu/record/187359 accessed 29/06/2024.

Makinde, O. A., Sule, A., Ayankogbe, O. & Boone, D. (2018). Distribution of health facilities in Nigeria: Implications and options for Universal Health Coverage. *International Journal of Health Planning Management*, 33, e1179–e1192. https://doi.org/10.1002/hpm.2603.

Mensah, J., Oppong, J. R. & Schmidt, C. M. (2010). Ghana's National Health Insurance Scheme in the context of the health MDGs: An empirical evaluation using propensity score matching. *Health Economics*, 19(S1), 95–106.

Michaud, J., Moss, K. & Kates, K. (2019). *The U.S. Government and Global Health Security.* Kaiser Family Foundation.

Moodie, A., Gerami, N. & D'Alessandra, F. (2021). *Rethinking Health Security after COVID-19*. University of Oxford.

Moon, S., Sridhar, D., Pate, M. A., Jha, A. K., Clinton, C., Delaunay, S., Edwin, V., Fallah, M., Fidler, D. P., Garrett, L., Goosby, E., Gostin, L. O., Heymann, D. L., Lee, K., Leung, G. M., Morrison, J. S., Saavedra, J., Tanner, M., Leigh, J. A., Hawkins, B., Woskie, L. R. & Piot, P. (2015). Will Ebola change the game? Ten essential reforms before the next pandemic. The report of the Harvard-LSHTM Independent Panel on the Global Response to Ebola. *Lancet*, 386(10009), 2204–2221.

Morrison, J. S. (2014). The Global Health Security Agenda: A Snowy Promising Start. CSIS.

Myagmar S, Lee AJ, Yurcik W. 2005. Threat modeling as a basis for security requirement available from https://people.cs.pitt.edu/~adamlee/pubs/2005/sreis-05.pdf accessed 29/06/2024

Nigeria Centre for Disease Control (2020). *Country-led Midterm Joint External Evaluation of* IHR Core Capacities. Nigeria Centre for Disease Control.

Norman RE, Byambaa M, De R, Butchart A, Scott J, Vos T. 2012. The long-term health consequences of child physical abuse, emotional abuse, and neglect: a systematic review and meta-analysis. PLoS Med. 9(11):e10

Nwakeze, N. M. & Kandala, N. (2011). The spatial distribution of health establishments in Nigeria. *African Population Studies*, 25(2), 681–696.

Peters, D.H., Garg, A., Bloom, G., Walker, D.G., Brieger, W.R. and Hafizur Rahman, M., 2008. Poverty and access to health care in developing countries. *Annals of the new York Academy of Sciences*, *1136*(1), pp.161-171.

Okoli, C., Hajizadeh, M., Rahman, M. M. & Khanam, R. (2020). Geographical and socio-economic inequalities in the utilization of maternal healthcare services in Nigeria: 2003–2017. *BMC Health Services Research*, 20(1), 849.

Oladimeji, E.A., Supakkul, S. and Chung, L., 2006, July. Representing security goals, policies, and objects. In *5th IEEE/ACIS International Conference on Computer and Information Science and 1st IEEE/ACIS International Workshop on Component-Based Software Engineering, Software Architecture and Reuse (ICIS-COMSAR'06)* (pp. 160-167). I

Onah, M. N. & Govender, V. (2014). Out-of-pocket payments, health care access and utilisation in south-eastern Nigeria: A gender perspective. *PLoS One*, 9(4), e93887. https://pubmed.ncbi.nlm.nih.gov/24728103/

Onwujekwe, O. E., Uzochukwu, B. S., Obikeze, E. N., Okoronkwo, I., Ochonma, O. G., Onoka, C. A., Madubuko, G. & Okoli, C. (2010). Investigating determinants of out-of-pocket spending and strategies for coping with payments for health-care in southeast Nigeria. BMC Health Services Research, 10(1), 67. https://doi.org/10.1186/1472-6963-10-67

Osei-Assibey, E., 2014. Nature and dynamics of inequalities in Ghana. Development, 57(3), pp.521-530.

Otu, E. (2018). Geographical access to healthcare services in Nigeria – A review. *International Journal of Integrative Humanism*, 10(1), 17–26.

Penchansky, R. and Thomas, J.W., 1981. The concept of access: definition and relationship to consumer satisfaction. *Medical care*, *19*(2), pp.127-140.

Republic of Ghana (2020). National Security Strategy. Ministry of National Security, Ghana.

Rushton, S. (2011). Global health security: Security for whom? Security from what? *Political Studies*, 59(4), 779–796.

Seery, E., Okanda, J. & Lawson, M. (2019). *A Tale of Two Continents: Fighting Inequality in Africa.*Oxfam.

Steven, J. & Peterson, G (2008) Defining misuse within the development process. IFEE Security and Privacy 4(6), 81-82.

Swiderski, F. and Snyder, W., 2004. *Threat modeling*. Microsoft Press.

United Nations (2003) Report on Human Security available at https://www.un.org/humansecurity/reports-resolutions/ accessed 30/06/2024

United Nations (1994) Human Development Report. Available at https://hdr.undp.org/content/human-development-report-1994. Aceesed 30/06/2024

USAID (2021). Global Health | Nigeria | U.S. Agency for International Development (usaid.gov).

World Health Organisation (2005). International Health Regulations. Available at https://www.who.int/health-topics/international-health-regulations#tab=tab_1accessed 30/06/24

World Health Organisation (2013). World Health Report ava https://www.afro.who.int/publications/world-health-report-2013-research-universal-health-coverage available at accessed 29/06/2024

World Health Organisation (2017) Joint external evaluation of the core capacities of the RepublicOf Ghana. Available at https://extranet.who.int/sph/sites/default/files/document-library/document/JEE%20Report%20Ghana%202017.pdf acessed 30/06/24

Yuk-ping, C. L. & Thomas, N. (2010). How is health a security issue? Politics, responses and issues. *Health Policy and Planning*, 25(6), 447–453.

PART 3

The Social Structures of Diseases and Health in Africa

Case Studies

11

PARTNERING TO ELIMINATE LEPROSY IN NIGERIA

What Do Our Religious Leaders Know? – A Case Study

Jennifer Tyndall

Introduction

Despite meeting the World Health Organization global elimination target for leprosy (less than 1 case per 10,000 population) at the national level in 1998, Nigeria is one of the few countries in the world where new cases of leprosy are still recorded (Daniel et al., 2016). In the last two decades, with the continued support of both national and international partners, there have been sustained efforts carried out by the National Tuberculosis and Leprosy Control Programme (NTBLCP) in Nigeria that have contributed to the rapid decline of the burden of leprosy in the country. Continuous efforts are made towards sustaining the current decline in the disease by targeting areas with a relatively high endemicity of the disease in Nigeria.

The Global Leprosy Strategy 2021–2030 emphasizes the mandate to reduce grade 2 disabilities among new cases (WHO, 2021). Thus, it is of great importance that patients present early for diagnosis and treatment and that they complete the course of their treatment in a timely manner so that they are cured. In many Nigerian communities, poor knowledge among leprosy patients highly contributes to the delay in seeking medical attention. Developing an effective referral service and increasing community awareness about leprosy will help to further reduce the burden of the disease, as being knowledgeable about it will encourage patients to present early for diagnosis and treatment. When patients seek medical care and treatment at an early stage of the disease, it is expected that issues related to stigmatization and discrimination will become easier to tackle through reducing disabilities and providing a more inclusive social and economic rehabilitation for leprosy patients. The Global Leprosy Strategy

DOI: 10.4324/9781003467601-14

2021–2030 also emphasizes the need to improve the capacity of general health-care workers in the diagnosis and treatment of leprosy, early detection of cases in the community and curing them through the provision of free multi-drug therapy (MDT) (WHO, 2021).

There has been a long-term collaboration between KIT Royal Tropical Institute and the Netherlands Leprosy Relief (NLR) aimed at working together to reduce leprosy and improve its study and evaluation methods. This collaboration has brought about a significant contribution to the detection and control of leprosy at the country-level as well as improvements in research, thereby promoting the global leprosy control agenda (KIT, n.d.).

Over the years, the NLR has been supported by KIT in their country-level projects, specifically in Brazil, Madagascar, India, Myanmar, Indonesia, Mozambique, Nigeria, the Mekong region, and Nepal. The collaboration between these two organizations has significantly contributed to global policy setting regarding leprosy control and its programme, as well as numerous other innovations. There have been advancements made in the area of research, systems of monitoring and evaluation, and processes of integration, proven in more than 40 peer-reviewed publications and shown in the form of three technical guidelines (KIT, n.d.).

In Nigeria, the NTBLCP was established in 1989 by the Nigerian government to co-ordinate efforts towards TB and leprosy control in the country. In 1991, the NTBLCP was implemented nationwide, and it has been working towards reducing the prevalence of leprosy in the country ever since. The programme aims to improve early detection of leprosy, provide free leprosy treatment for all leprosy patients according to WHO guidelines, prevent disabilities due to leprosy, and reduce social stigma associated with the disease (Ogbeiwi, 2005).

In Adamawa State, northeastern Nigeria, a leprosy programme was introduced in 1991 in line with the implementation of NTBCLP across the country. A decade later, in 2002, a tuberculosis (TB) component was added to the state's leprosy programme. This addition led to the renaming of the leprosy programme to the Adamawa state Tuberculosis and Leprosy Control Programme (ATBLCP) (ATBLCP, 2005). ATBLCP aims to provide TB and leprosy control services in Adamawa state and receives financial, technical, and logistic support from the NLR (John, 2008).

Some of the social problems faced in the control and management of leprosy include patients' delay in presenting for diagnosis and treatment, patients' lack of compliance with the complete course of MDT in a timely manner, lack of self-care, and stigmatization (Wong & Subramaniam, 2002). Reasons given for these social problems are mostly rooted in cultural beliefs, which have a tremendous effect on the healthcare-seeking behaviour of leprosy patients. Thus, in order to improve the effectiveness of leprosy control and management programmes, there is a need to better understand how socio-cultural beliefs and stigma associated with leprosy affect healthcare-seeking behaviour in people affected by leprosy. Stigma associated with leprosy, in particular, has been found to be a major factor that leads to the delay in patients presenting for diagnosis and treatment (Bekri et al., 1998).

People affected by leprosy face stigma and discrimination, normally due to the apparent effect leprosy has on their physical appearance and also due to the cultural beliefs and misconceptions surrounding the causes of leprosy. In many cultures, leprosy is viewed as a punishment from God (Browne, 1975; Jacob & Franco-paredes, 2008; Richards, 2000). For example, the Hindus in India consider any deformity from leprosy as a divine punishment (Muthankar, 1979). Similarly, in China, leprosy is considered to be a sexually transmitted disease caused by contact with a prostitute. Thus, the disease is a punishment for that immoral conduct (Skinsnes, 1964). In places such as India, Malaysia, China, and Africa, some people consider leprosy to be hereditary (Chen, 1986; Gussow 2021). During the beginning of the 12th century, in western Christendom, leprosy was associated with sin and regarded as a form of chastisement from God (Douglas, 1991). Biblical passages may have also played a role in promoting the perception that leprosy is associated with sin. Some verses in the Old Testament portray leprosy as a visible manifestation of transgression against God (Cochrane, 1961; Rao & Karthikeyan, 2020). In Botswana, some people believe that leprosy is a result of dirty blood, malnourishment, eating certain foods, charms, and affliction by evil spirits (Kumaresan & Maganu, 1994).

Additionally, in Nepal, a study carried out by De Stigter (2000) revealed that 18% of respondents believed that leprosy was contagious and a curse from God, 64% of the respondents believed that leprosy was contagious but not a curse from God, and 9% of the respondents believed that leprosy was a curse from God but not contagious. A study conducted in Nigeria showed that some community members might avoid exchanging greetings and even asking for anything from people affected by leprosy for fear of becoming infected with the disease (Alubo et al., 2003). In western Christendom, during the mid-12th century, being identified as a leper meant losing one's civic status. Leprosy patients – or the accused – are regarded as sinners, removed from public office, prohibited from inheriting any property or making legacies, and had to have their own churches and graveyards (Douglas, 1991).

Previous studies have found certain factors that play a significant role in the beliefs of leprosy patients regarding the cause and mode of transmission of the disease. Some of these factors include age, gender, educational level, and religion. For example, in Nigeria, religion greatly influences the general public's health-seeking behaviour and attitude towards disease. A study in Kano State revealed that some respondents believed that leprosy is God's will and others believed that leprosy is a curse or punishment for the sins they committed (Dahiru et al., 2022).

Due to the influence religion and traditional beliefs have on leprosy prevention and control, it is important that Nigeria, through its NTBLCP with the support of international partners, integrates religious leaders into their leprosy control programme and empower them to contribute to the fight against leprosy. This approach would also ensure that religious leaders are adequately educated on leprosy – what it is and how it is contacted, spread, and managed – to allow them to effectively play an active role in leprosy prevention and control. The WHO Global Leprosy Strategy recognizes the involvement of religious leaders in leprosy control programmes as a strategy that can promote societal inclusion through addressing all forms of discrimination and stigma (WHO, 2016).

The role played by religious leaders in leprosy prevention and control has not been extensively investigated in Northern Nigeria. This study sought to fill that knowledge gap by assessing the knowledge of Christian and Muslim religious leaders in Adamawa state, Nigeria, on leprosy transmission and control. It also investigated the role played by these religious leaders in the prevention of leprosy and the extent to which they contribute to creating awareness about leprosy in the state.

Objectives

The aim of this study was to

1 Investigate the knowledge of Christian and Muslim clergy in Adamawa State on leprosy transmission and control.
2 To investigate the role of religious leaders in the prevention of leprosy in Adamawa State, Nigeria;
3 To find out the extent to which religious leaders in Adamawa State contribute to leprosy awareness in Adamawa State.

Methodology

The study was conducted among randomly selected Christian and Muslim religious leaders in Adamawa State. Sixty respondents were selected from each religion, with 20 respondents from each of the three senatorial zones of the state. This restriction/standardization for 60 respondents was to control for selection bias in the study. Out of the 60 Muslim leaders, 40 were male and 20 were female. Out of the Christian leaders, 55 were male and 5 were female. A structured questionnaire was administered to respondents, requesting each of them to fill out the questionnaire within two days. The questionnaires were retrieved within the specified time (a few of them were retrieved a week later).

Demographics

The Statistical Package for the Social Sciences (SPSS) was used to generate frequency and descriptive statistics and charts (Tables 11.1–11.6).

TABLE 11.1 Age Category of Christian Leaders

		Frequency	Percent	Valid Percent	Cumulative Percent
Valid	25–30 yrs	2	2.2	3.3	3.3
	31–35 yrs	7	7.7	11.7	15.0
	36–40 yrs	19	20.9	31.7	46.7
	41–45 yrs	16	17.6	26.7	73.3
	46–50 yrs	11	12.1	18.3	91.7
	51–55 yrs	3	3.3	5.0	96.7
	56–60 yrs	1	1.1	1.7	98.3
	60–70 yrs	1	1.1	1.7	100.0
	Total	60	65.9	100.0	
Missing	System	31	34.1		
Total		91	100.0		

TABLE 11.2 Age Category for Muslim Leaders

		Frequency	Percent	Valid Percent	Cumulative Percent
Valid	25–30 yrs	16	17.6	26.7	26.7
	31–35 yrs	4	4.4	6.7	33.3
	36–40 yrs	13	14.3	21.7	55.0
	41–45 yrs	6	6.6	10.0	65.0
	46–50 yrs	10	11.0	16.7	81.7
	51–55 yrs	5	5.5	8.3	90.0
	56–60 yrs	3	3.3	5.0	95.0
	60–70 yrs	3	3.3	5.0	100.0
	Total	60	65.9	100.0	
Missing	System	31	34.1		
Total		91	100.0		

TABLE 11.3 Highest Academic Qualification among Christian Leaders

		Frequency	Percent	Valid Percent	Cumulative Percent
Valid	Primary school certificate	1	1.1	1.7	1.7
	SSCE	4	4.4	6.7	8.3
	OND	32	35.2	53.3	61.7
	NCE	3	3.3	5.0	66.7
	HND	4	4.4	6.7	73.3
	1st Degree	9	9.9	15.0	88.3
	Masters	7	7.7	11.7	100.0
	Total	60	65.9	100.0	
Missing	System	31	34.1		
Total		91	100.0		

TABLE 11.4 Highest Academic Qualification among Muslim Leaders

		Frequency	Percent	Valid Percent	Cumulative Percent
Valid	Primary School Certificate	5	5.5	8.3	8.3
	SSCE	9	9.9	15.0	23.3
	OND	5	5.5	8.3	31.7
	NCE	15	16.5	25.0	56.7
	HND	6	6.6	10.0	66.7
	1st Degree	15	16.5	25.0	91.7
	Master's Degree	3	3.3	5.0	96.7
	PhD	2	2.2	3.3	100.0
	Total	60	65.9	100.0	
Missing	System	31	34.1		
Total		91	100.0		

TABLE 11.5 Marital Status of the Christian Leaders Interviewed

		Frequency	Percent	Valid Percent	Cumulative Percent
Valid	Married	51	56.0	85.0	85.0
	Single	7	7.7	11.7	96.7
	Divorced/Separated	1	1.1	1.7	98.3
	Widow(er)	1	1.1	1.7	100.0
	Total	60	65.9	100.0	
Missing	System	31	34.1		
Total		91	100.0		

TABLE 11.6 Marital Status of the Muslim Leaders Interviewed

		Frequency	Percent	Valid Percent	Cumulative Percent
Valid	Married	37	40.7	61.7	61.7
	Single	18	19.8	30.0	91.7
	Divorced/Separated	4	4.4	6.7	98.3
	Widow(er)	1	1.1	1.7	100.0
	Total	60	65.9	100.0	
Missing	System	31	34.1		
Total		91	100.0		

Research Findings

The results of the study showed that all 60 (100%) Christian leaders indicated they were aware of the presence of leprosy as a disease. However, 6 (10%) Muslim leaders interviewed said they were not aware (Tables 11.7–11.19).

When asked whether they had talked to their congregations specifically on leprosy during worship time or during special programmes organized by them for their congregations for this purpose, 48 (80%) of Christian leaders and 48

TABLE 11.7 Christian Leaders' Response to: How Did You First Hear of Leprosy?

		Frequency	Percent	Valid Percent	Cumulative Percent
Valid	Through a friend	10	11.0	16.7	16.7
	In church	15	16.5	25.0	41.7
	Radio	9	9.9	15.0	56.7
	TV	8	8.8	13.3	70.0
	Newspaper	4	4.4	6.7	76.7
	At the hospital	14	15.4	23.3	100.0
	Total	60	65.9	100.0	
Missing	System	31	34.1		
Total		91	100.0		

TABLE 11.8 Muslim Leaders' Response to: How Did You First Hear of Leprosy?

		Frequency	Percent	Valid Percent	Cumulative Percent
Valid	Through a friend	5	5.5	8.3	8.3
	In Mosques	2	2.2	3.3	11.7
	Radio	28	30.8	46.7	58.3
	TV	6	6.6	10.0	68.3
	Newspaper	8	8.8	13.3	81.7
	At Hospital	5	5.5	8.3	90.0
	Other	6	6.6	10.0	100.0
	Total	60	65.9	100.0	
Missing	System	31	34.1		
Total		91	100.0		

TABLE 11.9 Christian Leaders' Response to: What Are the Causes of Leprosy?

		Frequency	Percent	Valid Percent	Cumulative Percent
Valid	parasite/germ/ pathogen	43	47.3	71.7	71.7
	A curse from God	5	5.5	8.3	80.0
	Eating goat meat	4	4.4	6.7	86.7
	Witches/wizards	1	1.1	1.7	88.3
	Other	7	7.7	11.7	100.0
	Total	60	65.9	100.0	
Missing	System	31	34.1		
Total		91	100.0		

TABLE 11.10 Muslim Leaders' Response to: What Are the Causes of Leprosy?

		Frequency	Percent	Valid Percent	Cumulative Percent
Valid	Parasite/pathogen/ germ	33	36.3	55.0	55.0
	A curse from God	3	3.3	5.0	60.0
	Eating goat meat	12	13.2	20.0	80.0
	Eating smoked fish	2	2.2	3.3	83.3
	Witches/wizards	5	5.5	8.3	91.7
	Other	5	5.5	8.3	100.0
	Total	60	65.9	100.0	
Missing	System	31	34.1		
Total		91	100.0		

TABLE 11.11 Christian Leaders' Response to: Leprosy Affects Which Organ of the Body?

		Frequency	Percent	Valid Percent	Cumulative Percent
Valid	Fingers	22	24.2	36.7	36.7
	Toes	22	24.2	36.7	73.3
	Mouth	8	8.8	13.3	86.7
	Nose	4	4.4	6.7	93.3
	Skin	4	4.4	6.7	100.0
	Total	60	65.9	100.0	
Missing	System	31	34.1		
Total		91	100.0		

TABLE 11.12 Muslim Leaders' Response to: Leprosy Affects Which Organ of the Body?

		Frequency	Percent	Valid Percent	Cumulative Percent
Valid	Fingers	13	14.3	21.7	21.7
	Toes	4	4.4	6.7	28.3
	Mouth	2	2.2	3.3	31.7
	Skin	32	35.2	53.3	85.0
	I don't know	9	9.9	15.0	100.0
	Total	60	65.9	100.0	
Missing	System	31	34.1		
Total		91	100.0		

TABLE 11.13 Christian Leaders' Response to: What Are the Symptoms of Leprosy?

		Frequency	Percent	Valid Percent	Cumulative Percent
Valid	Loss of sensation	13	14.3	21.7	21.7
	Loss of limbs/ body parts	15	16.5	25.0	46.7
	Discoloured patches on skin	20	22.0	33.3	80.0
	Itching of skin	12	13.2	20.0	100.0
	Total	60	65.9	100.0	
Missing	System	31	34.1		
Total		91	100.0		

TABLE 11.14 Muslim Leaders' Response to: What Are the Symptoms of Leprosy?

		Frequency	Percent	Valid Percent	Cumulative Percent
Valid	Loss of sensation	12	13.2	20.0	20.0
	Loss of limbs/ body parts	19	20.9	31.7	51.7
	Discoloured patches on skin	15	16.5	25.0	76.7
	Itching of skin	7	7.7	11.7	88.3
	Other	3	3.3	5.0	93.3
	I don't know	4	4.4	6.7	100.0
	Total	60	65.9	100.0	
Missing	System	31	34.1		
Total		91	100.0		

TABLE 11.15 Christian Leaders' Response to: Is There a Cure for Leprosy?

		Frequency	Percent	Valid Percent	Cumulative Percent
Valid	Yes	56	61.5	93.3	93.3
	No	1	1.1	1.7	95.0
	I don't know	3	3.3	5.0	100.0
	Total	60	65.9	100.0	
Missing	System	31	34.1		
Total		91	100.0		

TABLE 11.16 Muslim Leaders' Response to: Is There a Cure for Leprosy?

		Frequency	Percent	Valid Percent	Cumulative Percent
Valid	Yes	40	44.0	66.7	66.7
	No	10	11.0	16.7	83.3
	I don't know	10	11.0	16.7	100.0
	Total	60	65.9	100.0	
Missing	System	31	34.1		
Total		91	100.0		

TABLE 11.17A Christian Leaders' Response to: Who Can Cure Leprosy?

		Frequency	Percent	Valid Percent	Cumulative Percent
Valid	Doctor/healthcare personnel	48	52.7	80.0	80.0
	Prayer warrior	8	8.8	13.3	93.3
	4	4	4.4	6.7	100.0
	Total	60	65.9	100.0	
Missing	System	31	34.1		
Total		91	100.0		

TABLE 11.17B Muslim Leaders' Response to: Who Can Cure Leprosy?

		Frequency	Percent	Valid Percent	Cumulative Percent
Valid	Doctor/healthcare personnel	51	56.0	85.0	85.0
	Prayer warrior	5	5.5	8.3	93.3
	Traditional healer	4	4.4	6.7	100.0
	Total	60	65.9	100.0	
Missing	System	31	34.1		
Total		91	100.0		

TABLE 11.18 Christian Leaders' Response to: How Can Leprosy Be Prevented/ Controlled?

		Frequency	Percent	Valid Percent	Cumulative Percent
Valid	Prayer	4	4.4	6.7	6.7
	Avoid infected people	18	19.8	30.0	36.7
	Educate yourself	8	8.8	13.3	50.0
	Go for regular check-up/ treatment at hospital	14	15.4	23.3	73.3
	Other	16	17.6	26.7	100.0
	Total	60	65.9	100.0	
Missing	System	31	34.1		
Total		91	100.0		

TABLE 11.19 Muslim Leaders' Response to: How Can Leprosy Be Prevented/Controlled?

		Frequency	Percent	Valid Percent	Cumulative Percent
Valid	Prayer	11	12.1	18.3	18.3
	Avoid infected people	29	31.9	48.3	66.7
	Educate yourself	5	5.5	8.3	75.0
	Go for regular check-up/ treatment at hospital	5	5.5	8.3	83.3
	Other	10	11.0	16.7	100.0
	Total	60	65.9	100.0	
Missing	System	31	34.1		
Total		91	100.0		

TABLE 11.20 Christian Leaders' Response to: If No, Why Not?

		Frequency	Percent	Valid Percent	Cumulative Percent
Valid	No particular reason	20	22.0	37.0	37.0
	I don't know much about TB myself	31	34.1	57.4	94.4
	Other	3	3.3	5.6	100.0
	Total	s54	59.3	100.0	
Missing	System	37	40.7		
Total		91	100.0		

TABLE 11.21 Muslim Leaders' Response to: If No, Why Not?

		Frequency	Percent	Valid Percent	Cumulative Percent
Valid	No reason	16	17.6	33.3	33.3
	I don't know much myself	27	29.7	56.2	89.6
	No time during worship	2	2.2	4.2	93.8
	Other	3	3.3	6.2	100.0
	Total	48	52.7	100.0	
Missing	System	43	47.3		
Total		91	100.0		

TABLE 11.22 Christian Leaders' Response to: If Yes, What Did You Tell Them?

		Frequency	Percent	Valid Percent	Cumulative Percent
Valid	Go for regular check-up/early treatment	3	3.3	25.0	25.0
	Pray for infected people	3	3.3	25.0	50.0
	Show love to infected people	5	5.5	41.7	91.7
	Educate yourself on the disease	1	1.1	8.3	100.0
	Total	12	13.2	100.0	
Missing	System	79	86.8		
Total		91	100.0		

TABLE 11.23 Muslim Leaders' Response to: If Yes, What Did You Tell Them?

		Frequency	Percent	Valid Percent	Cumulative Percent
Valid	Abstain from pre/extra marital sex	2	2.2	15.4	15.4
	Practice mutual fidelity	7	7.7	53.8	69.2
	Don't discriminate against those infected	1	1.1	7.7	76.9
	Show love to those infected	3	3.3	23.1	100.0
	Total	13	14.3	100.0	
Missing	System	78	85.7		
Total		91	100.0		

(80%) of Muslim leaders indicated they had never before. Reasons given for not doing so are shown in Tables 11.20 and 11.21.

When it was enquired of them whether or not they had attended any training on leprosy before within or outside the state, 58 (96%) of Christian leaders and all 60 (100%) of Muslim leaders interviewed indicated that they had never attended any training on leprosy in Adamawa State. 56 (93%) of Christian leaders and 30 (50%) of Muslim leaders indicated they would attend training on leprosy if organized. 8 (13%) of Christian leaders and 30 (50%) of Muslim leaders were not sure if they would attend the training if organized (Tables 11.22–11.23).

Discussion

This chapter has explored the impact of religious leaders on collaborative partnerships working to eliminate leprosy, a condition that has impacted the health of individuals and their communities for centuries. It is evident that the social stigma and burden of leprosy have played a significant part in the hesitancy of affected individuals in terms of their health seeking behaviours. It is evident that stigmatizing approaches to leprosy increase vulnerability to any admission of living with the condition, where its impact can be perpetuated and worsen before the opportunity to intervene with treatment and appropriate management can be implemented.

As a direct response to this status quo, faith leaders have collaboratively challenged discriminatory practice and been very successful in advocating support, compassion, and human rights for those living with the condition within areas where leprosy is currently endemic. What these faith leaders have done is successfully put aside issues of religious doctrine, which may detract from the potential of collaborative working across differing faith perspectives. The existence of interfaith networks for the social acceptance of leprosy has meant a wider acknowledgement that this ancient disease is universal in its capacity to disable and ostracize people from society; there is no faith that is more affected than the other, so collaboration and shared vision for the eventual eradication of the disease ought also to be a universal aim.

The enhanced level of individual agency these people necessitate to improve levels of access to optimal leprosy assessment, diagnosis, and management is evident across affected countries across Africa. Illuminating the sociocultural beliefs of those living in contexts of endemic leprosy provides an insight into the reasons for the major delay in the initial presentation for formal diagnosis of the condition. The physical impact of delayed treatment is visually evident in the physical appearance of those who delay diagnosis; its impact is a permanent reminder of both the stigma and alienation individuals can experience because of living with the disease. What is apparent, though, is that the condition is not specific to the continent of Africa alone, but that the core characteristics of health-seeking behaviours towards leprosy share many similarities in terms of initial reluctance to receive a formal diagnosis. The potential for religious leaders to play a compassionate and educative role in raising awareness of both the impact of leprosy and the need for early diagnosis and management will be a pivotal means of reducing this social stigma and burden on what is still referred to as a biblical disease.

While none of these considerations pertain specifically to the fiscal implications of living with a stigmatizing condition such as leprosy, there are also evident similarities with the stigma of HIV/AIDs, which have become equally endemic and a source of discrimination for people in Africa, with comparisons being made to the impact of the disease across a continent already dealing with major communicable and non-communicable diseases. What remains true, across all these considerations, is that leprosy transcends faith and religiosity and that all are unduly impacted upon in losing people, loved, and cherished in their communities. Mobilizing central faith networks, as this chapter illustrates, has become a key means of changing centuries-old perceptions of a condition necessitating the earliest opportunity for assessment, diagnosis, and management if its devastating impact is to be in any way minimized.

Conclusions and Recommendations

A limitation of the study was that although the respondents were asked to be free to tick more than one option where they felt so, they did not. Consequently, the authors are of the opinion that the respondents selected the option they felt was of the highest priority in their order of thinking, for example, as it relates to the epidemiology, symptoms, and control of leprosy. A follow-up study where multiple selections of options are emphasized is strongly recommended.

References

Alubo, O., Patrobas, P., Varkevisser, C., & Lever, P. (2003). *Gender, leprosy and leprosy control: A case study in Plateau State, Nigeria.* Amsterdam: KIT.

ATBLCP (Adamawa State Tuberculosis and Leprosy Control Programme). (2005). Annual Report. Yola, Nigeria.

Bekri, W., Gebre, S., Mengiste, A., Saunderson, P. R., & Zewge, S. (1998). Delay in presentation and start of treatment in leprosy patients: A case-control study of disabled and non-disabled patients in three different settings in Ethiopia. *International Journal of Leprosy and Other Mycobacterial Diseases*, 66(1), 1–9.

Browne, S. G. (1975). *Some aspects of the history of leprosy: The leprosy of yesterday.* Journal of The Royal Society of Medicine. 68(8), 485–493

Chen, P. C. (1986). Human behavioral research applied to the leprosy control programme of Sarawak, Malaysia. *The Southeast Asian Journal of Tropical Medicine and Public Health*, 17(3), 421–426.

Cochrane, R. G. (1961). Biblical leprosy. *The Bible Translator*, 12(4), 202–203.

Dahiru, T., Iliyasu, Z., Mande, A. T., van't Noordende, A. T., & Aliyu, M. H. (2022). Community perspectives on leprosy and related stigma in northern Nigeria: A qualitative study. *Leprosy Review*, 93(1), 48–62.

Daniel, O. J., Adejumo, O. A., Oritogun, K. S., Omosebi, O., Kuye, J., & Akang, G. (2016). Spatial distribution of leprosy in Nigeria. *Leprosy Review*, 87(4), 476–485.

De Stigter, D. H., De Geus, L., & Heynders, M. L. (2000). Leprosy: Between acceptance and segregation. Community behavior towards persons affected by leprosy in eastern Nepal. *Leprosy Review*, 71(4), 492–498.

Douglas, M. (1991). Witchcraft and leprosy: Two strategies of exclusion. *Man NS 26 (4)*, 723–736.

Gussow, Z. 2021). *Leprosy, racism, and public health: Social policy in chronic disease control*. Routledge

Jacob, J. T., & Franco-Paredes, C. (2008). The stigmatization of leprosy in India and its impact on future approaches to elimination and control. *PLoS Neglected Tropical Diseases*, 2(1), e113.

John, S. (2008). *On factors contributing to differences in new leprosy cases detected in Adamawa State, Nigeria*. Amsterdam: Royal Tropical Institute (KIT).

KIT (KIT Royal Tropical Institute). (n.d.). Long term collaboration with Netherlands Leprosy Relief. https://www.kit.nl/project/long-term-collaboration-with-netherlands-leprosy-relief/

Kumaresan, J. A., & Maganu, E. T. (1994). Socio-cultural dimensions of leprosy in north-western Botswana. *Social Science & Medicine*, 39(4), 537–541.

Muthankar, R. K. (1979). *Society and leprosy*. Wardha: Gandhi Memorial Leprosy Foundation.

Ogbeiwi, O. I. (2005). Progress towards the elimination of leprosy in Nigeria: A review of the role of policy implementation and operational factors. *Leprosy Review*, 76(1), 65–76.

Rao, P. S., & Karthikeyan, G. (2020). Socio-medical perspectives on leprosy in Indian religions. *Leprosy Review*, 91(2), 190–199.

Richards, P. (2000). *The medieval leper and his northern. Martlesham:Suffolk. heirs.* Boydell & Brewer.

Skinsnes, O. K. (1964). Leprosy in society. *Leprosy Review*, 35(1), 13–15.

WHO (World Health Organization). (2016). Global Leprosy Strategy 2016–2020: Accelerating towards a leprosy-free world-Operational manual.

WHO (World Health Organization). (2021). Towards zero leprosy. Global leprosy (Hansen's Disease) strategy 2021–2030.

Wong, M., & Subramaniam, P. (2002). Socio-cultural issues in leprosy control and management. *Asia Pacific Disability Rehabilitation Journal*, 13, 85–94.

12

VACCINE-PREVENTABLE DISEASES

Exploring the Perspectives of the Nomadic Fulani Tribe

Kareem Olusegun Thompson, John Fulton and Catherine Hayes

Introduction

A nation's culture resides in the hearts and in the soul of its people.

Mahatma Gandhi (1869–1948)

Ethical and ethnic diversity are attributed to a comparatively elevated incidence and prevalence rates of vaccine-preventable disease in Nigeria (Afolabi et al., 2021). Evidence indicates that children of Igbo and Yoruba communities have the highest incidence of complete vaccination programmes, and the least are the Hausa/Fulani populations of Northern Nigeria. Studies provide a threefold attribution of the low immunisation coverage of vaccination in northern Nigeria to the belief that polio vaccines are contaminated with anti-fertility agents. Alongside a lack of knowledge regarding vaccination, religious factors, the positing that vaccines are used as an attempt to reduce population sizes, the fear of side effects, the unavailability of vaccine/personnel in healthcare facilities, and poor access to vaccination services, it is hardly surprising that avoidance and refusal of vaccines in children is common (Perieres et al., 2022).

Epidemiology

Nigeria is the most densely populous country on the continent of Africa and the seventh most populous country in the world (NBS, 2021). In 2021, the population of Nigeria was estimated to be 206 million, compared to 201 million in 2019 and 196 million in 2018 (NPC, 2020), with population levels rising exponentially. The population is projected to grow to 210 million by 2023 and

DOI: 10.4324/9781003467601-15

396 million by 2050, making Nigeria the third-largest global population, third only to India and China. The country has a young population structure wherein children aged under 15 years constitute 45% and young people (10–24 years) make up 33% of the population. Women in the reproductive age group, children under five, and the elderly (at least 65 years) make up 22%, 20%, and less than 5% of the population, respectively. Consequently, Nigeria has a high dependency ratio of 73.3%, which is worsened by the very high rate of youth unemployment and the high total fertility rate of 5.8 in 2017 (NPC, 2020).

Nigerian National Immunisation Policy

Extant research has ensured a body of rich information concerning the Fulani people, their history, and their traditional customs. Thousands of years of Fulani history in the context of African history provide an insight into their nomadic migration, jihad, and cultural domination in west Africa. Published evidence also provides information on the epidemiology of infectious disease spread because of the Fulani community's continual migration. Barriers and enablers of vaccine uptake in vaccine-preventable diseases such as polio in northern Nigeria are also well documented in the existing research. Vaccination hesitancy is high in northern Nigeria in comparison to other regions and reveals that the religion and culture of the major ethnic group in the north are major reasons for this low vaccination uptake. Similarly, studies have also established that the Fulani ethnic group is one of the groups with a low rate of vaccination uptake in children. Researchers have linked this poor immunisation to the nomadic tradition of the Fulanis, which means they often miss nationwide immunisation campaigns. This was also linked to the emergence of vaccine-preventable disease rates across Nigeria. The focus of this chapter is a report of research into the perceptions of the nomadic Fulani around vaccine-preventable diseases and their health-seeking behaviour in relation to common childhood diseases.

As an integral part of the infrastructure available for the prevention of infectious disease, the National Immunisation Programme (NIP) in Nigeria constitutes the administrative component of the Ministry of Health responsible for the prevention of disease, disability, and death from vaccine-preventable disease. Historically, the Expanded Programme on Immunisation (EPI) in Nigeria was initiated in 1976 with pilot projects organised and implemented with the assistance of the World Health Organisation (WHO) and the United Nations Children's Fund (UNICEF). The EPI was strategically modelled on the success of the global eradication of chicken pox, with almost 80% of operational delivery undertaken via mobile operations and travelling healthcare workers, whose roles entailed travelling within and between villages. The EPI focused specifically on vaccine uptake by parents for children aged from birth to two years of age and all pregnant women in accordance with formal immunisation schedules recommended by the WHO.

The National Primary Health Care Development Agency is responsible for the control of vaccine-preventable diseases in Nigeria via vaccine provision and focused health education surrounding immunisation. At a national level, responsibility for the development of communication interventions surrounding preventable disease vaccination programmes is given to the National Social Mobilisation Working Group, while state and Local Social Mobilisation committees are responsible for coordinating and implementing communication interventions at a local level. The national immunisation schedule formally recommends that all routine childhood vaccinations ought to be taken by nine months of age. Apart from the routine locally based immunisation schedules available across communities, several rounds of national supplementary mass campaigning take place annually as a mechanism of increasing the uptake of vaccinations against preventable disease. Despite these strategic interventions, from a metric perspective, the incidence of routine immunisation uptake in Nigeria is among the lowest in the world (Ifedilichukwu, 2022; Eze et al., 2021; Anorue et al., 2021; Adenike et al., 2017; WHO, 2017; Olorunsaiye and Degge, 2016; Ophori et al., 2014). Research from the last decade illustrates that across 40 districts, vaccine uptake rates persistently remain at 50% (Gunnala et al., 2016). The uptake of the third dose of diphtheria-pertussis-tetanus remains the lowest of all vaccines. Formal recorded uptake is documented as being below 1%. Attributed to the lack of knowledge of parents about vaccine-preventable diseases this deficit model still pervades.

The Epidemiology of Vaccine-Preventable Disease

The incidence and prevalence of vaccine-preventable disease in Nigeria have varied over the last century. Diphtheria was eliminated after the vaccine's introduction in the 1940–1950s, but there is currently global concern that the disease is once again re-emerging in terms of reported incidence and prevalence rates.

Southeast Asia and India have been the most significant contributors to increased global levels, while overall incidences across Nigeria have reportedly declined by 5,039 in 1989 to 3,995 in 2000. Similarly, in 2001, 2,468 cases were reported, and 790 in 2002 (WHO, 2009). In 2006, Nigeria reported 312 cases of diphtheria and since then, there have been sporadic cases in several different localities that have not been reported. No significant progress has been made in a global reduction of incidence and prevalence rates over the last decade.

In 2011, 107 probable cases of diphtheria were identified, with 24 deaths, giving a case-fatality ratio of 22.4%. In most cases, 62.4% were below ten years, and 38.5% of cases aged below five years died. Ninety-eight percent of the probable cases had never received any childhood immunisations. In addition, there were delays in seeking medical care and the absence of antitoxin and adequate antibiotic therapy (Sadoh and Oladokun, 2012).

A study by Abubakar et al. (2020) expresses the re-emergence of diphtheria in Nigeria as nine new cases were referred to the National Ear Care Centre, Kaduna, from various primary health centres in the state within six months. The cases were between children of ages 4 and 12 years, and all the patients presented a symptom of sore throat, odynophagia, bull neck, membrane in the throat, and fever.

Abubakar et al. (2020) identified that the eight cases had never been immunised and were of low socioeconomic status, which followed the previous studies. The immunisation rate in northern Nigeria is some of the lowest in the world, with coverage below 6% in the northeast. As a result, thousands of children are victims of vaccine-preventable diseases. The study also identified some of the reasons for the low rates of immunisation, including misconceptions about immunisation due to low confidence, lack of trust, religious influences, failure of the vaccines due to a poor cold chain, and a shortage of vaccine and immunisation supplies. Similarly, the primary care facilities or rural medical outlets had no expertise or facility to diagnose diphtheria and refer appropriately. Healthcare delivery is generally poor in Nigeria, due to factors such as poor management of human resources, inequitable and unsustainable healthcare financing, unpredictable economic and political relations, corruption, and illiteracy.

Paediatric Immunisation in Nigeria

Child immunisation in Nigeria is provided through routine immunisation and catch-up supplemental immunisation campaigns, which are also referred to as National Immunisation Days, and they are organised across the country or subrationally in selected areas (Antai, 2012; NPHCDA, 2009). In Nigeria, a fully immunised child is expected to have received one dose of Bacillus Calmette-Guerin (BCG) at birth or soon after, three doses each of Diphtheria, Pertussis, and Tetanus (DPT) and oral Polio vaccine(OPV) at 6, 10, and 14 weeks, and one dose of measles vaccine (at nine months or soon after) (NPC and ICF International, 2014). Yellow fever vaccination is also provided at nine months. Vaccines introduced more recently and administered before the first birthday of children include Hepatitis B, Pneumococcus, and Rotavirus vaccines (NPHCDA, 2009). Similarly, vitamin A is administered at nine and fifteen months, respectively (Ophori et al., 2014). As part of the Polio Eradication and End-Game Strategic Plan, inactivated polio vaccine was introduced in the routine immunisation schedule in 2015, and in 2016, Nigeria participated by switching from the trivalent to bivalent polio vaccine (WHO, 2013). As countries introduce a second dose of the measles vaccine and other booster doses, imposed coverage of routine immunisation is anticipated from the age of one year onwards, as this provides opportunities to catch up on any missed immunisation from the preceding twelve months of neonatal life (Ophori et al., 2014).

Belief about Childhood Preventable Diseases and their Causes

The Fulani are an animistic group that embraced Islam in addition to their traditional beliefs. To the Fulani, illness (*yau*) may be attributed to various ecological factors. In a general sense, any illness may be related to God's will *(toh Allah yerdi)*, who, to them, is the ultimate source of whatever happens in an individual's life. Sometimes, illness is associated with environmental factors such as cold (*jangol*) and hot (*gul dun*). Some participants also associated them with a personal attack (*be siri*), rivalry, spiritual attacks (*gin naji*), and witches (*mu to*). To the Fulani, the perception of wellness (*lafiya*) is a general state of physical and social well-being.

Fulani's term for medicine (*leki*) represents the totality of how man attempts to manipulate his mixed-up, conflict-ridden real world to bring it closer to health (*wi yebi jam*). The Fulani have an organised system of traditional medicine closely related to the Hausa people and originated from Islamic prophetic medicine. The practice of traditional medicine in the Fulani culture utilises both natural products (such as plants, animal parts, and some minerals) and spiritual/metaphysical aspects.

The charms containing Qur'anic verse*(layaru)* used to bring good fortune and protection against spirit-induced illness are as much medicine (*leki*) as an herbal remedy used to treat the symptoms of a particular illness.

Traditional health practitioners among the Fulani are referred to as the *Jemo leki*, or *yan dibbu*, which is of Arabic origin, according to the responses the word dibbu means medicine or curing diseases, and *yan dtsibbu* or *Moddibo* d refers to as the scholars or holy men and talisman

The *Bude* refers to an herbalist with good knowledge who supports the ng some verses or chapters from the Quran, either recites to expirate *(tofi)*, write to drink (*rubutun sha*), incantation Fulani community by collecting and selling herbs, advice, and treatment. The Bude uses herbs to treat minor ailments such as colds, headaches, or stomach upsets.

The Fulani animism is called yan *Bòòríí* and is the most known practitioner in the Fulani communities. The *yan bori* are spiritual and heal by praying and performing rituals to the spirit based on the child or person's ailment. The belief in spiritual possession and having different names for the spirit in the world of illness and that the spirits could possess a child and must be cleansed from their body.

Pulaaku – The Basis of the Fulani Conservative Worldview

Pulaaku is an essential concept for the Fula people. It is an ethical and moral code of conduct based on humility, respect, honesty, courage, and moderation. It is the cornerstone of Fula culture and values and helps maintain the

Fula people's social cohesion. Pulaaku is the basis for all Fula people's moral and social conduct. It is the foundation of their identity and helps ensure their culture's survival. The *Fula* people use *pulaaku* to govern their behaviour, relationships, and interactions within their communities. It is their culture's foundation and helps maintain their social cohesion. Pulaaku is also a source of respect and unity among the *Fula* people. It is used to promote mutual understanding and harmony among community members. It is also used to encourage cooperation and collaboration among community members. The Fula people adhere to pulaaku through mutual respect, honest communication, and respect for the opinions of others. They also respect their elders, the elderly, and the disabled. The *Fula* people also have a strong sense of justice derived from their adherence to *pulaaku. Pulaaku* is also the source of protection and well-being for the Fula people. Respect and kindness are extended to all community members, regardless of age, gender, or class. This type of treatment is unique to the *Fula* people and is seen to maintain their cultural identity.

The importance of *pulaaku* to the Fulani cannot be overstated. In the face-to-face interview with Fulani women and FGD with the men, they all mentioned that *Pulaaku* is the cornerstone of their social and cultural identity and is the foundation for their values and beliefs.

They emphasise that respect, justice, and integrity are essential to the Fulani way of life. These values are passed down from generation to generation and are integral to their culture and identity. When treating a child's infectious disease instead of immunising them, the Fulani value of pulaaku would suggest that the most important consideration is the child's health. The Fulani would seek the best possible treatment for the child, regardless of the cost or difficulty involved, as their focus would be on the child's well-being. They would likely seek advice from the community leader, *Ardo*, to ensure the child receives the best care possible. In addition, they would likely also seek support from their community, as the Fulani emphasise the importance of communal support and cooperation as this quotation from the interviews illustrates:

…Pulaaku is a major problem for men as expressed in masculinity and the patriarchal society. There are certain things we men believe people should not know us for. Most of the time if you are not feeling all right, you charge or motivate yourself to be strong because your wife and children are observing you. you would not want to present yourself as a Sickler because the whole family would be disturbed. It is not a thing of pride for the head of the family to be complaining. It is a sign of weakness…so we pretend as if nothing is happening…

(Representative of the Fulani Community, 2021)

Methods

Situational analysis provided the focused ability to focus on the specific context and culture of the Nomadic Fulani community (Clarke, 2005) and to acknowledge researcher positionality (Charmaz, 2014) as a research insider and then research outsider to issues of health behaviour. During the initial planning of this study, the methodological positions of phenomenology, narrative research, grounded theory, ethnography, and case study research all potentially offered mechanisms of articulating an approach offering a degree of constructive alignment in relation to the ontological and epistemological origins of the study. While each offered distinctive approaches to gaining rich, thick description through This approach has significant similarities, but each offers the distinctive feature of gaining a thick description and understanding of people's perspectives.

Methodologically, situational analysis was aligned with the need to be able to:

• Generate knowledge in an area of research about which little is known.
• Consider the individual perspectives as well as the structural background of the individual in society, and explore their social world.
• Acknowledge researcher reflexivity and positionality.
• Encompass the analysis of diverse perspectives and circumstantial elements surrounded by the situation.
• Guarantee thoroughness so that the salience of findings can be established due to stringent mechanisms of data analysis.

Clarke (2005) acknowledges messy mapping for its somewhat systematic and technical qualities, though she contends that plotting all the possible positions enables a view of what 'could be'. It may be that there exists a position that remains 'unarticulated' in the data, with the insinuation being that it represents a 'silenced' space. Clarke (2005) emphasised that these mapping techniques are an aid to analysis rather than a replacement for the analysis and coding processes described by Strauss and Corbin (1990). According to Clarke, the maps themselves may, or may not, become part of the final findings of the research process. Therefore, constructing these maps can assist a researcher in achieving a more detailed consideration of the bigger picture of the situation of interest, mainly when used alongside memos as encouraged in grounded theory approaches. Relating this idea to this present study, the complexities that are aimed at being captured are those related to how the Nomadic Fulani comprehend issues of vaccine-preventable disease in children. When applied to studying Nomadic Fulani communities, the context of migration and cattle rearing is of central importance since this acknowledges how their applied cultural parameters are designed and endorsed, which in themselves can be related to the outcome of active discourse.

Research Findings

Theme A: Knowledge and Perception of Childhood Diseases by the Fulani Community

Based on the data generated from the in-depth interview with the Fulani and health officials, this finding revealed the overall knowledge and perception of childhood preventable disease, alongside information generated in relation to childhood preventable disease in men.

Awareness about the Childhood Preventable Disease

Awareness of childhood preventable disease amongst the Fulani was revealed to be from previous experience of illness amongst the childhood community. The majority of women interviewed admitted they had minimal knowledge until they became mothers of their own children, for example:

> …I was told of some of this illness and the sign and symptoms to check out for when I had my child, and some herbal medications were also given to me as prevention of illness. Some of the prevention was used to bathe the child, and others were laya (Hamlet and beads) ….

Several men and women attributed illness to spiritual power or an act of God, while others to environmental factors such as cold weather. Illness was also seen by some men as a means of predicting the future of their children; for example, when they stated,

> …these illnesses that you are asking us about are the will of God most time, and in some cases, it is iska and we have some good medication for them. ….

Sources of Information about Childhood Illness

Women also noted intergenerational wisdom across the community between those who had already experienced the incidence and prevalence of childhood illness. Far fewer relied on their own experiential learning experiences.

> …I learned more from the older women as they share their experiences and stories about childhood illness…and times when we are together, we ask questions or share experiences….

Perception of Childhood Preventable Diseases

The belief of the nomads in childhood preventable diseases was also founded on their experience of the process; for example,

> …We don't have much traditional/ cultural reason to avoid immunisation is just that the pain our children goes through after the treatment is too much and we don't see the health officer to complain to and you know I told you the distance of the cottage is too far to start taking a child to and it may be at night I would return…

Theme B: Fulani Health Seeking behaviour for Childhood Preventable Disease

Findings revealed that health-seeking behaviour refers to the actions taken by people who, in their perception, are ill or in need of healthcare intervention. It was apparent that various structural, socioeconomic, cultural, psychological, and demographic factors can impact health-seeking behaviour among the Fulani community.

Influences on Decision-Making by the Fulani Community

Diagnosis was seen as a structural process aligned with the Pulaaku, which is in itself the motivation to seek care, the role of the family members/community network, and the treatment options available.

The Fulani report experiencing several different arenas as they navigate childhood-preventable diseases.

Recognising the Signs and Symptoms of Childhood Illness

Specific triggers and predisposing factors that influence children with illness were considered here. Most parents reported noticing signs and symptoms such as weight loss, sweating, coughing, high temperature, loss of appetite or ability to eat, not sleeping, and body weakness, the relative severity of which led them to seek care, stating that:

> …You know that when the temperature rises at night, it makes the child weak, in the afternoon they feel better, but at night it becomes a problem… but when herbs are given, they get all right… but this is usually in both male and female child.

In some cases, where the signs and symptomology of illness are less acute in onset, parents and family adopt a more conservative approach, acknowledging,

> …A times, we first wait and see for the child's condition before we give them herb or even know what to administer.

The importance of public awareness and knowledge about the type of childhood illness in the decision to seek care was highlighted by Fulani men. According to them, decisions on where to seek care were regarded as family affairs involving members of the family and their wider social networks. These have a powerful influence on decision-making processes in relation to whether they are advised to opt for the advice of a traditional healer/herbalist or a chemist. Decisions as to whether formal intervention by outside sources are also influenced at this stage. There is a tendency to wait and see whether signs and symptoms spontaneously improve, and rushed decisions to seek care are advised against,

> ...when I see these signs and we are not sure, I ask the older women or tell my husband who discusses it with the men...and we will wait and see... maybe it is not what it looks like or maybe it is this illness or other ... let wait and see...

Prioritising Preferred Treatments for Childhood Diseases

When there is a degree of ambiguity in relation to signs and symptoms, traditional healers or herbalists are usually prioritised in preference of chemists, until signs and symptoms fail to be relieved by traditional methods.

The Fulani men indicated that there is a clear categorisation of methods of treatment intervention into prevention and cure. Preventative interventions can take the form of amulets such as the Layaru, which are leather pouch charms containing folded pieces of paper on which Quranic verses and symbols have been written. Individual charms are made to protect from specific childhood illnesses or misfortunes. Notably, this amulet is used to ward off spiritual attacks (*iskoki*). Infants and children often wear dozens of layaru, reflecting the need for protection or the aim to bring good fortune by the prevention or cure of diseases or other protective purposes.

Among the Fulani, the traditional birth attendant is usually the old women of the community who specialise in all aspects of child delivery. The post-partum care of the mother and infant the Fulani tradition is similar to the Hausa tradition, which prescribes 40 days of special care under the supervision of the traditional attendant, during which the mother of the infant is asked to stay indoors in a heated bed, take hot herbal baths (*shawara*), and also drink. They are also fed food containing potash (*Kanwa*). The mothers interviewed mentioned that the essence of the treatment is to ensure that the mother produces sufficient breast milk for breastfeeding and also to protect the child from cold (*Sanyi*). The traditional birth attendant also performs surgical procedures during delivery or treats neonatal conditions such as heart palpitations. She usually has considerable knowledge of herbal medicines used to treat women's and children's illnesses. *Hande ke je* is a preventive boiled herbal mixture produced from the bark of a tree. The mixture is given to a child by the birth attendant in their first 40 days to prevent common childhood diseases.

Collective Decision-Making within a Patriarchal Society

Fulani men's level of compliance with masculinity beliefs and health-seeking behaviour.

From a cultural perspective, the traditional patriarchy of Fulani men has a significant influence on children's access to healthcare treatment and the health-seeking behaviour of the community within the context of infectious disease. Fulani men are the patriarchal heads of their families and, as such, have the greatest influence on leading decision making in the family. As such, they influence whether a child should receive medical treatment, the choice of medical provider, and the type of medical treatment. Their leadership also influences the health behaviour of the children, such as whether they practice proper hygiene habits, are vaccinated, and whether they seek medical attention when necessary. Understanding this culture is essential for health practitioners since these social and cultural norms influence the capacity of the Fulani men to understand better and address the health needs of children with infectious diseases.

Within the focus groups and interviews, Fulani men expressed a degree of masculine sentiment that men ought not to be sick, as illustrated by the following statement:

> ...It is a known fact within our culture that women cannot just take a child for treatment ...except in an adverse condition where no one is around so this is only the condition a woman can take charge of...Pulaaku does not allow me to go to chemist...and the woman will be attending to you as a man... No oh...

Fulani Women

After interviewing the Fulani women about their autonomy when a child is sick or has a childhood disease, they highlighted three extents related to women's right to seek treatment for their child. These are women's roles, *Actors controlling the decision-making process*, decision-making *when seeking treatment* and economic *autonomy*.

Most women interviewed are petty traders who travel long distances or go to the market to sell milk, but they all said the man manages the rights and income of a family. The nomadic community is made up of men, women, and children with clearly defined roles (*Pulaaku*) in terms of who takes care of the cattle, the home, and even the health needs of the family. During the FGD, the men interviewed stated their roles and what is expected of women.

Generally, when the Fulani nomads form a community, they tend to remain there for a considerable length of time. They particularly state that they have settled here for more than five years. The young men move out with the cattle and could go as far as down to other states. When asked if they have their child immunized, the majority said no, or that it is rarely a priority for them:

> ...of all my children (five) only one was immunised but not completely... It was in our former settlement before we arrived here, and I have four more children here and non-have been immunised....

Agency in Decision-Making Processes

Fulani women reported that processes of decision-making are controlled by a collective group of men and not only their husband as an individual. This can even be extended to the wider community, especially the Ardo (head of the camp), who takes responsibility for the management of the problem and proposes a solution for the husband. Elderly women are invited to contribute and have major agency in terms of their wisdom in decision-making.

Financial Autonomy

Payments related to child healthcare are an obligation for men. The cost of care is sometimes a source of discouragement for the men in relation to sending their children to health centres:

> ...our husband pay for care even when the traditional healer visit he talks to the husband and he(husband) relates to us...

Theme C: Fulani Coping and Management of Childhood Preventable Disease

Subthemes generated provided an insight into the structural barriers of access to care, which pose challenges for the Fulani using the health facilities.

The Fulani Social Structure and Perceptions of Healthcare and Immunisation

Nomadic Fulanis, much like other populations in Nigeria, live with a myriad of health issues ranging from communicable to non-communicable diseases. The major causes of mortality and morbidity appear to be preventable infectious diseases. The data revealed that malaria, fever, anaemia, skin diseases, and snake and insect bites occurred very frequently among the Fulani community, which they attribute to the environments within which they live.

One man revealed:

> …as we are in the bush many things bite us, especially the women but if it is a snake, we know the medicine for snakes but the other insects we do not know, and they give women rashes on their body.

The general understanding of the Fulani participants in relation to immunisation and preventative healthcare was well established, and as a general consensus, they agreed that immunisation was a good thing to do in terms of preventative healthcare. Trust is clearly an issue, with one Fulani community member asking, "Did you not say we can have one of our own trained to be going to the government to collect our own share of drugs?"

Structural Barriers

Structural barriers refer to social and environmental conditions that affect the Fulani people's functional access to healthcare interventions such as immunisation. The data revealed language barriers to be a key reason why, as a community, many do not accept immunisation or visits to the hospital.

Language Compatibility and Communication with Healthcare Workers

Most participants said they did not understand the health worker in terms of what is needed, especially since they do not follow up on treatment and are left unsupported to care for children who had treatment.

They are faced with the challenge of telling the health workers about the problem or illness of a child:

> … health worker just gives us medication not waiting to hear from us the mother, some time.

Some women identify the increased temperature of the children after the visitation to the clinic, and in some situations, they must administer local treatment to normalise the situation of the child.

Some women mention children's high temperatures:

> … Their body is usually hot, and you know we walk a long distance to the clinic … this condition keeps us awake all night and it is a big challenge some….

Community Involvement in Planning

Men stressed their active wish to be involved in decision-making:

> ...why will we not want it? Is it not for our health and that of our children... In the name of Allah, we want it" ....

Relationship of Fulani with Healthcare Professionals/Healthcare Services

The Fulani lack good representation during the immunisation activities with the health workers, which generally results in poor health among them. They complain that, apart from the leader, Ardo, some men and women should be involved in the process.

Representation

> ...Through our leader Ardo, they inform our camp elders that they are coming to give such immunization and our elders inform us to stay at home because they are coming. We are not involved in administering the drugs.

Conclusion

The integration of situational analysis as a methodology provided a contextual insight into a complex and ambiguous culture and setting and served to capture the uniquely situated nature of Fulani living in relation to vaccine-preventable disease. Rhizomes quickly became authentic metaphorical models for reflection and the modelling of reflexive interventions in relation to complex human systems, which have no fixed hierarchical structure but continue to grow and spread in a decentralised and non-linear manner. Applying the process of rhizomatic analysis to the study of Fulani perceptions and their health behaviour towards vaccine-preventable diseases highlighted the importance of interconnectedness, fluidity, and flexibility in being able to authentically understand beliefs and practices related to health and disease prevention, beyond tokenism. The Fulani have a complex and dynamic network of cultural, historical, social, economic, and environmental factors influencing their perceptions, attitudes, and behaviours in health and disease prevention processes. These social epidemiological factors are intrinsically interconnected and in a dynamic state of flux, with no clear hierarchical structure to influence the concept or potential for societal change.

Viewing Fulani health behaviour as a rhizome permitted the illumination of how different nodes or points of influence interact and how the system adapts, flexes, and evolves over time. Fundamental examples of this include the Fulani's cultural practices, such as their nomadic lifestyle and their use of traditional medicines, which may in turn intersect with modern medical practices and external factors such as global health initiatives, climate change, and political instability. These interactions have the potential to create new forms of 'becoming' as different nodes or points of influence merge and transform into new prospective configurations. Rhizomes also facilitated and enabled emphasis to be placed on the importance of diversity and multiplicity in understanding complex and ambiguous human systems and infrastructures. The Fulani's perceptions, attitudes, and behaviours towards vaccine-preventable diseases are not homogenously constructed but rather shaped by a multiplicity of both intrinsic and extrinsic factors, alongside individual perspectives on them. Acknowledging and respecting this diversity has the potential to influence the development of more subtly nuanced and appropriately pitched context-specific approaches to advocacy for disease prevention and health promotion.

The process of territorialisation has resonance in relation to the process by which individuals or groups establish a sense of identity, belonging, and control over a particular space or territory. Deterritorialisation, conversely, involves the disruption of these established identities and control, leading to the potential for the loss of capacity for meaning-making coupled with a corresponding potential loss of any sense of societal belonging. Reterritorialisation occurs when new forms of identity and control are established, often in response to the disruptions caused by deterritorialisation. Since the Fulani have a distinct cultural identity and a strong attachment to their nomadic lifestyle, it is clear how the process of territorialisation plays a crucial role in their perception of vaccine-preventable disease in children. Their cultural beliefs and practices related to both health, well-being and disease prevention are deeply rooted in their cultural identity and territoriality.

Deterritorialisation has also impacted the Fulani due to ongoing exposure to external forces such as globalisation, modernisation, and the concept of Westernisation. These forces have typically disrupted traditional ways of life and introduced new beliefs and practices related to health and disease prevention. Territorialisation entails establishing new progressive forms of identity and control, which may be a fusion of traditional and modern praxis. In this context, encounters between the Fulani and external agents, such as healthcare workers, can be crucial in shaping the future of Fulani health and wellbeing.

'Becoming', as a concept, refers to the process of transformational change in perspective lens that occurs because of encounters and interactions between different actors. In the case of the Fulani and their perception of vaccine-preventable diseases in children, encounters with healthcare workers and modern medical practices have the potential to lead to new forms of becoming, which, in turn, may either provide a raft of challenges in the acceptance of what is new or simply reinforce existing historical beliefs and practices. Overall, territorialisation, deterritorialisation, territorialisation, encounter, and becoming offer a valuable framework for studying the complex interplay between culture, identity, and health behaviour within the Fulani community, with a specific focus on their thinking and practice surrounding vaccine-preventable disease in childhood populations. By understanding these concepts, it is possible to gain a strategic insight into the dynamics of perspective transformation that are shaping Fulani perceptions, attitudes, and behaviour towards prospective health and disease prevention.

The deficit-based approach is an approach to understanding health disparities that focuses on the underlying socio-economic and environmental factors that contribute to health disparities. It has been used to better understand health disparities within certain populations, such as the Fulani people in West Africa. This approach can be used to identify and address the existing gaps in immunisation coverage among Fulani populations. The deficit-based approach considers the cultural and social norms that influence health-seeking behaviours, as well as the historic and ongoing socio-economic disparities that prevent access to immunisation services. By understanding the unique challenges faced by the Fulani people, healthcare providers and policymakers can develop and implement tailored interventions that are culturally sensitive and promote equitable access to immunisation services. Such interventions can include increasing awareness of immunisation services, providing transportation assistance, and offering incentives to ensure that all children in Fulani communities have access to immunisation services. Through the deficit-based approach, healthcare providers and policymakers can better understand and address the underlying challenges faced by Fulani populations and ensure that all children have equitable access to immunisation services.

An asset-based intervention is an approach to public health that focuses on building and reinforcing existing resources, skills, and knowledge to improve health. It recognises that many individuals and communities have valuable assets and seeks to build on these strengths to create sustainable, health-promoting environments. Asset-based interventions focus on creating support networks, promoting community collaboration, and providing education and training to help individuals and communities reach their health goals. Examples of asset-based interventions include community gardens, health education workshops, and peer health coaching. These interventions can be tailored to meet the specific needs of a given community and can be used to address a wide range of health issues, including chronic diseases, obesity, mental health, and substance use disorders. When implemented correctly, asset-based interventions can have a significant impact on public health and the well-being of individuals and communities.

One asset-based intervention for improving the health-seeking behaviour of Fulani on vaccine-preventable diseases is the introduction of mobile health clinics. Mobile health clinics are a cost-effective and convenient way to provide healthcare services to communities that are difficult to access or are underserved. By providing mobile health clinics to Fulani nomadic populations, healthcare services can be brought directly to them, making it easier for them to access the services. Additionally, these mobile clinics can provide education and awareness about vaccine-preventable diseases, as well as provide immunisation services for those who require them. Furthermore, this asset-based intervention can also provide access to other healthcare services, such as antenatal care, maternal and child health services, and general health screenings.

Overall, a situational analysis study on nomads' health-seeking behaviour provides valuable insights for research and policy development. Researchers and policymakers can develop more effective interventions and policies tailored to this population's unique needs by understanding the cultural and social factors that influence health behaviour.

Research focused specifically on the Nomadic Fulanis was relatively limited in the context of public health generally and vaccine-preventable disease specifically until this work. By applying the theoretical framework of Deleuze and Guattari, it was possible to reveal issues of salience in this field of social epidemiology. The conceptual basis of rhizomatic analysis in relation to territorialisation, deterritorialisation, reterritorialisation, encounter, and becoming, as advocated by Deleuze and Guattari's seminal work, offered the opportunity to provide valuable insights into the perception and health behaviour of the Fulani kinsmen towards both vaccine-preventable disease and vaccination in childhood populations.

References

Abubakar, Y. M., Lawal., J., Dadi, H., and Grema, U. S. (2020). Diptheria: A Re-Emerging Public Health Challenge. *International Journal of Otorhinolaryngology and Head Surgery*. DOI: 10.18203/issn.2454-5929.ijohns20195713.

Adenike, O. B., Adejumoke, J., Olufunmi, O., and Rilwan, O. (2017). Maternal Characteristics and Immunisation Status of Children in North Central of Nigeria. *Pan African Medical Journal*, 26, 159. DOI: 10.11604/pamj.2017.26.159.11530.

Afolabi, R. F., Salawu, M. M., Gbadebo, B. M., Salawu, A. T., Fagbamigbe, A. F., and Adebowale, A. S. (2021). Ethnicity as a Cultural Factor Influencing Complete Vaccination among Children Aged 12–23 Months in Nigeria. *Human Vaccines Immunotherapeutics*, 17(7), 2008–2017. DOI: 10.1080/21645515.2020.1870394. Available on: https://www.ncbi.nlm.nih.gov/pmc/articles/PMC8189114/.

Anorue, L. I., Ugwu, C. A., Ugboaja, U. S., Nwabunze, O. U., Ugwulor-Onyiyechi, C., and Njoku, C. (2021). Communicating COVID-19 Vaccine Safety: Knowledge and Attitude among Residents of South East, Nigeria. *Infection and Drug Resistance*, 1, 3785–3794. DOI: 10.2147/IDR.S329183.

Antai, D. (2012). Gender Inequalities, Relationship Power, and Childhood Immunization Uptake in Nigeria: A Population-Based Cross-Sectional Study. *International Journal of Infectious Diseases*, 16(2). DOI: 10.1016/j.ijid.2011.11.004.

he SAGE H harmaz, K. (2014). *Constructing Grounded Theory: A Practical Guide Through Qualitative Analysis*. London: Sage.

Clarke, A. (2005). *Situational Analysis: Grounded Theory after the Postmodern Turn*. Thousand Oaks, CA: Sage.

Eze, P., Agu, U. J., Aneibo, L. C., Agu, S. A., Lawani, L. O., and Acharya, Y.(2021). Factors Associated with Incomplete Immunisation in Children Aged 12–23 Months at subnational Level, Nigeria: A Cross-Sectional Study. *BMJ Open*, 11, e047445. DOI: 10.1136/bmjopen-2020–047445.

Gunnala, R., Ogbuanu, I. U., Adegoke, J. O., Scoibe, H. M., Uba, B. V.,Wannemuehler, K. A., Ruiz, A., Elmousaad, H., Ohuabunwo, J. C., Mustafa, M., Nguku, P., Waziri, E. N., and Vertefeuille, J. F. (2016). Routine Vaccination Coverage in Northern Nigeria: Results from District-Level Cluster Survey, 2014–2015. *PLOS ONE*. DOI: 10.1371/journalpone.0167835.

Ifedilichukwu, I. (2022). Scaling Up Routine Immunisation Coverage in Nigeria: Critical Months Ahead. *Save the Children*. Available on: https://www.savethechildren.org.uk/blogs/2022/scaling-up-routine-immunisation-coverage-in-nigeria.

National Population Commission, (NPC) Nigeria (2020) available at https://national population.gov.ng/ accessed 30/06/202

National Population Commission (NPC) (Nigeria) and ICF International. (2014). Demographic and Health Survey 2013, Abuja, Nigeria, and Rockville, MD.

National Primary Health Care Development Agency. (2009). National Immunization Policy (rev.). Abuja, Nigeria: Federal Ministry of Health. Available on: https://polioeradication.org/wp-content/uploads/2016/07/7.5_6IMB-1.pdf.

Nigerian National Bureau of Statistics (2020). available https://nigerianstat.gov.ng/ accessed 30/06/2024

Olorunsaiye, C. Z., and Degge, H. (2016). Variation in the Uptake of Routine IMMUNIZATION in Nigeria: Examining Determinants of Inequalities Access. *Global Health Communication*, 2(1). DOI: 10.1080/23762004.2016.1206780.

Ophori, E. A., Tula, M. Y., Azih, V. A., Okojie, R., and Ikpo, P. (2014). Current Trends of Immunization in Nigeria: Prospect and Challenges. *Tropical Medicine and Health*, 42(2), 67–75. DOI: 10.21149/tmh.2013-13. Available on: https://www.ncbi.nlm.nih.gov/pmc/articles/PMC4139536/.

Perieres, L., Seror, V., Boyer, S., Sokha, C., and Watel., P. (2022). Reasons Given for Non-Vaccination and Under-Vaccination of Children and Adolescents in Sub-Saharan Africa: A Systematic Review. *Human Vaccines & Immunotherapeutics*, 18(5). DOI: 10.1080/21645515.2022.2076524.

Sadoh, A. E., and Oladokun, R. E. (2012). Re-emergence of Diphtheria and Pertussis Implications for Nigeria. *Vaccine*. DOI: 10.1016/j.vaccine.2012.10.014.

Strauss, A. L., and Corbin, J. (1990, 1998). *The Basis of Qualitative Analysis: Grounded Theory Procedure and Techniques* (1st and 2nd Ed.). Newbury Park, CA: Sage.

World Health Organisation, (2009). World Health Statistics available at https://www.who.int/publications/i/item/9789241563819 accessed 30/06/2024

World Health Organisation (2013). World Health Report available at https://www.afro.who.int/publications/world-health-report-2013-research-universal-health-coverage accessed 30/06/2024

World Health Organisation(WHO). (2017). Seventy Seven Percent (77%) of Children 12–23 Months in Nigeria Did Not Receive All Routine Immunisation-Survey Findings. Available on: https://www.afro.who.int/news/seventy-seven-percent-77-children-12-23-months-nigeria-did-not-receive-all-routine.

World Health Organisation (2022). Immunization Coverage. Available on: https://www.who.int/news-room/fact-sheets/detail/immunization-coverage.

13

A FRAMEWORK TO DESCRIBE HOW SOCIOCULTURAL FACTORS INFLUENCE INFORMAL DEMENTIA CAREGIVING

Candidus Nwakasi

Introduction

There is a prediction that, compared to developed countries, developing countries such as those in Sub-Saharan Africa (SSA) will be more affected by the burden of Alzheimer's disease and related dementias (ADRD – also referred to as dementia in this chapter) and other types of burden soon (Prince, 2000). This chapter describes Nigeria's inadequate readiness to address a growing dementia burden, gaps in formal long-term care and the need for informal caregiving, the stress of informal dementia caregiving, and findings from a study on the experiences of Nigerian women who identify as informal dementia caregivers. Further, this chapter includes a proposed sociocultural framework that explains the influence of sociocultural factors on dementia caregiving in Nigeria. This chapter also highlights some of the socio-structural factors in the field of social epidemiology that have been identified to determine health and well-being including gender, race/ethnicity, discrimination (e.g., dementia-related stigma), social network, socioeconomic status, and social policy (Honjo, 2004).

Nigeria's Demography, Health System, and Long-Term Care

In 2020, Nigeria's older population is ranked 19th largest and is projected to be ranked 11th by 2050—it has an older adult population of about 10.9 million that may triple to 33.2 million by 2050 (He et al., 2020). Nigeria's high fertility rate has long masked its rapidly aging population, and despite demographic

DOI: 10.4324/9781003467601-16

change, Nigeria's weak health system and lack of long-term care policies indicate an unpreparedness and incapacity to address the increasing demands of an aging population, such as the increased risk of chronic diseases and dementia (George-Carey et al., 2012; Nwakasi et al., 2019; Velkoff & Kowal, 2006). The challenges of its health system are summarized as: high health inequity and an underfunded health system (George-Carey et al., 2012; Welcome, 2011); lack of responsive health programs (Muhammad et al., 2017); weakening health infrastructure and high migration rate of specialized health workers (Abosede & Sholeye, 2014; Kress et al., 2016; Welcome, 2011); and extremely high out-of-pocket health expenses (Olugbenga, 2017).

Given the situation of Nigeria's health system, it should not be surprising that functional formal-long-term care policies are scarce (Tanyi et al., 2018). However, this lack of formal long-term care policies may be a product of the views of many Nigerians that caregiving for older adults should be within the family and/or from the government's neglect of the implications for a rapidly aging population (Togonu-Bickersteth & Akinyemi, 2014). Conceivably, it is because Nigerians are far from accepting the concept of formal long-term care (Okoye, 2012). These descriptions explain why informal long-term care remains the most accessible type of long-term care for most older adults.

Cultural and Informal Caregiving

Most Nigerian families are structured such that older adults are supported by their adult children and relatives (Ogunniyi et al., 2005; Togonu-Bickersteth & Akinyemi, 2014)—women provide most of the direct informal care while men are expected to provide financial support (Okoye, 2012; Uwakwe, 2006). Utilizing formal long-term care facilities such as nursing homes is not culturally acceptable, and this is a barrier to accessing the scarcely available formal long-term care facilities. Moreover, while caring for a person living with dementia who may be exhibiting symptoms associated with dementia (e.g., aggression, sleep disorder, and communication issues) can be demanding and difficult, informal caregivers tend to not seek external or professional support. Therefore, dementia care in Nigeria is substantially worse compared to developed countries (Ogunniyi et al., 2005). To add to the complicated situation, many adult children on whom families depend for care are also experiencing economic hardships such as lower income and unemployment (Akinyemi, 2014; Okoye, 2014), which add to the stress of providing informal care for older relatives with dementia and other chronic conditions. To further understand the context of dementia and familial caregiving in Nigeria, this chapter examines the possible intersections of caregiving, perceptions of dementia, gender-based violence, and economic hardship in Nigeria.

Findings from a Qualitative Study of Nigerians in Nigeria and the U.S.

The findings in this chapter are based on a qualitative descriptive research approach used to explore caregivers' perceptions of dementia, stigma, and care in Nigeria. Semi-structured interviews were conducted with a purposive sample of 12 adult informal female caregivers in Anambra, Nigeria. The data were then analyzed for themes. Afterwards, focus groups involving 21 adult Nigerians residing in Ohio, US, were conducted to offer more insight on the findings. The details of the research method are available (Nwakasi, 2019). The findings from Nwakasi (2019) and Nwakasi (2021) are briefly described.

Perceptions of dementia symptoms. In the study, dementia symptoms were viewed as normal aging, madness, the results of sorcery or witchcraft, and/ or wickedness (Nwakasi, 2019; Nwakasi et al., 2021). Although participants described dementia symptoms as part of being older, some attributed the symptoms to witchcraft and sorcery, while others saw them as madness. These views are conflicting, as others think, "…it is what she [person with dementia] did when she was young that is affecting her." Therefore, people with dementia may be viewed as victims of other people's evil acts or victims of their own previous evil acts.

Caregiving challenges and supports. The participants described their challenges of dementia caregiving and what they found to be supportive. These challenges and supports are related to the cost of caregiving and financial support, the sharing of caregiving responsibilities, and their faith as Christians. The issue of the availability of financial resources for dementia caregiving was common to all caregivers. Dementia caregiving can be expensive because most caregivers have to provide medical expenses, special needs (e.g., specific meals), personal care, and round-the-clock care. Some talked about the availability of financial and physical support from family members, while others complained of non-support from family members who are supposed to share part of the caregiving responsibilities.

Sometimes, this abandonment of the caregiver is due to dementia-related stigma—family members dissociate themselves from relatives with dementia to reduce the impact of the stigma on themselves. In extreme cases, family members (e.g., husbands) may become barriers to caregiving as they have certain expectations from their wives, which conflicts with adequately providing dementia care. Thus, there is a conflict between cultural expectations of being a wife to a husband, a mother to children, and a child to an older parent with dementia. This could result in caregivers becoming victims of physical violence by their spouses or imposing strain on their marriage.

Caregiving endures regardless of the stress. Even with the challenges identified, the participants continued to provide care. Some believe that caregiving is the obligation of the family, especially the woman, and she must attend to her responsibility as the caregiver despite the stress involved. Others think caregiving serves as protection for people with dementia who are vulnerable. They also believe that caregiving protects the family from shame—as people may laugh or speak badly about you and your family due to the stigma associated with dementia symptoms or because they see you as irresponsible for not providing informal care to a relative in need. Most of the caregivers explained that there is reward from caregiving as "good begets good." For example, the view that their children would provide care for them when they are older and need care, and the belief that they will be blessed by God for being a good daughter and caregiver. Some provided care because of the strong bond shared with the person with dementia when the person was younger.

Framework to Describe Sociocultural Factors Influencing Dementia Caregiving

Before proposing a framework to describe how sociocultural factors influence caregiving experiences in Nigeria, this chapter first used the life course principle of linked lives and family stress theory to describe the Nigerian context of dementia caregiving.

The life course perspective provides a framework for understanding the socio-structural, psychological, and physiological experiences of people within historical and cultural contexts over the course of their lives (Elder et al., 2003; Settersten, 2018). This perspective includes the principle of linked lives, which suggests that individuals are part of social networks such as their families, friendships, peers, work colleagues, and communities, and these relationships serve as sources of potential capital through the provision of social support (Cornwell & Schafer, 2016). The principle of linked lives highlights the importance of Nigerian families as the social safety net for catering to the expectations of informal care access for older parents/relatives with dementia. The emphasis on familial interdependence is especially crucial for older persons in need of care when other care alternatives (e.g., formal long-term care), if at all available, may be undesirable or unaffordable (Nwakasi et al., 2021).

Family stress theory, like the concept of linked lives, emphasizes the role of family as the primary social support provider for its members (McCubbin, 1979; McCubbin et al., 1980). It also highlights how some interruptions or shocks, such as dementia onset, may disrupt seemingly normal life routines, impose huge demands on family members as caregivers, and overstretch limited family resources (McCubbin, 1979; McCubbin et al., 1980). Both the life course principle of linked lives and the family stress theory offer critical lenses to explore the gendered nature of caregiving for older adults with dementia in

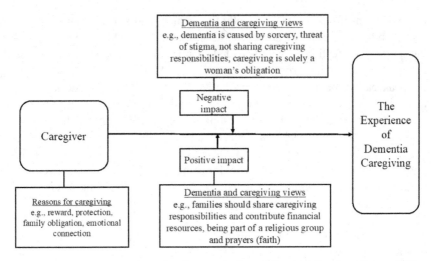

FIGURE 13.1 "Factors Influencing Dementia Caregiving by Nigerian Woman." The box at the top of the diagram is entitled Dementia and Caregivers Views, e.g., dementia is caused by sorcery, the threat of stigma, not sharing caregiving responsibilities, and caregiving is solely a woman's obligation. This box leads to a feature of negative impact in the diagram, which is straddled by the main protagonists, caregiver, and the experience of dementia caregiving. The caregiver is explained further as having reasons for the activity such as reward, protection, family obligation, and emotional connection. Also feeding into the protagonists is their positive impact. Positive impact is further expanded into dementia and caregiving views; e.g., families should share caregiving responsibilities, contribute financial resources, be part of a religious group, and offer prayers (faith).

a developing country and the influence of culture on the health and wellbeing of caregivers and those receiving care, thus adding to the literature on social epidemiology in SSA.

Based on the earlier reported study findings, the principle of linked lives, and family stress theory, Figure 13.1 is a diagrammatic representation of how sociocultural factors may influence dementia caregiving experiences in Nigeria. The women in the study setting provided caregiving for their older relatives (e.g., parent, grandparent, spouse) due to the belief that there was a reward for their actions. This perceived reward includes blessings from God or good karma from being a caregiver. Good karma refers to believing that one good turn deserves another – "my children will take good care of me like I took good care of my parents." Sometimes caregiving is primarily done by women because of a sense of family obligation resulting from the cultural expectation that women should be the caregivers for older adults in the family. It may be done to protect the vulnerable older adult and the family from stigmatizing views in the community, or they may be providing caregiving out of the strong emotional bond (e.g., love) they share with the person with dementia.

There are some factors identified as helpful to the person providing care for a person with dementia. For example, sharing dementia caregiving responsibilities, including the financial aspects, with family members may reduce the stress of dementia caregiving on the primary caregiver. Other sociocultural factors, such as religion/faith – having people pray for you, praying over a stressful caregiving situation, and social support from fellow church members—may help the caregiver cope with the burden of dementia caregiving.

However, some factors were identified as having negative effects on dementia caregiving. Negative attitudes about dementia symptoms and persons with dementia by family members, friends, and other members of the community may add to the difficulty of providing dementia caregiving. For example, the erroneous assumption that people with dementia are sorcerers or under a sorcerer's spell and the stigma associated with viewing older adults with dementia as mad or mentally insane may limit access to specialized care and support for people with dementia. Additionally, the cultural expectation that caregiving is solely a woman's obligation may limit access to caregiving support from male family members. In worse-case scenarios, a lack of support may result in abuse of the person with dementia, especially when the caregiver becomes overstressed from caregiving. Overall, dementia caregiving is impacted by sociocultural factors in the caregiver's community, and this has implications for the quality of dementia caregiving provided for the person with dementia and the quality of life of the primary caregiver.

Conclusion

Nigeria's rapidly aging population, increasing risk of ADRD, dearth of aging-related studies, and lack of long-term care policies may be resulting in an increasing need for informal dementia caregiving. This chapter offers insight on Nigerians' attitudes toward dementia symptoms, people with dementia, and dementia caregiving. It also described how some of these factors may be impacting women's dementia caregiving. Caregivers have access to informal support through their families and communities. However, poor dementia awareness, such as the belief that dementia is associated with sorcery or madness (dementia stigma), the view that caregiving is solely a woman's responsibility, and non-support from other family members, may negatively impact dementia caregiving. Regardless of these issues and burdens from caregiving, women were providing caregiving because they believed their role was a family obligation, that there was reward for caregiving, and because of the emotional connection shared with the person with dementia.

References

Abosede, O. A., & Sholeye, O. F. (2014). Strengthening the foundation for sustainable primary health care services in Nigeria. *Primary Health Care*, 4(167). https://doi.org/10.4172/2167-1079.1000167

Akinyemi, A. (2014). Ageing and national development in Nigeria: Costly assumptions and challenges for the future. Retrieved February 9, 2018, from https://www.researchgate.net/publication/289428065_Ageing_and_national_development_in_Nigeria_Costly_assumptions_and_challenges_for_the_future

Cornwell, B., & Schafer, M. H. (2016). "Social networks in later life." Pp. 181–201 in *Handbook of aging and the social sciences*. Elsevier, London, UK.

Elder, G. H., Jr., Johnson, M. K., & Crosnoe, R. (2003). "The emergence and development of life course theory." Pp. 3–19. In DeLamater, John (ed.) *Handbooks of sociology and social research*. Boston, MA: Springer.

George-Carey, R., Adeloye, D., Chan, K. Y., Paul, A., Kolčić, I., Campbell, H., & Rudan, I. (2012). An estimate of the prevalence of dementia in Africa: A systematic analysis. *Journal of Global Health*, 2(2). https://doi.org/10.7189/jogh.02.020401

He, W., Aboderin, T., & Adjaye-Gbewonyo, D. (2020). U.S. Census Bureau, International Population Reports, P95/20–1 Africa Aging: 2020 U.S. Government Printing Office, Washington, DC. https://www.census.gov/content/dam/Census/library/publications/2020/demo/p95_20-1.pdf

Honjo, K. (2004). Social epidemiology: Definition, history, and research examples. *Environmental Health and Preventive Medicine*, 9(5), 193–199. https://doi.org/10.1007/BF02898100

Kress, D. H., Su, Y., & Wang, H. (2016). Assessment of primary health care system performance in Nigeria: Using the primary health care performance indicator conceptual framework. *Health Systems and Reform*, 2(4), 302–318.

McCubbin, H. I. (1979). Integrating coping behavior in family stress theory. *Journal of Marriage and the Family*, 41(2), 237.

McCubbin, H. I., Joy, C. B., Cauble, A. E., Comeau, J. K., Patterson, J. M., & Needle, R. H. (1980). Family stress and coping: A decade review. *Journal of Marriage and the Family*, 42(4), 855.

Muhammad, F., Abdulkareem, J. H., & Chowdhury, A. A. (2017). Major public health problems in Nigeria: A review. *South East Asia Journal of Public Health*, 7(1), 6–11. https://doi.org/10.3329/seajph.v7i1.34672

Nwakasi, C. C. (2019). Exploring the experiences of Nigerian female dementia caregivers [Doctoral dissertation, Miami University]. OhioLINK Electronic Theses and Dissertations Center. http://rave.ohiolink.edu/etdc/view?acc_num=miami1574869417297074

Nwakasi, C. C., de Medeiros, K., & Bosun-Arije, F. S. (2021). "We are doing these things so that people will not laugh at us": Caregivers' attitudes about dementia and caregiving in Nigeria. *Qualitative Health Research*, 31(8), 1448–1458. https://doi.org/10.1177/10497323211004105

Nwakasi, C., De Medeiros, K., & Kafayat, M. (2021). Poverty, domestic violence or both. *Comparative Sociology*, 20(5), 615–632. https://doi.org/10.1163/15691330-12341541

Nwakasi, C. C., Hayes, C., Fulton, J., & Roberts, A. R. (2019). A pilot qualitative study of dementia perceptions of Nigerian migrant caregivers. *International Journal of Africa Nursing Sciences*, 10, 167–174. https://doi.org/10.1016/j.ijans.2019.03.003

Nwakasi, C. C., de Medeiros, K., & Bosun-Arije, F. S. (2021). "We are doing these things so that people will not laugh at us": Caregivers' attitudes about dementia and caregiving in Nigeria. *Qualitative Health Research, 31*(8), 1448-1458.

Olugbenga, E. O. (2017). Workable social health insurance systems in Sub-Saharan Africa: Insights from four countries. *Africa Development / Afrique et Développement, 42*(1), 147–175.

Okoye, U. (2012). Family care-giving for ageing parents in Nigeria: Gender differences, cultural imperatives and the role of education. Retrieved December 20, 2017, from https://www.researchgate.net/publication/233762967_Family_care-giving_for_ ageing_parents_in_Nigeria_gender_differences_cultural_imperatives_and_the_role_ of_education

Okoye, U. (2014). Financial incentives to support family caregivers of older adults in Nigeria: A policy consideration. Retrieved December 20, 2017, from https://www. researchgate.net/publication/267868227_Financial_Incentives_to_Support_Family_ Care-Givers_of_Older_Adults_in_Nigeria_a_Policy_Consideration

Ogunniyi, A., Hall, K. S., Baiyewu, O., Gureje, O., Unverzagt, F., Gao, S., & Hendrie, H. C. (2005). Caring for individuals with dementia: The Nigerian experience. *West African Journal of Medicine, 24*(3), 259–262.

Prince, M. (2000). Dementia in developing countries. A consensus statement from the 10/66 Dementia Research Group. *International Journal of Geriatric Psychiatry, 15*(1), 14–20. https://doi.org/10.1002/(SICI)1099-1166(200001)15:1<14::AID-GPS 70>3.0.CO;2-8

Settersten, R. (2018). *Towards new understandings of later life.* New York, NY: Routledge.

Tanyi, P. L., André, P., & Mbah, P. (2018). Care of the elderly in Nigeria: Implications for policy. *Cogent Social Sciences, 4*(1), 1555201. https://doi.org/10.1080/23311886. 2018.1555201

Togonu-Bickersteth, F., & Akinyemi, A. I. (2014). Ageing and national development in Nigeria: Costly assumptions and challenges for the future. *African Population Studies, 27*(2), 361–371.

Uwakwe, R. (2006). Satisfaction with dementia care-giving in Nigeria – A pilot investigation. *International Journal of Geriatric Psychiatry, 21*, 296–297.

Velkoff, V. A., & Kowal, P., R. (2006). Aging in Sub-Saharan Africa: The changing demography of the region. Retrieved December 6, 2016, from http://www.nap.edu/ read/11708/chapter/5#55

Welcome, M. O. (2011). The Nigerian health care system: Need for integrating adequate medical intelligence and surveillance systems. Retrieved April 12, 2017, from https:// www.ncbi.nlm.nih.gov/pmc/articles/PMC3249694/

14

UNDERSTANDING THE SOCIAL, POLITICAL, AND CULTURAL DIMENSIONS OF LOWER LIMB AMPUTATION EXPERIENCES AMONG PEOPLE LIVING WITH DIABETES MELLITUS

Joseph Sunday

Introduction

This chapter provides a first-hand insight into the experiences of lower limb amputation (LLA) for those living with one of the chronic complications of poor glycaemic control within the context of West Africa (WA). Using social epidemiology as a mechanism of theoretically framing a contextual understanding of the interplay of socio-political factors, the role of culture in how individuals manage an acquired disability and a chronic disease condition will be the central focus of this chapter. The justification of the qualitative research paradigm within this context provides a more authentic opportunity to integrate constructivist grounded theory so that global audiences can reflect on and potentially understand the experience of people living in WA with a LLA attributable to the underlying pathophysiological changes attributable to poor glycaemic control and systemic management of the condition.

Lower Limb Amputation and Diabetes Mellitus

Amputation can be operationally defined as "The surgical removal of the whole or part of a limb..." (International Standards Organisation (ISO), 2014). While focusing specifically on the lower limb, within this chapter, amputation will refer to the loss of any limb or extremity of the human anatomical structure. Amputation of the limb is undertaken for a diverse variety of reasons, which can be broadly grouped as either traumatic or non-traumatic depending on the underlying pathology and aetiology of the condition that is clinically presented (Esquenazi and DiGiacomo, 2001).

DOI: 10.4324/9781003467601-17

Diabetes mellitus remains one of the most exponentially increasing public health conditions, which, when poorly managed, can result in a complex series of complications, all of which are micro-vascular or macro-vascular in origin. (Papatheodorou et al., 2018). What is significant about these complications is their potential to be avoided altogether through optimal control of glycaemic index, blood pressure, and serum triglycerides. Normalising these measures is a fundamental part of ensuring that long-term complications do not have the opportunity to develop in the first place. Often, the specific changes that can be made hinge on lifestyle modification and timely health interventions such as the assessment, diagnosis, and management of complications to the microvascular and macrovascular systems of the body. constant eye and limb. However, within the context of developing countries such as those within WA, the lack of physical healthcare infrastructure means that multi-disciplinary team approaches to the avoidance of long-term complications in diabetes mellitus are not yet either physically possible or financially feasible (Levitt, 2008; Atun et al., 2017).

The Global Epidemiology of Diabetes Mellitus

The Global Burden of Disease (GBD) Study 2017 provided an estimate of the burden of diabetes mellitus across 195 countries (Lin et al., 2020). The study illustrated a 129.7% increase in the global prevalence of diabetes mellitus, from circa 211.2 million in 1990 to circa 476.0 million in 2017. Inferential statistics provide a predicted prevalence of diabetes mellitus to increase to 570.9 million between 2018 and 2025 in the absence of effective clinical interventions to assess, diagnose, and manage potential and actual complications 'in situ' (Lin et al., 2020). Another systematic review comprehensively estimated that there were 451 million adults (18–99 years) living with diabetes mellitus globally in 2017 (Cho et al., 2018). The International Diabetes mellitus Federation (IDF, 2022) have estimated that globally 537 million adults (20–79 years) were living with diabetes mellitus, a number that equates to one in ten people.

In addition to lower limb pathology attributable to the long-term complications of diabetes mellitus, McDonald et al. (2020) estimated that in 2017, there were 57.7 million people living with limb amputations associated with traumatic origins globally, with just over one third of these amputations (36.2%) directly associated with falls. On the other hand, Zhang et al. (2020), using data from the GBD 2016, estimated that of 131 million people (1.8% of the world's population) living specifically with diabetes mellitus-related lower-extremity complications, 6.8 million people were living with amputations (4.3 million who are without prosthetics and 2.5 million without.). This highlights the significant number of people living with amputations globally and the significant contributory role played by suboptimally managed diabetes mellitus in the global burden of LLA.

Diabetes Mellitus and Africa

Africa bears a significant burden of the global prevalence of diabetes mellitus in terms of morbidity and mortality. As a consequence, the growth in the number of people diagnosed with the condition is a significant cause for concern. The prevalence rate of diabetes mellitus in the early 1960s was less than 1% in most African countries (Abbas and Boulton, 2022), but now an estimated 24 million adults (1 in 22) are living with diabetes mellitus, with an estimated 54% as yet undiagnosed. In addition to this, there is a projected population increase of 129% to 55 million people by 2045. Diabetes mellitus has been associated with 416,000 deaths in 2021 alone (International Diabetes Mellitus Federation (IDF), 2022). This highlights a significant public health issue as Africa's health as a nation is further characterised by inordinate levels of deprivation and poverty, coupled with the challenges of infectious/communicable diseases, which in turn add to the strain on relatively scarce resources. All serve to ensure diabetes mellitus remains a challenging clinical condition to optimally manage across societies where its incidence and prevalence rates are increasing on an annual basis (Atun et al., 2017). WA is a demographic region characterised by significant levels of poverty, poor healthcare systems, and public health infrastructure. Therefore, it is important to understand the impact of living with amputations associated with diabetes mellitus from broader, socio-political, and cultural perspectives, which can be contextualised and framed beyond an individual perspective as the rise in the condition in this region transcends any simplistic or tokenistic explanation.

Demographic changes, urbanisation and an accompanying increase in sedentary lifestyle, changing dietary trends due to access to less healthy or processed foods, smoking and alcohol use, and Westernisation have all been identified as contributory factors to the rise in incidence and prevalence rates of diabetes mellitus in WA (Azevedo and Alla, 2008; Atun et al., 2017; Zimmermann et al., 2018; Abbas and Boulton, 2022).

Diabetes Mellitus, Amputation, and Africa

Diabetes mellitus is responsible for the majority of non-traumatic amputations globally (Zhang et al., 2020). An individual with Diabetes mellitus is 22 times more likely to undergo a non-traumatic amputation than an individual without the condition (Buckley et al., 2012). It is estimated that 6.8 million people are living with the impact of amputation globally (Zhang et al., 2020). However, the specific number of people living with amputation within Sub-Saharan Africa (SSA), especially WA, remains unknown. This has been attributed to several issues, such as poor monitoring and surveillance (Esquenazi and DiGiacomo, 2001; Abbas and Boulton, 2022). Estimates of amputation rates associated with diabetes mellitus within this region vary from 15% to as high as 52% among

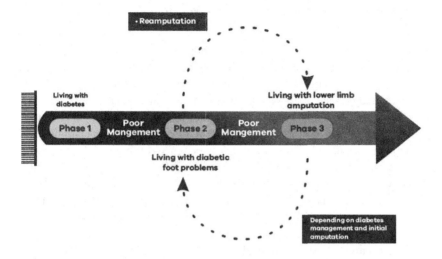

FIGURE 14.1 The three phases of living with diabetes with lower limb amputation due to poorly managed diabetes.

people with foot ulcers attributable to the condition (Edo et al., 2013; Rigato et al., 2018; Ugwu et al., 2019; Adeleye et al., 2020).

Historically, traumatic amputations have been the leading cause of amputation in SSA (Dada and Awoyomi, 2010). However, studies on foot complications due to diabetes mellitus show marked increases in relation to rates of amputation (Opedele et al., 2007; Dada and Awoyomi, 2010; Rigato et al., 2018; Ugwu et al., 2019; Khan et al., 2020).

Undergoing an amputation is a traumatic process that parallels experiencing bereavement (Spiess et al., 2014). Living with amputation due to diabetes mellitus within WA is further exacerbated due to the additional negative impacts of undergoing the process, such as medical costs, the rate of progressive re-amputation, and mortality, which are higher in this population (Dillingham et al., 2005; Kono and Muder, 2012; Adeleye et al., 2020; Liu et al., 2021). These additional factors beyond the direct control of the individual are external factors, which are covered within the field of social epidemiology (Honjo, 2004).

Active discussion around the experiences of living with amputations due to diabetes mellitus has the potential to elucidate some of the unique socio-political and cultural factors impacting situated experiences within the WA. context. This can be framed across three distinct phases of an individual living with amputation experience, namely: (i) living with diabetes mellitus; (ii) living with foot pathology as a consequence of diabetes mellitus[1]; and (iii) living post-surgically with the implications of LLAs.

Socio-political Factors in Living with Lower Limb Amputations Associated with Poorly Managed Diabetes Mellitus

Social epidemiology is predicated on the notion that social conditions have a tangible impact on the health of a population. It "focuses particularly on the effects of socio-structural factors on states of health" (Honjo, 2004, p. 193). As a field of study, social epidemiology transcends the individual context and captures the social contexts where public health issues, resistant to intervention, prevail. Among people living with LLAs that are associated with complications due to poorly managed diabetes mellitus, experiences of living with an acquired disability are preceded by the poor management of a chronic disease condition. While it is not uncommon to shift the responsibility of glycaemic control onto the individuals themselves, there are various socio-political factors that influence the management of diabetes mellitus that are beyond their control. Diabetes mellitus (Bosun-Arije et al., 2019).

Understanding the socio-political factors influencing the experience of living with LLA requires a contextual understanding of the continuum of care from being diagnosed and living with diabetes mellitus to living with the impact of post-surgical amputation. It is important to highlight that, from a public health perspective, the relevance of diabetes mellitus prevention and interventions strategically designed to address this ought to remain a priority. Hu et al. (2015) provide an extensive review of various examples of policy modifications to aid in the prevention of diabetes mellitus in SSA. Nonetheless, the discussion will focus on addressing socio-political factors along the three major phases, as shown in Figure 14.1.

Living with Diabetes Mellitus

Managing optimal control of diabetes mellitus for individuals living in WA can be challenging. This is in addition to ensuring the avoidance of other prevailing communicable diseases with high incidence and prevalence rates that individuals face on a daily basis within WA (Azevedo and Alla, 2008; Atun et al., 2017). Most studies suggest that management of diabetes mellitus rests at an individual level, incorporating a form of *victim-blaming* for any inability to adequately manage the condition (Bosun-Arije et al., 2019). An argument can be made for the high level of responsibility of the individual for diabetes mellitus self-management, and in many cases, this responsibility is not yet apparent among this population (Abbas, 2017; Stephani et al., 2018). However, the level of poverty and other wider socio-political issues that directly affect the self-management of this condition, in addition to the influence of other external factors beyond the control of the individual, cannot be disregarded. For example, common at an individual level is the use of traditional healers or other sources of alternative medicine for the management of diabetes mellitus (Ogbera et al.,

2010; Aaron et al., 2021). However, there are many factors beyond the individual that inform this pattern of health-seeking behaviour among individuals, such as family customs, traditions, belief systems, proximity, affordability, and availability of medication, among many others (Ogbera et al., 2010; Tuei et al., 2010; Abbas, 2017). Adequate management of Diabetes mellitus needs to transcend attributing blame to the individual and acknowledging external factors beyond the individual level, while at the same time dissolving the case for management at individual levels.

The optimal management of diabetes mellitus is greatly influenced by several socio-political factors (Levitt, 2008; Atun et al., 2017). The lack of a robust healthcare infrastructure is typical of this, with limited resources and systems that are stretched as organisations and individuals continue to tackle the challenges of communicable/infectious diseases prevalent in the regions, which most of these health systems have been set-up to do (Whiting et al., 2003; Atun et al., 2017).

Healthcare systems are integral to diabetes mellitus management (Atun et al., 2017). People with diabetes mellitus are faced with a multi-faceted condition requiring multi-professional specialist care, adequate patient information and education, long-term patient care and follow-up, and regular screening of the microvascular and macrovascular systems, which readily avails them to efficient intervention by healthcare systems that employ specialist clinicians (Delea et al., 2015). The lack of adequate healthcare systems in this region means the amount of care needed to manage the condition is not met. Furthermore, medical expenses, including medications such as insulin, are dominated by out-of-pocket (OOP) payment systems (Chinenye and Ogbera, 2013). The long-term implications of these issues are notable, as people living with diabetes mellitus are left in a position of self-management, even though their lack of capacity to control glycaemic levels may be attributable to their post-surgical amputation status.

Funding for the healthcare system in WA and other policy strategies needed in the management of diabetes mellitus are closely linked to the political situation and lie predominantly within the domain of the government and other key players (Hu et al., 2015). For example, Pastakia et al. (2017, p. 247) outline six broad areas that need to be evaluated for the improvement of diabetes mellitus care in SSA: policy, epidemiology, pathophysiology, care protocols, medication access, and healthcare systems. Of these six areas, five primarily sit within the domain of the government, which does not provide the attention and infrastructure needed to address these issues, such as lack of funding.

Funding continues to be one of the major reasons for the poor management of diabetes mellitus in this region, which translates to the state of the health systems already discussed. (Pastakia et al., 2017). Limited funds are often focused more on communicable or infectious diseases, with less attention paid to non-communicable diseases (NCDs). Inadequate funding for managing NCDs is observed from funding support from international organisations and nationally. Countries in the SSA continue to spend the least on healthcare compared to other regions of the world. Additionally, most of these countries spend less than the Chatham House goal of 5% of their GDP on health, compared to 12.4% by countries of the Organisation for Economic Cooperation and Development (Dieleman et al., 2016).

The need for government intervention goes beyond only funding to improved policies and national interventions aimed at tackling diabetes mellitus and, more broadly, chronic disease conditions (Pastakia et al., 2017). Beran and Yudkin (2006) have pointed out that many countries in the SSA *lack policy frameworks* for NCDs and diabetes mellitus that cover the necessary building blocks for the management of these conditions. Policy initiatives can potentially improve the overall experience of diabetes mellitus management at individual levels and, as a result, reduce the issue at the population level (Hu et al., 2015). Political interventions are needed beyond care to cover other factors such as the availability of food and agricultural products, which will potentially create an environment from which individuals can make healthier dietary choices or infrastructure or urban planning initiatives to enhance physical activity levels or address the challenges associated with urbanisation and other factors that could affect the management of diabetes mellitus in WA (Mbanya et al., 2010).

Living with Diabetic Foot Problems

Diabetic foot problems are commonly reported among people with poorly managed diabetes mellitus. They account for more hospital admissions compared to any other complications associated with diabetes mellitus (Ahmad, 2016). Around 10% of people living with diabetes mellitus will develop foot problems at some point (Abbas and Archibald, 2007). The correlation between diabetic foot ulcers and death is very strong (Walsh et al., 2016). In a cohort study conducted in the United Kingdom, Walsh et al. (2016) showed that 5% of people with ulcers died within 12 months of their first foot ulcer visit, and 42.2% died after 5 years from their population-based study. Considering the quality of healthcare in the UK, outcomes are likely to be more severe among members of this population in WA. Rigato et al. (2018) estimated the average hospital mortality rates in Africa at 14.2%, with other studies reporting higher from 14.3% to 40.5% in Nigeria (Ekpebegh et al., 2009; Edo et al., 2013; Adeleye et al., 2020) and 38.1% in Burkina-Faso (Sano et al., 1998). There is also a high level of mortality, with a five-year mortality rate comparable to that of cancer (Armstrong et al., 2020). Armstrong et al. (2020) reported that the five-year mortality for diabetic foot ulcers could be as high as 30.5%. Additionally, even when successfully treated, the recurrence of diabetic foot ulcers is high, with about 40% within one year and 90% within ten years. Such a potential for recurrence further adds to the complexity associated with living with diabetic foot problems for these individuals (Armstrong et al., 2017).

Crucial to the issue of diabetic foot complications is the *lack of awareness* of the relationship between diabetes mellitus and foot problems (Abbas, 2017). This informs the pattern of health-seeking behaviour displayed by individuals who have diabetes mellitus (Abbas and Boulton, 2022). Abbas (2017) identifies education as the most important tool towards preventing foot problems in Africa, in addition to proper foot care. Additionally, many people seek treatment late, and this can be associated with other wider issues such as distance to health centres and the influence of cultural factors, which will be discussed subsequently in this chapter. When prevention of diabetic foot complications fails, the management of diabetes mellitus-related foot problems becomes more important towards preventing amputation.

The management of diabetic foot problems in WA has challenges more pronounced than in developed countries of the world due to the unique contextual challenges of this region (Abbas, 2017). One of the greatest challenges associated with managing diabetic foot problems is the **financial burden** associated with treatment at both individual and societal levels, resulting in losing functional abilities in many cases (Abbas, 2017; Armstrong et al., 2020).

Unlike the management of diabetes mellitus, which entails diverse, broad health interventions that are beyond the immediate medical setting, managing diabetic foot problems sits predominantly within the auspices of clinical interventions (Ahmad, 2016; Armstrong et al., 2017; Mishra et al., 2017). This means that attention is on the quality of the healthcare system, which is significantly lacking in many countries in WA. It is beyond the scope of this work to discuss the specific clinical interventions in the management of diabetic feet. Readers are referred to studies (Ahmad, 2016; Abbas, 2017; Mishra et al., 2017; Abbas and Boulton, 2022) that have delineated the management of diabetic foot problems.

Beyond the clinical setting, the establishment of a monitoring system and more localised health centres or hospitals with the capability of managing foot complications have also been suggested as issues that can be addressed from a broader, socio-political landscape (Pastakia et al., 2017; Abbas and Boulton, 2022). This is important in preventing major amputations, which have been reported to be feared more than death by people dealing with diabetic foot problems (Wukich et al., 2018).

Living with Lower Limb Amputations

Following amputation due to complications associated with diabetes mellitus, individuals must deal with having acquired a physical disability alongside managing the chronic disease condition that caused the amputation. There are additional concerns that can further complicate the experiences of these individuals beyond these two significant challenges: acquired physical disability and managing diabetes mellitus. For example, the post-amputation mortality rate is very high, with a five-year mortality rate among people with major amputations more than 50% (Izumi et al., 2009; Morbach et al., 2012; Huang et al., 2018). Furthermore, the chances of undergoing a further amputation are about 19% within a year (Liu et al., 2021). This is in addition to the mental, emotional, and psychological issues associated with this experience, akin to bereavement (Spiess et al., 2014). Notwithstanding the challenges that individuals in this population must deal with, there are other socio-political factors that affect their experiences, which at this stage are as much within the challenges of being physically disabled as having diabetes mellitus.

At a socio-political level, disabled people experience significant additional challenges compared to their non-disabled counterparts. There are issues of **social exclusion** and high levels of **poverty,** which are associated with a **lack of employment,** as many jobs within these countries are physically demanding, such as agriculture and farming (Amoah et al., 2019). Disabled people face significant challenges in competing with non-disabled people for employment. Furthermore, WA is not structured to meet the needs of disabled people, in addition to other **barriers.** There are no accessible roads, buildings, transport provisions, or a welfare system to meet the needs of people with disabilities (Lang and Upah, 2008). Lang and Upah highlighted key socio-political issues affecting the experiences of disabled people in Nigeria, which is likely to be like the reality of this population across WA. They highlighted **environmental, institutional,** and **attitudinal issues.** These are socio-political factors that need to be addressed at all levels of government (local, national, and international) and by other institutions such as charity organisations and other NGOs.

The problem of **prosthesis and rehabilitation** (Edomwonyi and Onuminya, 2014) is another key issue at a socio-political level impacting the experiences of this population. Prostheses play a significant role in recovery for members of this population as they augment some of the functional limitations due to the amputation (Columbo et al., 2018). Proper fitting of prostheses can help improve the post-amputation quality of life of people who have had amputations (Udosen et al., 2009). However, these services are rarely available, and when available, the quality of these prostheses is poor or substandard and may restore a few functional capabilities. Furthermore, the geography of many WA countries makes ambulation difficult due to a lack of accessible roads. This therefore highlights the need for government attention towards addressing the availability and use of assistive technologies to improve the quality of life and wellbeing of these people (Liu et al., 2010).

Cultural Factors Associated with Living with LLA Attributable to Poorly Managed Diabetes Mellitus

The UNESCO Declaration on Cultural Diversity (2001) explains culture as "the set of distinctive spiritual, material, intellectual and emotional features of

society or a social group, and that it encompasses, in addition to art and literature, lifestyles, ways of living together, value systems, traditions and beliefs". It
can also "be thought of as a set of practices and behaviours defined by customs,
habits, language, and geography that groups of individuals share" (Napier et al.,
2014). Napier et al. (2014) argue that an understanding of cultures is equally as
important as addressing political and socioeconomic inequalities and is key to
improving the overall health and wellbeing of societies.

The major cultural factors impacting the experiences of this population will
now be addressed. Parallel to the layout of the socio-political factors influencing
the experiences of this population, the cultural factors will be discussed along
the three important phases in the lives of these individuals: living with diabetes
mellitus, living with diabetic foot problems, and living with amputations (see
Figure 14.1).

Living with Diabetes Mellitus

Several cultural factors affect the experiences of living with diabetes mellitus
in WA. Relatively recently, diabetes mellitus was uncommon in Africa and
commonly perceived as a 'disease of affluence' due to its prevalence in the
developed Western countries of the world (Azevedo and Alla, 2008; Abbas and
Boulton, 2022). Another reason for the widely held perception could be related
to people with higher socioeconomic status, living largely in urban areas, to
afford processed foods, which were once generally very expensive and beyond
the day-to-day access of ordinary citizens. This is before the global changes due
to globalisation and urbanisation that have allowed processed foods to be more
within the reach of many more Africans (Azevedo and Alla, 2008). There is also
the cultural **perception of obesity,** which provides another dimension to the
cultural aspects of living with diabetes mellitus.

Obesity, a significant risk factor for diabetes mellitus, has generally been culturally acceptable among people in this region and perceived as a sign of good
living (Chinenye and Ogbera, 2013). For example, there has been a reported
practice among the Calabar people of Nigeria with women kept in fattening
rooms (Chinenye and Ogbera, 2013). The practice of *Leblouh*, or force-feeding,
continues to be practiced in parts of Africa where young girls are force-fed to
gain weight for marriage. There is also another dimension to the cultural acceptance of being obese, which can be tied to the HIV/AIDS pandemic that has
plagued SSA. At the height of the HIV/AIDS pandemic, being infected with the
virus meant a very depreciated body size, and for many, having a big body was
a way to show one was not infected. There are also issues around malnutrition
and malnourishment with diseases such as kwashiorkor that cause depreciation
in body size. Therefore, to be obese was an acceptable public sign (Mogre et al.,
2019), a sign that one does not have any of the aforementioned, hence adding to

the notion of diabetes mellitus being a 'disease of opulence' (Azevedo and Alla, 2008) or 'disease of the wealthy' (Aikins, 2003).

Due to the poor state of health systems in WA, many cases of diabetes mellitus remain undiagnosed, and when an individual becomes medically aware that they have diabetes mellitus, the **use of traditional or alternative medicine** as a management option is common (Chinenye and Ogbera, 2013). Self-medicating is also widespread in the diagnosis and management of diabetes mellitus. There are also some **superstitious beliefs** about diabetes mellitus. Studies have reported individuals with diabetes mellitus associating their conditions to witchcraft, ancestral interventions, or other forms of sorcery (Aikins, 2003; Awah and Phillimore, 2008; Zimmermann et al., 2018). It is important to note that the use of traditional healers is further complicated as many people do not rely solely on these healers, but rather consult them alongside seeking professional medical advice and potentially self-medicating – the hybridity of diabetes mellitus care (Ogbera et al., 2010; Zimmermann et al., 2018). This pattern of health-seeking behaviour is predicated on the belief that a **cure for diabetes mellitus** can be found (Zimmermann et al., 2018). This combination of orthodox medical treatment and traditional or alternative medicine further complicates the health-seeking pattern of this population (Ogunlana et al., 2021). Closely linked to the superstition are the religious beliefs of many people in WA, which also inform how people live with diabetes mellitus.

The WA region is deeply **religious,** predominantly divided into Christianity, Islam, and traditional beliefs. This informs the management of diabetes mellitus, as many people seek care from non-medical sources or believe that they could be healed from the condition through their faith (Zimmermann et al., 2018). Other religious practices, such as fasting during Ramadan, further impact the management of diabetes mellitus (Abdulrehman et al., 2016). The review by Zimmerman et al. (2018) outlines the common religious beliefs among people in SSA and, by implication, many parts of WA. According to the authors, in seeking a cure for diabetes mellitus, many will attribute the success of their quest to God's will and identify God's intervention as the only way out of the condition. Furthermore, some aspects of Christian practices are observed in what has been described as "special Diabetes mellitus prayers, taking communion, being anointed with holy water, and visiting dedicated faith healers" (Zimmermann et al., 2018, p. 8).

Dietary patterns in many countries in WA have also been identified as key cultural factors in living with diabetes mellitus among people in this region. Many African foods within this region have been reported to have high caloric content with little source of protein, which could make the dietary modifications needed to manage diabetes mellitus very difficult or unrealistic due to scarce financial resources (Chinenye and Ogbera, 2013; Abdulrehman et al., 2016).

Family customs and traditions have also been reported to have an impact on living with diabetes mellitus. Although not a West African country, a study conducted in Kenya (Abdulrehman et al., 2016) can shed more light on this, as the authors reported patterns in the study that are applicable to WA. The authors outlined practices such as eating large food portions, eating at social events that individuals are obligated to attend, and difficulty adjusting the dietary intake of an entire family for one person. According to the findings of the study by Mogre et al. (2019) in Ghana, the polygamous setting of many African families means meeting the specific dietary needs of people with diabetes mellitus is unrealistic. This is because in many households, the entire, relatively large family of about 10 members eats from a single cooked source. Any alteration needed for one person within a setting with scarce resources, among other external factors, is difficult (Mogre et al., 2019).

Living with Diabetic Foot Problems

Few studies have qualitatively investigated the experience of living with diabetic foot problems in WA. The few studies that have reported on this issue have been mostly quantitative and retrospectively gathered information post-amputation (Opedele et al., 2007; Dada and Awoyomi, 2010; Edomwonyi and Onuminya, 2014; Adeleye et al., 2020; Abbas and Boulton, 2022). One of the reasons for this pattern could be associated with the delay in seeking medical assistance, and by the time the individual seeks professional help, things have deteriorated beyond managing the diabetic foot problem to offering amputation as an intervention (Abbas and Archibald, 2007). Therefore, it is difficult to gather the experiences of these individuals, as they live with diabetic foot problems. Nevertheless, an understanding of cultural factors impacting the management of wounds among the general public in this setting can provide an insight into what living with diabetic foot problems entails (Builders and Builders, 2016).

Superstitious beliefs around wounds and diabetic foot ulcers are commonly reported. Many believe that wounds are a result of supernatural beings or spirits, charms, or other forms of causes that are beyond modern medicine and will require traditional healers or interventions (Koka et al., 2016). Consequently, cultural practices such as seeking alternative sources of treatment, visiting faith healers, and self-medicating using natural remedies are often reported (Abdulrehman et al., 2016).

In the Ghana study by Koka et al. (2016) investigating cultural practices and beliefs around wound management, some respondents reported beliefs such as that severe wounds would not heal if treated by a pregnant woman or if more than one person attended to the wound treatment – something more likely within a hospital setting. Therefore, these individuals with such beliefs will prefer to visit traditional healers rather than seek modern medical attention. Cultural beliefs and practices that directly impact the management of diabetic foot ulcers need to be explored further through studies towards creating awareness, addressing misconceptions, and improving the overall health and wellbeing of the members of this population.

One of the major challenges associated with living with diabetic foot problems is the pattern of health-seeking behaviour among this population. A common cultural factor impacting the experiences of living with diabetic foot problems in this phase is the use of **traditional healthcare providers** (solely or complemented with orthodox medicine) linked to superstitious beliefs about the origins of the diabetic foot problems, in addition to self-treatment and the use of informal healthcare providers (IHP) (Ogbera et al., 2010; Ogunlana et al., 2021), commonly referred to as *chemist*.

In cases where an individual seeks medical attention and is advised not to weight bear on the affected limb, other cultural practices due to **gender roles** may make this medical advice less likely to be adhered to (Abbas, 2017). The man will be expected to continue to provide for his family, which may entail physically demanding jobs, while the woman, on the other hand, would be tasked with looking after the home through chores such as cooking, cleaning, and looking after the children. These societal gender norms make the management of diabetic foot problems difficult.

There is also a common practice of **walking barefoot** or without appropriate shoes (Abbas, 2017) among many people in the WA region of Africa, which is another cultural practice that is associated with living with diabetes mellitus and significantly informs the prevalence of diabetes mellitus foot problems. These practices are associated with religious and traditional beliefs, such as walking on sacred grounds, while in some cases, the hot weather conditions of the tropics make wearing shoes less likely (Abdulrehman et al., 2016).

Living with Lower Limb Amputations

LLA is not generally perceived as an intervention aimed at saving the life of an individual, with many people preferring death rather than undergoing a major amputation (Wukich et al., 2018). While many people about to undergo amputation are intellectually aware that the surgical procedure is aimed at saving their lives, they will be willing to accept the procedure (Udosen et al., 2009; Aaron et al., 2021). However, there are cultural factors impacting the experiences of living with LLAs, which may make the acceptance of this decision difficult for individuals.

Udosen et al. (2009) report that although intellectual awareness is there, when it comes to practically carrying out the procedure, individuals are reluctant, with statements such as "*I would rather die than lose my limb*" or "*that is not my portion*" reported among people informed of the need for amputation as a surgical intervention (p. 256). In WA, the cultural factors impacting living with amputations attributable to diabetes mellitus are predominantly associated with attitudinal responses from others and society at large due to the physical disability caused by undergoing the amputation. This fear of being rejected by other members of society continues to inform the hesitancy of many people to undergo amputation (Aaron et al., 2021).

There is a common superstitious belief that individuals with amputated limbs are at risk of returning in the next life without a complete body (Aaron et al., 2021). Other commonly held beliefs reported in the study by Aaron et al. also include the fear of being regarded as outcasts in the community, being considered cursed, and being buried in the evil forest (p. 793). There are other beliefs held among many people, such as the amputation being a curse from God; the person may have trespassed against traditional, societal, or ancestral beliefs, attacks from supernatural beings that may or may not be instigated by jealousy. These cultural beliefs result in stigmatisation, discrimination, and societal exclusion due to the disability.

A fear or experience of stigmatisation and discrimination among people with LLA has been commonly reported in several studies (Opedele et al., 2007; Aaron et al., 2021; Ogunlana et al., 2021). People living with LLAs have also reported the worry of *self-pity* from members of society and being pigeonholed into the *charity box* and becoming members of the population that "*need our help*". These individuals are seen as having less bodily worth and are now perceived as issues to be tackled by charity or welfarism rather than those of human right issue (Lang and Upah, 2008). There is frequent discussion about how disabled people should be treated. Readers are referred to these works and the doctoral work of the author for further discussion of this issue within the context of a developing country (Thomas, 2012; Macdonald, 2017; Shakespeare, 2017). While the individual contends with the adverse impacts of becoming disabled after amputation, cultural perceptions of the disabled body further exacerbate the negative impact associated with amputation.

These persistent cultural beliefs inform many practices that further make the lives of these individuals difficult and need to be addressed through disabling barriers, creating awareness and education among people, and implementing context-specific interventions that will elevate the overall experiences of these individuals (Lang and Upah, 2008; Thomas, 2012; Shakespeare, 2017).

Methodological Approach

There are complexities associated with living with amputations due to poorly managed diabetes mellitus. These issues have been discussed within this chapter, highlighting the socio-political and cultural factors impacting these experiences, consistent with social epidemiology. The experiences of people living vary widely (Hamill et al., 2010). Studies carried out, particularly from a qualitative perspective, to highlight the unique socio-political and cultural factors impacting this population in WA along the journey from living with diabetes mellitus to living with the amputations underlined by the condition. However, there is a paucity of studies in Africa, especially in SSA. For example, in the systematic review by Rigato et al. (2018) on diabetic foot ulcers, the authors reported that only 55 full-text papers from 19 African countries on 56,173 people living with diabetes mellitus were retrieved. This is low when compared to the estimated number of 24 million people living with diabetes mellitus (International Diabetes mellitus Federation (IDF), 2022). Furthermore, the authors reported only 16 studies in WA, 12 of which were in Nigeria, with Senegal, Burkina Faso, Mali, and Benin reporting one study (Rigato et al., 2018). The paucity of studies is even more dire when only qualitative studies are considered. For example, in the scoping review by Zimmermann et al. (2018) investigating the experiences of people living with diabetes mellitus in SSA, only 21 studies were included in the review, all from eight countries in SSA. Only six (6) of these studies – five from Ghana and one from Senegal qualitatively reported the experiences of people living with diabetes mellitus. In a presently ongoing meta-synthesis by this author and colleagues registered with PROSPERO (Sunday et al., 2021), only two peer-reviewed studies have qualitatively explored the experiences of living with LLAs in SSA, with only one conducted in WA, Ghana.

The doctoral research of this author is one of the very few studies that have qualitatively explored the experiences of living with LLAs attributable to poorly managed diabetes mellitus in a WA context – in Lagos, Nigeria. The work adopted a constructivist grounded theory approach towards exploring the aim of the study. Grounded theory is the most appropriate methodological approach as it explores issues in areas that have not been previously explored (Charmaz, 2014).

The findings of the doctoral research study provided insight into the experiences of these individuals. Data analysis highlighted commonalities from these experiences towards developing a theory themed – *regaining some order* – which described the experiences of people within this context. It is therefore pertinent that more studies adopting a qualitative approach are conducted within this population through the three major phases that have been discussed – living with diabetes mellitus, living with diabetic foot problems, and living with amputations. Although this chapter has elucidated some of the major socio-political and cultural factors impacting this population (Figure 14.2), more studies adopting a qualitative approach are needed to provide further insight into the experiences of this population, with the aim of informing policy and improving the overall quality of life for members of this population.

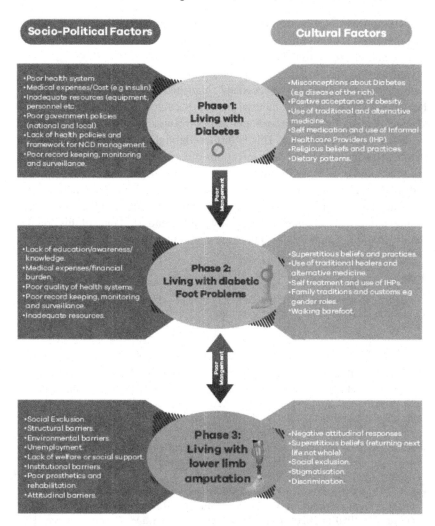

FIGURE 14.2   Summary of the major socio-political and cultural factors impacting the experiences of this population in WA.

Conclusion

This chapter has taken a social epidemiological lens to provide insight into the experiences of living with LLAs associated with poorly managed diabetes mellitus within a WA context. The socio-political and cultural factors impacting individuals living with amputations were outlined along the three major phases in the journey towards living with amputations underlined by Diabetes mellitus. These are living with diabetes mellitus, living with diabetic foot problems, and living with amputations. These phases share commonalities in terms of socio-political factors such as quality and access to healthcare and cultural factors such as superstitious beliefs. However, there are also unique factors that have been outlined across the three major phases.

Considering the predictions made on the increase in prevalence of diabetes mellitus and other NCDs if not adequately managed in Africa, it is important that the major socio-cultural and cultural factors discussed in this work are tackled adequately using evidence-based approaches towards improving the health and wellbeing of this population. This is further highlighted by the reality that this region will continue to deal with infectious diseases such as malaria, diarrhoea, and tuberculosis, along with the emerging burden of NCDs – double burden of disease. Additionally, more studies, especially those from a qualitative paradigm, need to be conducted to provide contextual insights into the experiences of these individuals and improve the quality of life and wellbeing of this population by providing contextually applicable interventions.

Note

1 Diabetic foot problems will be used in this chapter to cover all complications related to lower limbs due to poorly managed diabetes.

References

Aaron, F., Ijah, R. and Obene, T. (2021) 'The orthopedic patient and limb amputation: impact of traditional beliefs on acceptance in Port Harcourt, Nigeria', *International Surgery Journal*, 8, p. 789. doi:10.18203/2349–2902.isj20210907.

Abbas, Z. and Archibald, L. (2007) 'The diabetic foot in sub- Saharan Africa: a new management paradigm', *South Africa*, 10(3), p. 5.

Abbas, Z.G. (2017) 'Managing the diabetic foot in resource-poor settings: challenges and solutions', *Chronic Wound Care Management and Research*, 4, pp. 135–142. doi:10.2147/CWCMR.S98762.

Abbas, Z.G. and Boulton, A.J.M. (2022) 'Diabetic foot ulcer disease in African continent: "From clinical care to implementation" – Review of diabetic foot in last 60 years – 1960 to 2020', *Diabetes mellitus Research and Clinical Practice*, 183. doi:10.1016/j.diabres.2021.109155.

Abdulrehman, M.S. et al. (2016) 'Exploring cultural influences of self-management of Diabetes mellitus in Coastal Kenya: an ethnography', *Global Qualitative Nursing Research*, 3. doi:10.1177/2333393616641825.

Adeleye, O.O. et al. (2020) 'Predictors of intra-hospital mortality in patients with diabetic foot ulcers in Nigeria: data from the MEDFUN study', *BMC Endocrine Disorders*, 20(1), p. 134. doi:10.1186/s12902-020-00614-4.

Ahmad, J. (2016) 'The diabetic foot', *Diabetes & Metabolic Syndrome*, 10(1), pp. 48–60. doi:10.1016/j.dsx.2015.04.002.

Aikins, A.D.-G. (2003) 'Living with Diabetes mellitus in rural and Urban Ghana: a critical social psychological examination of illness action and scope for intervention', *Journal of Health Psychology*, 8(5), pp. 557–572. doi:10.1177/13591053030085007.

Amoah, V.M.K. et al. (2019) 'A qualitative assessment of perceived barriers to effective therapeutic communication among nurses and patients', *BMC Nursing*, 18(1), p. 4. doi:10.1186/s12912-019-0328-0.

Armstrong, D.G. et al. (2020) 'Five year mortality and direct costs of care for people with diabetic foot complications are comparable to cancer', *Journal of Foot and Ankle Research*, 13(1), p. 16. doi:10.1186/s13047-020-00383-2.

Armstrong, D.G., Boulton, A.J.M. and Bus, S.A. (2017) 'Diabetic foot ulcers and their recurrence', *The New England Journal of Medicine*, 376(24), pp. 2367–2375. doi:10.1056/NEJMra1615439.

Atun, R. et al. (2017) 'Diabetes mellitus in sub-Saharan Africa: from clinical care to health policy', *The Lancet Diabetes mellitus & Endocrinology*, 5(8), pp. 622–667. doi:10.1016/S2213–8587(17)30181-X.

Awah, P.K. and Phillimore, P. (2008) 'Diabetes mellitus, medicine and modernity in Cameroon', *Africa*, 78(4), pp. 475–495. doi:10.3366/E0001972008000405.

Azevedo, M. and Alla, S. (2008) 'Diabetes mellitus in Sub-Saharan Africa: Kenya, Mali, Mozambique, Nigeria, South Africa and Zambia', *International Journal of Diabetes mellitus in Developing Countries*, 28(4), pp. 101–108. doi:10.4103/0973–3930.45268.

Beran, D. and Yudkin, J.S. (2006) 'Diabetes mellitus care in sub-Saharan Africa', *The Lancet*, 368(9548), pp. 1689–1695. doi:10.1016/S0140–6736(06)69704-3.

Bosun-Arije, F.S. et al. (2019) 'A systematic review of factors influencing Type 2 Diabetes mellitus mellitus management in Nigerian public hospitals', *International Journal of Africa Nursing Sciences*, 11, p. 100151. doi:10.1016/j.ijans.2019.100151.

Buckley, C.M. et al. (2012) 'Trends in the incidence of lower extremity amputations in people with and without Diabetes mellitus over a five-year period in the Republic of Ireland', *PloS One*, 7(7). doi:10.1371/journal.pone.0041492.

Builders, P.F. and Builders, M.I. (2016) *Wound care: traditional African Medicine approach, worldwide wound healing - innovation in natural and conventional methods*. IntechOpen. doi:10.5772/65521.

Charmaz, K. (2014) *Constructing Grounded Theory*. SAGE.

Chinenye, S. and Ogbera, A. (2013) 'Socio-cultural aspects of Diabetes mellitus mellitus in Nigeria', *Journal of Social Health and Diabetes mellitus*, 1, p. 15. doi:10.4103/2321–0656.109833.

Cho, N.H. et al. (2018) 'IDF Diabetes mellitus Atlas: global estimates of Diabetes mellitus prevalence for 2017 and projections for 2045', *Diabetes mellitus Research and Clinical Practice*, 138, pp. 271–281. doi:10.1016/j.diabres.2018.02.023.

Columbo, J.A. et al. (2018) 'Patient experience of recovery after major leg amputation for arterial disease', *Vascular and Endovascular Surgery*, 52(4), pp. 262–268. doi:10.1177/1538574418761984.

Dada, A.A. and Awoyomi, B.O. (2010) 'Is the trend of amputation in Nigeria changing? A review of 51 consecutives cases seen at Federal medical centre Ebute Metta, Lagos, Nigeria', *Nigerian Medical Journal*, 51(4), p. 167.

Delea, S. et al. (2015) 'Management of diabetic foot disease and amputation in the Irish health system: a qualitative study of patients' attitudes and experiences with health services', *BMC Health Services Research*, 15, p. 251. doi:10.1186/s12913-015-0926–9.

Dieleman, J.L. et al. (2016) 'National spending on health by source for 184 countries between 2013 and 2040', *The Lancet*, 387(10037), pp. 2521–2535. doi:10.1016/S0140–6736(16)30167-2.

Dillingham, T.R., Pezzin, L.E. and Shore, A.D. (2005) 'Reamputation, mortality, and health care costs among persons with dysvascular lower-limb amputations', *Archives of Physical Medicine and Rehabilitation*, 86(3), pp. 480–486. doi:10.1016/j.apmr.2004.06.072.

Edo, A.E., Edo, G.O. and Ezeani, I.U. (2013) 'Risk factors, ulcer grade and management outcome of diabetic foot ulcers in a Tropical Tertiary Care Hospital', *Nigerian Medical Journal: Journal of the Nigeria Medical Association*, 54(1), pp. 59–63. doi:10.4103/0300-1652.108900.

Edomwonyi, O.E. and Onuminya, E.J. (2014) 'An update on major lower limb amputation in Nigeria', *Journal of Dental and Medical Sciences*, 13(10), pp. 90–96.

Ekpebegh, C.O. et al. (2009) 'Diabetes mellitus foot ulceration in a Nigerian hospital: in-hospital mortality in relation to the presenting demographic, clinical and laboratory features', *International Wound Journal*, 6(5), pp. 381–385. doi:10.1111/j.1742-481X.2009.00627.x.

Esquenazi, A. and DiGiacomo, R. (2001) 'Rehabilitation after amputation', *Journal of the American Podiatric Medical Association*, 91(1), pp. 13–22. doi:10.7547/87507315-91-1-13.

Hamill, R., Carson, S. and Dorahy, M. (2010) 'Experiences of psychosocial adjustment within 18 months of amputation: an interpretative phenomenological analysis', *Disability and Rehabilitation* [Preprint]. doi:10.3109/09638280903295417.

Honjo, K. (2004) 'Social epidemiology: definition, history, and research examples', *Environmental Health and Preventive Medicine*, 9(5), pp. 193–199. doi:10.1007/BF02898100.

Hu, F.B., Satija, A. and Manson, J.E. (2015) 'Curbing the Diabetes mellitus pandemic: the need for global policy solutions', *JAMA*, 313(23), pp. 2319–2320. doi:10.1001/jama.2015.5287.

Huang, Y.-Y. et al. (2018) 'Survival and associated risk factors in patients with Diabetes mellitus and amputations caused by infectious foot gangrene', *Journal of Foot and Ankle Research*, 11(1), p. 1. doi:10.1186/s13047-017-0243-0.

International Diabetes mellitus Federation, IDF (2022) *Diabetes mellitus in Africa*. Available at: https://idf.org/our-network/regions-and-members/africa/ (Accessed: 21 February 2022).

International Standards Organisation, ISO (2014) *ISO 8549-4:2014(en), Prosthetics and orthotics — Vocabulary — Part 4: Terms relating to limb amputation*. Available at: https://www.iso.org/obp/ui/#iso:std:iso:8549:-4:ed-1:v1:en (Accessed: 22 February 2022).

Izumi, Y. et al. (2009) 'Mortality of first-time amputees in diabetics: a 10-year observation', *Diabetes mellitus Research and Clinical Practice*, 83(1), pp. 126–131. doi:10.1016/j.diabres.2008.09.005.

Khan, M.Z. et al. (2020) 'Evolving indications for lower limb amputations in South Africa offer opportunities for health system improvement', *World Journal of Surgery*, 44(5), pp. 1436–1443. doi:10.1007/s00268-019-05361-9.

Koka, E. et al. (2016) 'Cultural understanding of wounds, buruli ulcers and their management at the obom sub-district of the Ga South municipality of the greater accra region of Ghana', *PLOS Neglected Tropical Diseases*, 10(7). doi:10.1371/journal.pntd.0004825.

Kono, Y. and Muder, R.R. (2012) 'Identifying the incidence of and risk factors for reamputation among patients who underwent foot amputation', *Annals of Vascular Surgery*, 26(8), pp. 1120–1126. doi:10.1016/j.avsg.2012.02.011.

Lang, R. and Upah, L. (2008) *Scoping study: disability issues in Nigeria. DFID.*, *doczz. net.* Available at: http://doczz.net/doc/7982675/scoping-study--disability-issues-in-nigeria-final (Accessed: 22 February 2022).

Levitt, N.S. (2008) 'Diabetes mellitus in Africa: epidemiology, management and healthcare challenges', *Heart*, 94(11), pp. 1376–1382. doi:10.1136/hrt.2008. 147306.

Lin, X. et al. (2020) 'Global, regional, and national burden and trend of Diabetes mellitus in 195 countries and territories: an analysis from 1990 to 2025', *Scientific Reports*, 10, p. 14790. doi:10.1038/s41598-020-71908-9.

Liu, F. et al. (2010) 'The lived experience of persons with lower extremity amputation', *Journal of Clinical Nursing*, 19(15–16), pp. 2152–2161. doi:10.1111/j.1365–2702.2010.03256.x.

Liu, R. et al. (2021) 'Lower extremity reamputation in people with Diabetes mellitus: a systematic review and meta-analysis', *BMJ Open Diabetes mellitus Research & Care*, 9(1). doi:10.1136/bmjdrc-2021–002325.

Macdonald, S.J. (2017) 'Five models of disability', in Deacon, L. and Macdonald, S. J. (eds.). London: SAGE Publications, pp. 174–186. Available at: https://uk.sagepub. com/en-gb/eur/social-work-theory-and-practice/book249422 (Accessed: 22 February 2022).

Mbanya, J.C.N. et al. (2010) 'Diabetes mellitus in sub-Saharan Africa', *The Lancet*, 375(9733), pp. 2254–2266. doi:10.1016/S0140–6736(10)60550-8.

McDonald, C.L. et al. (2020) 'Global prevalence of traumatic non-fatal limb amputation', *Prosthetics and Orthotics International*. doi:10.1177/0309364620972258.

Mishra, S.C. et al. (2017) 'Diabetic foot', *BMJ (Clinical research ed.)*, 359. doi:10.1136/ bmj.j5064.

Mogre, V. et al. (2019) 'Barriers to diabetic self-care: A qualitative study of patients' and healthcare providers' perspectives', *Journal of Clinical Nursing*, 28(11–12), pp. 2296–2308. doi:10.1111/jocn.14835.

Morbach, S. et al. (2012) 'Long-term prognosis of diabetic foot patients and their limbs: amputation and death over the course of a decade', *Diabetes mellitus Care*, 35(10), pp. 2021–2027. doi:10.2337/dc12–0200.

Napier, A.D. et al. (2014) 'Culture and health', *The Lancet*, 384(9954), pp. 1607–1639. doi:10.1016/S0140–6736(14)61603-2.

Ogbera, A.O. et al. (2010) 'Complementary and alternative medicine use in Diabetes mellitus mellitus', *West African Journal of Medicine*, 29(3), pp. 158–162. doi:10.4314/ wajm.v29i3.68213.

Ogunlana, M.O. et al. (2021) 'Qualitative exploration into reasons for delay in seeking medical help with diabetic foot problems', *International Journal of Qualitative Studies on Health and Well-being*, 16(1). doi:10.1080/17482631.2021.1945206.

Opedele, T.O. et al. (2007) 'Emerging indications for lower limb amputation in Abuja, Nigeria', *Nigerian Journal of Orthopaedics and Trauma*, 6(1), pp. 6–7. doi:10.4314/ njotra.v6i1.29280.

Papatheodorou, K. et al. (2018) 'Complications of Diabetes mellitus 2017', *Journal of Diabetes mellitus Research*, 2018. doi:10.1155/2018/3086167.

Pastakia, S.D. et al. (2017) 'Diabetes mellitus in sub-Saharan Africa – from policy to practice to progress: targeting the existing gaps for future care for Diabetes mellitus', *Diabetes mellitus, Metabolic Syndrome and Obesity: Targets and Therapy*, 10, pp. 247–263. doi:10.2147/DMSO.S126314.

Rigato, M. et al. (2018) 'Characteristics, prevalence, and outcomes of diabetic foot ulcers in Africa. A systematic review and meta-analysis', *Diabetes mellitus Research and Clinical Practice*, 142, pp. 63–73. doi:10.1016/j.diabres.2018.05.016.

Sano, D. et al. (1998) '[Management of the diabetic foot, apropos of 42 cases at the Ouagadougou University Hospital Center]', *Dakar Medical*, 43(1), pp. 109–113.

Shakespeare, T. (2017) *Disability: the basics*. London: Routledge. doi:10.4324/9781315624839.

Spiess, K.E. et al. (2014) 'Application of the five stages of grief to diabetic limb loss and amputation', *The Journal of Foot and Ankle Surgery*, 53(6), pp. 735–739. doi:10.1053/j.jfas.2014.06.016.

Stephani, V., Opoku, D. and Beran, D. (2018) 'Self-management of Diabetes mellitus in Sub-Saharan Africa: a systematic review', *BMC Public Health*, 18, p. 1148. doi:10.1186/s12889-018-6050-0.

Sunday, J., Morgans, S. and Onuoha, J. (2021) 'The experience of living with non-traumatic lower limb amputations: a meta-synthesis.' Available at: https://www.crd.york.ac.uk/prospero/display_record.php?ID=CRD42021296153 (Accessed 17 February 2022).

Thomas, C. (2012) 'Theorising disability and chronic illness: where next for perspectives in medical sociology?', *Social Theory & Health*, 10(3), pp. 209–228. doi:10.1057/sth.2012.7.

Tuei, V.C., Maiyoh, G.K. and Ha, C.-E. (2010) 'Type 2 Diabetes mellitus mellitus and obesity in sub-Saharan Africa', *Diabetes mellitus/Metabolism Research and Reviews*, 26(6), pp. 433–445. doi:10.1002/dmrr.1106.

Udosen, A. et al. (2009) 'Attitude and perception of patients towards amputation as a form of surgical treatment in the University of Calabar teaching hospital, Nigeria', *African Health Sciences*, 9(4), pp. 254–257.

Ugwu, E. et al. (2019) 'Burden of diabetic foot ulcer in Nigeria: current evidence from the multicenter evaluation of diabetic foot ulcer in Nigeria', *World Journal of Diabetes mellitus*, 10(3), pp. 200–211. doi:10.4239/wjd.v10.i3.200.

UNESCO (2001) *UNESCO universal declaration on cultural diversity: UNESCO.* Available at: http://portal.unesco.org/en/ev.php-URL_ID=13179&URL_DO=DO_TOPIC&URL_SECTION=201.html (Accessed: 22 February 2022).

Walsh, J.W. et al. (2016) 'Association of diabetic foot ulcer and death in a population-based cohort from the United Kingdom', *Diabetic Medicine*, 33(11), pp. 1493–1498. doi:10.1111/dme.13054.

Whiting, D.R., Hayes, L. and Unwin, N.C. (2003) 'Challenges to health care for Diabetes mellitus in Africa', *European Journal of Cardiovascular Prevention and Rehabilitation*, 10(2), pp. 103–110. doi:10.1177/174182670301000205.

Wukich, D.K., Raspovic, K.M. and Suder, N.C. (2018) 'Patients with diabetic foot disease fear major lower-extremity amputation more than death', *Foot & Ankle Specialist*, 11(1), pp. 17–21. doi:10.1177/1938640017694722.

Zhang, Y. et al. (2020) 'Global disability burdens of Diabetes mellitus-related lower-extremity complications in 1990 and 2016', *Diabetes mellitus Care*, 43(5), pp. 964–974. doi:10.2337/dc19-1614.

Zimmermann, M. et al. (2018) 'Experiences of type 2 Diabetes mellitus in sub-Saharan Africa: a scoping review', *Global Health Research and Policy*, 3(1), p. 25. doi:10.1186/s41256-018-0082-y.

15

CHALLENGES AND IMPLICATIONS OF LIVING WITH RETINOPATHY

Florence Oseji and Catherine Hayes

Introduction

> When you lose your vision, you lose contact with things. When you lose your hearing, you lose contact with people.
>
> *Helen Keller (1880–1968)*

Diabetic retinopathy (DR) is a common micro-vascular complication in the eyes of individuals with Diabetes mellitus (DM) and may have a sudden and debilitating impact on vision and visual acuity, leading to functional impairment and blindness (Ciulla et al., 2003). DR is also commonly termed 'diabetic eye disease' in contexts where people may be unfamiliar with the microvascular changes occurring as a consequence of the systemic impact of DM. Advanced stages of DR (proliferative DR) are characterised by the growth of abnormal retinal blood vessels secondary to ischaemia, in which the blood vessels, in an attempt to supply oxygenated blood to the hypoxic retina, cause damage. DR is generally asymptomatic at early stages but requires pharmacological therapies, emphasising the need for early detection through regular ocular checks and screening programmes (Yau et al., 2012).

The prevalence of DR in individuals with DM is higher than previously reported; this is due to poor data collection and an increased incidence of DM (Ashaye et al., 2008). About 30 years ago, DR was said to be rare amongst Nigerians as it was indicated to be a condition of the affluent, but recent studies have shown otherwise (Ashaye et al., 2008). This change could potentially be attributed to several causes. Typically, it could be explained by the process of globalisation, such as population displacement through increased

DOI: 10.4324/9781003467601-18

international migration. More debatably, it could be attributed to climate change, technological improvement, ageing, improved communication mechanisms, the concentration of capital and economic power, increasing levels of chronic conditions, free trade methods, neo-liberalism, the spread of Western consumer culture in the world and rising levels of inequality between and within countries.

Diabetic Retinopathy in Nigeria

The prevalence of diminished sight as a consequence of DR in Nigeria is increasing annually. It has been indicated that only about 19% of care providers in Nigeria examine the eyes of all people with DM, and less than 3% of the doctors referred all such patients for eye care, while the majority (73%) of health care professionals only referred DM patients after the onset of visual complaints (Yau et al., 2012). Patterns of care and referrals are consistent across all disciplines of health care professionals, indicating that there is a need to create awareness among people with DM about the need for routine ocular examinations (Omolase et al., 2010). Non-attendance at ocular screening was first reported by Agarwal et al. (2005), and as a result of this, it was advised that this high non-attendance rate called for creating more awareness programmes for the consequential ocular effects of DM. Onakpoya et al. (2010) indicated that the attendance of individuals with DM in Nigeria for dilated eye examinations was low, stating that inadequate knowledge about DR as well as low referral rates were contributory factors. Several factors have constrained progress in the prevention of DR, including underestimation of the effectiveness of intervention, belief in a long delay in achieving measurable impacts, commercial pressures, institutional inertia and inadequate resources. As the incidence of DM increases, there is a possibility that more people will suffer from DR (WHO, 2013). If not properly managed, the condition leads to a permanent loss of vision (WHO, 2013). Early detection of retinopathy in people with DM is critical in preventing visual impairment, but there is no evidence to suggest that current methods of screening are effectively identifying all patients at risk of the development of DR.

Research Aims

The aim of this research was to ascertain the level of knowledge of DR among people with a known diagnosis of DM and to see whether the level of knowledge they had could be associated with an increased motivation to avoid DR development. A secondary aim of the study was to ascertain whether an increased awareness of DR necessarily leads to an increased ability to identify the signs and symptomology of the condition. This was carried out by assessing the attitude and behaviour of people with DM with regard to their ocular status using invited research subjects who attended a Community Hospital in Lagos, Nigeria, for eye care and who had given their informed consent to participate in the investigation. Formal ethical approval was ensured prior to the commencement of the investigation.

Research Methods

This study adopted an interpretive phenomenological perspective. The process of exploring behaviours, perspectives, experiences, feelings and the in-depth quality and complexity of a situation is an integral part of the qualitative paradigm. The method involved collecting a thick description of human experience, which was then interpreted from a theoretical perspective using a phenomenological approach. The overall aim was to understand the phenomenon by allowing the data to speak for itself and by the researcher suspending any known preconceptions about the subject. It also aimed to understand the 'constructs' people use in everyday life to make sense of their world by uncovering meanings contained within conversation or text (Ritchie and Lewis, 2004).

The investigation of modes of awareness was used because it was an efficient means of determining the perceptions, behaviours, opinions and reactions of the participants involved (Thorne, 2000). The aim of this method was to portray phenomena through description and relationships between behaviours, individuals and/or events (Thorne, 2000). The decision to collect data through a questionnaire or interview required careful consideration of factors such as available resources, time constraints of the individuals, sample size and the geographical location of the research participants (Wilhot, 2009). To increase the rigour of the study, data was triangulated from two sources: interviews and questionnaires.

Sampling Techniques, Ethical Issues and Data Collection

A purposive sampling technique was adopted as a type of non-probability sampling that would be most effective since there was a need to study a specific cultural domain (Tongco, 2007). It involved deliberately choosing people on the basis of their lived experience, although it still necessitates a rigorous process so that the sample could be subject to independent scrutiny (Ritchie and Lewis, 2004). There was enhanced critical thinking about the parameters of the population for inclusion (Silverman, 2000). Although several patients from the GOPD of the Community Hospital had DM and other co-morbid conditions, the participants selected were only diagnosed with DM and had no other co-existing medical conditions. This was a means of ensuring that the sample population was homogeneous. Although there are no rigid rules for the number of sample sizes in qualitative research, 15 individuals with DM were contacted via the purposive sampling method and 10 responded positively. According to Kuzel (1992), about 6–8 data units are needed when the sample studied comprises a homogenous group, while 12–20 units are required for a heterogeneous group. For this study, the sample used was homogenous. Choosing the purposive sample was fundamental to the quality of the data gathered; thus, the capability, trustworthiness and authenticity of the respondent had to be ensured (Tongco, 2007). The age range for participants was 18–74 years. Interpreters were made available for further communication barriers in Ibo, Yoruba and Hausa languages. Of the total population, 5 male and 5 female respondents were used to create a gender-balanced review.

The respondents were identified by a Medical Director and a General Physician and contacted directly to explain the purpose of the study and to formally invite them to take part. Those interested received an information sheet and signed an informed consent form. All participants were informed that their consent could be withdrawn at any time during the study without any impact on their future care pathways. Data collection was dialogical, with the participants taking a significant role in determining what was being said (Willig and Stainton-Rogers, 2008). Confidentiality of information was a fundamental priority for the investigation process (Denzin and Lincoln, 2003). The data given were not linked in any way to the participants. Codes were used for each participant as an alternative to names in the questionnaire sheets to ensure anonymity between all those involved in the study. Data was managed, stored and protected appropriately in order to ensure that participants were not identifiable. For this research, interviews were the primary source of data collection, with the questionnaire as a secondary means of triangulating the data source.

Data Analysis

Data analysis refers to the interaction of the researcher and the participants as the process of interpretation proceeds (Osborne, 1990). It is an iterative inductive process, beginning with several close, detailed readings to provide a holistic perspective that notes points of interest and significance (Willig and Stainton-Rogers, 2008). Suspending personal beliefs and preconceived ideas about the subject was a fundamental part of this process (Snow, 2009).

Since this phenomenological research aimed to illuminate the meaning and understanding of awareness, a thematic approach to data analysis was implemented. Thematic analysis is a method for identifying, analysing and reporting patterns (themes) within data (Braun and Clarke, 2006). One of the benefits of thematic analysis was the flexibility it afforded the analysis phase of the research

(Braun and Clarke, 2006). It also enabled a clear description of phenomena and followed a logical sequence (Snow, 2009). This analysis involves:

- Transcribing and reading all descriptions and answers given by participants during the interview process and questionnaires. Transcription refers to the process by which spoken discourse is represented as written text.
- Extracting significant statements
- Creating formulated meanings
- Forming themes from collected, formulated meanings
- Clustering the themes and representing them as superordinate themes
- Writing a very thorough description
- Identification of the fundamental structure of the research concept
- Returning to participants for validation

This process also contributed to the overall authenticity of the study, as suggested by Colaizzi (Snow, 2009). Quotes from participants were analysed in relationship with their behaviour (Cresswell, 2013). This afforded participants the opportunity to reject a researcher's interpretations, even though they were valid. It had to be recognised that such situations could result from participants' defensiveness. For this reason, data collection was triangulated with questionnaires.

Ensuring Trustworthiness and Authenticity

Unlike quantitative research, where concepts of scientific rigour are validity, reliability and the capacity for generalisation, qualitative research has trustworthiness built on the concepts of credibility, dependability, transferability and conformability (Lincoln and Guba, 1985). Credibility aims to evaluate the integrity and confidence in how well the data collection and analysis phases are addressed. To ensure that the study was credible and conformable, the transcribed data was reviewed with the participants to ensure that the information given correlates to their experience of being aware of DR (content validity check). Dependability is a parallel term to reliability in quantitative research and seeks to understand the factors of phenomena (Shenton, 2004). To ensure dependability, all documents and data were available for external scrutiny. Transferability refers to the extent to which the findings can be transferred to other groups or settings (Given, 2008).

Findings

The results convey the participants' responses, behaviour, perceptions and level of awareness of their ocular status in relation to the potential development of DR.

Invitations were sent to a total of 15 participants, but only 10 of them participated in the study, representing about 70% of the intended number of participants.

The data analysis demonstrated that participants were able to talk on issues as widely as possible about their awareness of DR in relation to their perceived beliefs and attitudes. This led to the formation of three superordinate themes: knowledge about DM, focus on DR and focus on eye checks. The first theme looked at issues concerning causes of DM, types of DM, sense organs affected and insulin injections. Focus on DR considers matters relating to awareness of DR and whether ocular diseases from DM can be treated. The third theme focused on regular eye checks, how often eyes should be examined and referrals for diabetic eye conditions.

Knowledge about DM

What causes DM?: Most of the participants had good knowledge about the cause of DM except participants 2 and 3, who said refined sugar and hereditary factors are causal factors, respectively.

Interviewer:	Alright, what do you think is the cause of DM
2:	…excess sugar in my system like when I drink tea or ogi (palp)
3:	…runs in the family blood line

Other participants, like 5 and 6, had a good grasp of the causes of DM:

5:	I think insulin resistance, insufficiency and problems from the pancreas
6:	….hereditary and insufficiency of insulin produced by the pancreas

Type of DM: All except participant 3 knew about the type of DM they had, although some couldn't differentiate if they were on insulin injections as they claim they are usually injected during follow-up visits

Interviewer:	What type of DM do you have (done with the aid of an interpreter)
3:	I don't know. Was just told I have DM

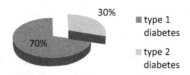

FIGURE 15.1 Percentage of participants with Type 1 and Type II DM.

Sense Organs Affected: Participant 6 was more familiar than the rest in regards to the effects of DM to the eyes. Others mentioned breathing and sexual activity.

Interviewer: Ok, so which sense organ do you think is affected by DM
6:   I think the eyes because my grandma had cataract and retinopathy from DM. She had a laser surgery done in India. I also think it affected her weight....

Focus on Diabetic Retinopathy

Awareness of DR: Only participants 4, 5, 6 and 7 knew about DR. Others, like participant 8, had been counselled about it but couldn't explain.

Interviewer: what about DR
Interviewee: hmmm, heard about it once before and again while reading the information sheet. What's that....

Can ocular diseases from DM be treated: All participants except participant 6 were not aware if eye complications from DM can be treated.

Interviewer: Do you think eye diseases from DM can be treated
6:   yes, from my grandma's experience

Focus on Regular Eye Examinations: Different perspectives were given for when eye checks should be done. This varied from six months to yearly checks except for participant 2 who specified that eye checks should be done based on finance and presence of signs and symptoms of visual impairment.
   Behaviour and attitude toward ocular examination:

Interviewer: What do you know about eye checks, when do you think you should check your eyes
2:   how
Interviewer: 6 months, 1year or....
2:   when I'm not seeing my farm well. Besides, I don't read. They said it's worse if you read too much

Perceived cultural beliefs:

Interviewer: what do you think causes blindness in Nigeria?
3:   hereditary eye diseases, spiritual beliefs
Interviewer: any other causes....
3:   children playing and causing injury to their selves...

Interviewer: do you think poor nutrition causes blindness
3: I think so especially after drinking garri (cassava) for children

Financial Affordability

Most of the participants did not see finances as a hindrance to visiting an eye specialist for regular eye examinations. Participant 2, however, indicated that eye check-ups should be done when patients can financially afford to pay.

Interviewer: what do you know about eye check, when do you think you should your eyes...
2: how
Interviewer: 6 months, 1 year or when you have symptoms like not seeing ....
2: when I'm not seeing my farm well. Besides I' don't read
Interviewer: ...for other people...
2: depends on when they have the money ....

Implications of the Study to Social Epidemiology

According to pre-existing published literature, some of the barriers to awareness of DR are unrealistic expectations, poor educational backgrounds, apathy and a lack of internal motivation. The major findings from this study were grouped into knowledge on DM, focus on DR and regular ocular examinations. These findings are related to the level of awareness of DR. Based on these findings, some participants had poor general knowledge of DM, like its causal factors and type of DM. This shows that inadequate knowledge in terms of biomedical factors on causes of DM can contribute to the poor awareness of DR amongst the same participants. This is confirmed by Ogden (2012), who indicated that knowledge plays a role in how people behave. Others who were aware of the causes and type of DM were professionals and semi-skilled participants with tertiary education but still had poor awareness of DR. This can be attributed to a lack of regular ocular examinations where there would have been avenues for an eye specialist to educate them on the condition (Brown et al., 2000; Omolase et al., 2010). Long intervals between ocular follow-up visits may lead to an increase in the prevalence of DR (Omolase et al., 2010). Some had poor awareness of other ways of glycaemic control. Glycaemic control, however, depends not only on proper glucose-lowering medications but also on patient adherence to diet and physical activity programmes (Axer-Siegel et al., 2006). Health promotion and health education perspectives emphasise the role of knowledge in predicting health behaviours towards awareness of DR and aim to change behaviour by improving what people know (Ogden, 2012).

There are different theoretical perspectives that can be linked to the perception and awareness of the participants in relation to DR and the research findings. Hence, the application of these theories in relation to the results of this study reveals the reasons why most of the participants are not aware of DR. The health belief model HBM, the theory of reasoned action TRA, symbolic interactionism and social constructionism have an impact on the way a person perceives ill-health.

Understanding the role of behaviour in DM and DR allows unhealthy behaviours to be targeted (Ogden, 2012). In HBM, the likelihood that an individual will take preventive action to perform health protective behaviour, like seeking knowledge on DM and DR, depends directly on the outcome of the threat and the pros and cons of taking the action (Sarafino, 2006). In response to previous HBM criticisms like the role of emotions such as fear and denial, the model has been revised to add the construct 'health motivation' to reflect an individual's readiness to be concerned about his ocular health (Ogden, 2012). Using the revised HBM, if applied to a health-related behaviour like screening for DR, the HBM predicts regular screening for DR if the individual perceives that he or she is highly susceptible to DR, that DR is a severe ocular threat, that the benefits of regular screening and ocular checks are high, and that the costs of such action are comparatively low. This will also be true if the individual is subjected to cues to action that are external, such as a leaflet in the GP's waiting room, or internal, such as an ocular symptom perceived to be related to DR (whether correct or not), such as blurry vision or seeing halos. It is important to note that a person's cognitive state influences their symptom perception (Ogden, 2012). Studies have provided support for the role of cues to action in predicting health behaviours, especially external cues such as informational input (Ogden, 2012). Health promotion models can use these cues to action a change in beliefs and consequently promote future health behaviours by improving awareness of DR. This model would also predict participants who would attend screenings, if they were confident and motivated to maintain good ocular health. Although Ogden has indicated that several studies have reported conflicting findings about HBM in relation to the level of perceived severity of ill-health, its importance cannot be overemphasised. RA predicts on the assumption that an individual's intention to act on preventing DR is the most important factor in behaviour change and that other external factors influencing such acts will be mediated through his/her beliefs and intention to behave (Nutbeam et al., 2010). Here, intention is determined by attitudes towards health-protective behaviour and perceived subjective norms. Attitude towards the behaviour is, in turn, determined by behavioural beliefs, specifically the perceived outcomes of the behaviour for ocular examinations and the value placed on those outcomes, while perceived subjective norms are determined by normative beliefs, which include perceptions of significant referents' beliefs about whether one should engage in a behaviour and motivation to comply with those referents.

Social constructionism theory from a cultural perspective can be attributed to beliefs (Blum et al., 2004). This was related to the participants' responses, as one of the participants claimed that DR cannot cause loss of vision except if blindness was in the lineage. Social construction perspectives, from family and cultural perspectives, are in play here. By studying how illness is socially constructed, we examine how social forces shape our understanding of and actions towards health, illness and healing. Poverty and the unavailability of health resources shape people's construction of the meaning of their health and their control, or lack thereof, over how healthy or ill they are. In most parts of rural and some urban Nigerian settings, cultural health beliefs, knowledge, lay perceptions, and health behaviour interact strongly (Mbanya et al., 2010). Owing to social construction and misconceptions indicated by popular health beliefs, many people fail to take appropriate measures for the prevention of DM and DR (Mbanya et al., 2010). Obesity is still viewed, in some parts of Nigeria, as a sign of good living because it confers respect and influence. Such lay perceptions are borne out of a contextual environment in which most people are poor, hungry, and deprived and, therefore, view obesity as an obvious social marker for affluence (Mbanya et al., 2010). One of the male participants mentioned poor sexual activity as a complication from DM and can be regressed by local herbs. Although the relationship between local herbs and sexual activity is socially constructed, it has been indicated that DM causes sexual function impairment, especially in females (Issa and Baiyewu, 2006; Olarinoye and Olarinoye, 2007). Here, it was indicated that individuals with DM with sexual function impairment had poor health satisfaction, physical health, psychological domain and social relationships (Issa and Baiyewu, 2006).

In symbolic interaction, the individual's specific action taken to tackle the prevention of DR is determined by cues to taking the action and a consideration of the perceived benefits and barriers, where actions with many benefits and few barriers are most likely to be chosen (Rutter and Quine, 2002). From this perspective, individuals with DM act on the basis of the meaning they have for eye examination and the prevention of DR. Here, individuals with DM who adhere greater meanings to their ocular health would have regular eye examinations and be aware of DR, which in turn would decrease the incidence of DR (Benzies and Allen, 2008).

Furthermore, apart from theoretical perspectives that can explain the participants' health behaviour towards prevention of DR, level of education, health literacy, socio-economic status (SES) and urban unsustainability have relationships with awareness of DR (Namperumalsamy et al., 2004). To develop effective patient education and improve patients' diabetic control and own complications, it is important to consider their health literacy (Tang et al., 2008). Low health literacy levels, even in educated participants, are a significant contributing factor to non-compliance with treatment, which ultimately leads to worse glycaemic control and higher rates of retinopathy (Zheng et al., 2012). There is therefore a need to develop materials and tools to facilitate DM education and management in patients with low health literacy. Adequate patient outreach and reminder programmes may be useful to improve awareness of DR. Adding incentives to eye care programmes further helps in enhancing awareness of regular ocular checks, DR and its treatment as well, though the effectiveness and sustainability of such interventions are rarely evaluated in Nigeria (Zheng et al., 2012). Overall, the study revealed that poor awareness of the existence or development of DR is a key factor in its development and prevention.

There is a relationship between urbanisation and health, as Papadopoulos et al. (2007) indicated that urbanisation affects the prevalence of DR, with higher rates in urban areas than rural communities. Alder and Snibbe (2003) also indicated that urban unsustainability causes inequitable access to social, educational and material resources and has both direct and indirect effects on health status through its influence on stress, psychosocial resources and positive and negative emotions. Historically, in urban regions of Nigeria, wealthy individuals with a high level of education were more likely to be obese and overweight than poorer or less educated people (Mbanya et al., 2010). However, the increase in obese and overweight people over the past decade has been more substantial in poor urban dwellers than in their richer counterparts (Mbanya et al., 2010). With urban unsustainability in Lagos State, there would be gaps existing in reliable population-based data, especially when relating to health issues (Ruta et al., 2013). In an increasingly globalised and urbanised city like Lagos, the struggle against poverty and amenities, focused on reconstructing communities and creating relationships, is most played out in the city (Girard et al., 2003). This affects the quality of life (QOL) of individuals with DM. Lower income, lower education, low-rated employment, and physical complications adversely affect the QOL of these patients (Issa and Baiyewu, 2006). In other words, urban unsustainability in the state results in poor and unequal access to adequate eye specialist health care facilities (Girard et al., 2003). It has also been indicated that persistent poverty and deprivation, which are associated with urban unsustainability, means that traditional perceptions and cognitive imagery about lifestyle risk factors for DM and DR are unlikely to alter in any significant way unless socio-culturally appropriate health promotion campaigns are implemented (Mbanya et al., 2010). This is where policies that affect the social determinants of health should be encouraged (Whitehead, 2001).

The gradient between SES and health has been well established from previous studies, which demonstrate that ideal health increases as SES increases (Adler and Snibbe, 2003). Although the mechanisms underlying this association are not well understood, behavioural, cognitive and affective tendencies develop in response to the greater psychosocial stress encountered in low-SES environments, and this may partially mediate the impact of SES on awareness of

DR. There were SES differences between participants, which were traditionally measured by income, education and occupation. SES is associated with the physical and social environments in which individuals work and live. They encounter more social conflict, less social support and decreased access to means for restoring and maintaining good ocular healthcare (Adler and Snibbe, 2003). The root causes of health disparities are numerous and relate to individual behaviour, provider knowledge and attitudes, the health system and societal and cultural values (Thomas et al., 2004). These are related to the SES of individuals with DM and their awareness of DR. Disparities have been well documented, even in Nigeria, with its encumbered access to health care, suggesting factors like culture and health communication other than access to healthcare are responsible (Oso and Pate, 2011). Brown et al. (2004) and a substantial amount of literature reveals that material and social deprivation are directly related to DR incidence and prevalence.

Collier et al. (2010) indicated that enticement proves abortive in a long-term campaign of awareness programmes, but in the short term, it provided a slight change. This is where incentives for regular ocular examinations come in. There is high-quality evidence available relevant to the prevention of DR and care that needs to be translated into practice (Williams et al., 2002). Although some critics indicate the disadvantages of evidence-based practice, like that the evidence needed is not always available, accessible or always of the highest quality, its advantages should be strongly advocated (Williams et al., 2002). Attendance at screening programmes should be encouraged, as it has been indicated that there is a very high non-attendance level of people with DM at ocular screening camps (Agarwal et al., 2005). It was also indicated that a lot of female patients with DM do not go for the recommended eye examination annually, which is necessary for the early detection of retinopathy (Pasagian -Macaulay et al., 1997). Ocular screening is a form of secondary prevention of DR, and it refers to interventions aimed at detecting ill-health at an asymptomatic stage of development so that its progression can be halted or retarded (Ogden, 2012). As a result of this, it is advisable that this high non-attendance rate should create more awareness programmes for the consequential effects of DR (Agarwal et al., 2005). Access to adequate treatment is also a concern because, even if basic eye screening is available, many patients with DR still have no adequate access to laser treatment in Nigeria (Zheng et al., 2012). Therefore, efforts must be made to ensure that any regional or national DR eye care programme does not exacerbate health inequalities (Zheng et al., 2012). DR conforms to the cardinal principles of screening recommended by the WHO (Vashist et al., 2011). Patients' health beliefs and attitudes are also known to have an important influence on participation in screening and follow-up, and these effects vary significantly between socioeconomic classes and ethnic groups (Zheng et al., 2012). This research claimed that any regional or national DR eye care programme in the country does not exacerbate health inequalities. One key health belief that people hold relates to their perception of risk and their sense of whether or not they are susceptible to any given health problem (Ogden, 2012). This is the case of the participant, who claimed that she was not at risk of blindness from DR because blindness is not in her lineage. In contrast, others may overestimate their risk of DR, believing that reoccurring ocular complications from DM mean that it is inevitable and that there is little they can do to prevent these complications (Ogden, 2012). This is similar to the 17-year-old participant whose grandmother had undergone surgery for cataracts and DR. In such cases, the individuals should be motivated to either start a new behaviour or change an existing one (Ogden, 2012).

One of the participants reported that she expects her GP to tell her about eye conditions and referrals. This is in tune with the doctor–patient relationship and health communication. It is a two-way street where both parties are accountable to each other. The challenge of improving physicians' compliance with recommended guidelines is not new (Zheng et al., 2012). Non-adherence to these guidelines in Nigeria may be due to the physicians' lack of awareness of the rationale behind referral guidelines, a lack of time for communication, especially in busy health settings, a lack of reimbursement, a lack of resources or a combination of these factors (Zheng et al., 2012). Many residency projects and continued medical education programmes in Nigeria offer limited education about effective communication. Training health professionals to improve their communication skills and to carry out interventions may help to improve awareness and prevention of DR (Ogden, 2012). There should also be clinician sharing of the therapeutic responsibility with patients to improve glycaemic control and complications of DR (Axer-Siegel et al., 2006). Education on the potential risk of vision loss will motivate individuals with DM to comply with medical treatment, recommended lifestyle and ocular checks. This is in support of findings from Ogden (2012) and previous literature that recommended that patient-centredness is the preferred style of doctor-patient communication, which is also a means of improving patient outcomes. Health workers should be made aware of the QOL of individuals with DM, especially those with physical complications that result in poor functional impairment. Lower socio-demographic status, medical conditions, and disabilities confound the relationship between visual impairment from DR and QOL (Chia et al., 2004). Although past research has shown that the QOL of individuals with DM is better than that of people with other chronic illnesses, it is also important to note that people with DM have a worse QOL than people with no chronic diseases (Issa and Baiyewu, 2006). Without organisational involvement, support, reimbursement mechanisms and computerised tracking systems, effective physician-patient communication may be difficult to attain. To further conceptualise the communication process, it is important to understand not only the health professional's preconceived ideas, stereotypes or prejudices but also to consider the processes involved in any communication between the health professional and patient as an interaction that occurs in the context of these beliefs and cultural aspects (Kreuter and McClure, 2004; Ogden, 2012). Efforts to eliminate health disparities can be enhanced by health communication and must be informed by the influence of culture on the attitudes, beliefs, and practices of not only the minority populations with DM but also public health policy makers and the health workers responsible for the delivery of medical services and public health interventions designed to close this gap (Thomas et al., 2004). There is also no doubt that, in Nigeria, lack of coordination among the various organs of government involved in health communication has been one of the greatest impediments to the promotion of health issues generally (Oso and Pate, 2011). Thus, the need to harmonise various efforts by these sectors of government cannot be overemphasised.

Although there is general agreement about the relevance of transferring awareness into action, there is a still lack of quality information about what works, in which health settings and with whom (Ward et al., 2009). This is especially so in developing nations like Nigeria, where individuals have varying educational and cultural diversity. Although there are a lot of models and theories for knowledge transfer interventions, most are untested, meaning their applicability and relevance are largely unknown (Ward et al., 2009). The role of cultural contexts in successful implementation of programmes is sometimes omitted, even though there's evidence that culture is a central feature in health behaviours and decisions, particularly in behaviours that may predispose people to have DR from DM (Airhihenbuwa and Obregon, 2000). It is therefore inevitable that the integration of knowledge about the relevance of culture in health behaviour will become a critical component of DR prevention and care.

Conclusion

The goal of this research was to affect the behaviours of individuals with DM in regards to awareness of DR. The qualitative methodology used enhanced the objectivity of the study. The aim of this research was achieved since there was a measured positive response by the participants and corresponding levels of awareness observed. The results of this study are comparable with previous research done in the West and Africa. They thus confirm that poor awareness is a major factor in the increased prevalence of DR and can be used as an aspect of solving public health problems in Nigeria. It was hoped that through this research, more significant changes would be encouraged in creating awareness of the ocular complications of DM. However, since DR is an irreversible DM ocular complication, the creation of awareness programmes would go a long way towards decreasing visual impairment.

Public health initiatives will be required to provide affordable DR screening, and initiatives into education will be needed to improve patient compliance with ophthalmic examinations and encourage follow-ups. Low-cost interventions should be provided to encourage compliance. The current management of DR eye care networks lacks a scientific basis and measurable key performance indicators; electronic media records may represent an effective approach to monitor performance and accountability. Efforts are needed to strengthen the capacity of existing national and local institutions to provide screening services, train eye care workers, and develop low-cost interventions to improve compliance and awareness.

The world today is much more interconnected, and the emerging issues of today are different from those we faced in the past. However, on the basis of the past success of health promotion strategies in addressing social determinants and health issues, the multi-level and multi-faceted nature of these approaches and the attention to social context, health promotion strategies have a great potential to address other preventive modes of DR, especially when they are strengthened and integrated with other actions like partnerships, community engagement decisions, attention to socio-environmental context, political commitment and the use of multiple strategies in various settings, levels and sectors. Such awareness programmes can have long-term benefits for the knowledge and psychosocial functioning of individuals.

A process requiring both improved technology and interdisciplinary co-operation between health workers caring for patients with DM is required for effective screening programmes and therapies for DR in Nigeria. A multidisciplinary, politically driven and co-ordinated approach in all areas related to health can contribute to the prevention of DR.

Research programmes on early HbA1c screening for effective blood glucose control should be done. In addition to poverty elimination programmes in the nation, new healthcare delivery strategies should be promoted to meet the demand for DR eye care. Telemedicine, the use of telecommunication and information technologies to provide clinical healthcare at a distance, should be encouraged, as it is a major way to reach rural areas.

Delivering optimal ophthalmic care at the appropriate time to individuals with DM can provide eye care programmes with huge cost savings, besides decreasing the personal suffering caused by visual impairment and blindness. It is important to increase awareness regarding DR in Nigeria and to transform this increased awareness into actual utilisation of services.

References

Adler, E. and Snibbe, A.C. (2003) The Role of Psychosocial Processes in Explaining the Gradient between Social Economic Status and Health. *Current Directions in Psychological Science*, 12(4), pp. 119–123.

Agarwal, S., Mahajan, S., Rani, P.K., Raman, R., Paul, P.G., Kumaramanickavel, G. and Sharma, T. (2005) How High is the Non Response Rate of Patients Referred for Eye

Examination from Diabetic Screening Camps? *Ophthalmic Epidemiology*, 12(6), pp. 393–394.

Airhihenbuwa, C.O. and Obregon, R. (2000) A Critical Assessment of Theories/Models Used in Health Communication for HIV/AIDS. *Journal of Health Communication*, 5, pp. 5–15.

Ashaye, A., Arije, A., Kuti, M., Olusanya, B., Ayeni, E., Fasanmade, A., Akinlade, K., Obajimi, M. and Adeleye, J. (2008) Retinopathy among Type2 Diabetic Patients Seen at a Tertiary Hospital in Nigeria: A Preliminary Report. *Clinical Ophthalmology*, 2(1), pp. 103–108.

Axer-Siegel, R., Herscovici, Z., Gabbay, M., Mimouni, K., Weinberger, D. and Gabbay, U. (2006) The Relationship between DR, Glycaemic Control, Risk Factor Indicators and Patient Education. *The Israel Medical Association Journal*, 8, pp. 523–526.

Benzies, K.M. and Allen, M.N. (2008) Symbolic Interactionism as a Theoretical Perspective for Multiple Method Research. *Journal of Advanced Nursing*, 33(4), pp. 541–547.

Blum, L.S., Pelto, G.H. and Pelto, P.J. (2004) Coping with a Nutrient Deficiency: Cultural Models of Vitamin A Deficiency in Northern Niger. *Medical Anthropology: Cross-Cultural Studies in Health and Illness*, 23(3), pp. 195–227.

Braun, V. and Clarke, V. (2006) Using Thematic Analysis in Psychology. *Qualitative Research in Psychology*, 3(2), pp. 77–101.

Brown, A.F., Ettner, S.L., Piette, J., Weinberger, M., Gregg, E., Shapiro, M.F., Karter, A.J., Safford, M., Waitzfelder, B., Prata, P.A. and Beckles, G.L. (2004) Socioeconomic Position and Health among Persons with Diabetes mellitus: A Conceptual Framework and Review of Literature. *Epidemiologic Reviews*, 26(1), pp. 63–77.

Brown, G.C., Brown, M.M., Sharma, S., Brown, H., Gozum, M. and Denton, P. (2000) Quality of Life Associated with Diabetes mellitus in an Adult Population. *Journal of Diabetes and Its Complications*, 14(1), pp. 18–24.

Chia, E., Wang, J.J., Rochtchina, E., Smith, W., Cumming, R.R. and Mitchell, P. (2004) Impact of Bilateral Visual Impairment in Health Related Quality of Life: The Blue Mountains Eye Study. *Investigative Ophthalmology and Visual Science*, 45(1), pp. 71–76.

Ciulla, T.A., Amador, A.G. and Zinman, B. (2003) DR and Diabetic Macular Edema. *DM Care*, 26(9), pp. 2653–2664.

Collier, A., Cotterill, A., Everett, T., Muckle, R., Pike, T. and Vanstone, A. (2010) Understanding and Influencing *Behaviours: A Review of Social Research, Economics and Policy Making in Defra*. DEFRA, London.

Cresswell, J.W. (2013) *Qualitative Inquiry and Research Design: Choosing among Five Approaches*. London: Sage Publications.

Denzin, N.K. and Lincoln, Y.S. (2003) *Strategies of Qualitative Inquiry*. 2nd edn. London: Thousand Oaks.

Girard, L.S., Forte, B., Cerreta, M., De Toro, P. and Forte, F. eds (2003) *The Human Sustainable City: Challenges and Perspectives from the Habitat Agenda*. Aldershot: Ashgate Publishing Limited.

Given, L.M. ed (2008) *Qualitative Research Methods*. 2nd edn. England Sage Publications, Oxford, UK.

Issa, B.A. and Baiyewu, O. (2006) Quality of Life of Patients with DM mellitus in a Nigerian Teaching Hospital. *Hong Kong Journal of Psychiatry*, 16(1), pp. 27–33.

Kreuter, M.W. and McClure, S.M. (2004) The role of Culture in Health Communication. *Annual Review of Public Health*, 25, pp. 439–455.

Kuzel, A.J. (1992) *Doing Qualitative Research*. Thousand Oaks: Sage Publications.

Lincoln, Y.S. and Guba E.G. (1985) *Naturalistic Inquiry*. London: Sage Publications.

Mbanya, J.N., Motala, A.A., Sobngwi, E., Assah, F.K. and Enoru, S.T. (2010) DM in Sub-Saharan Africa. *The Lancet*, 375(9733), pp. 2254–2266.

Namperumalsamy, P., Kim, R., Kaliaperumal, K., Sekar, A., Karthika, A. and Nirmalan, P.K. (2004) A Pilot Study on Awareness of DR among Non-medical Persons in South India: The Challenge for Eye Care Programmes in the Region. *Indian Journal of Ophthalmology*, 53(3), pp. 247–251.

Nutbeam, D., Harris, E. and Wise, M. (2010) *Theory in a Nutshell: A Practical Guide to Health Promotion Theories*. 3rd edn. North Ryde: McGraw Hill.

Ogden, J. (2012) *Health Psychology: A Textbook*. 5th edn. Maidenhead: Open University Press.

Olarinoye, J. and Olarinoye, A. (2007) Determinants of Sexual Function among Women with Type 2 DM in a Nigerian Population. *The Journal of Sexual Medicine*, 5(4), pp. 878–886.

Omolase, C. O., Adekanle, O., Owoeye, J. F. A., & Omolase, B. O. (2010). Diabetic retinopathy in a Nigerian community. *Singapore medical journal*, 51(1), 56.

Onakpoya, H.O., Adeoye, A.O. and Kolawole, A.B. (2010) Determinants of Previous Dilated Examination among Type2 Diabetics in South Western Nigeria. *European Journal of Internal Medicine*, 21(3), pp. 176–179.

Osborne, A. (1990) Some Basic Existential-Phenomenological Research Methodology for Counsellors. *Canadian Journal of Counselling*, 24(2), pp. 79–91.

Oso, L. and Pate, U. (2011) *Mass Media and Society in Nigeria*. Surulere, Lagos: Malthouse Press Limited.

Papadopoulos, A.A., Kontodimopoulos, N., Frydas, A., Ikonomakis, E. and Niakas, D. (2007) Predictors of Health-related Quality of Life in Type 2 Diabetic Patients in Greece. *Bio-medical Central Public Health*, 7(186), pp. 1–9.

Pasagian-Macaulay, A., Basch, C. E., Zybert, P., & Wylie-Rosett, J. (1997). Ophthalmic knowledge and beliefs among women with diabetes. *The Diabetes Educator*, 23(4), 433-437.

Ritchie, J. and Lewis, J. eds (2004) *Qualitative Research Practice: A Guide for Social Science Students and Researchers*. London: SAGE Publications.

Ruta, L.M., Magliano, D.J., LeMesurier, R., Taylor, H.R., Zimmet, P.Z. and Shaw, J.E. (2013) Prevalence of DR in Type 2 DM in Developing and Developed Countries. *Diabetic Medicine*, 30(4), pp. 387–398.

Rutter, D.R. and Quine, L. (2002) *Changing Health Behaviour: Intervention and Research with Social Cognition Models*. Maidenhead: McGraw Hill.

Sarafino, E.P. (2006) *Health Psychology*. 5th edn. Danvers: John Wiley and Sons.

Shenton, A.K. (2004) Strategies for Ensuring Trustworthiness in Qualitative Research Projects. *Education for Information*, 22, pp. 63–75.

Silverman, D. (2000) *Doing Qualitative Research: A Practical Handbook*. London: SAGE Publications.

Snow, S. (2009) Nothing Ventured, Nothing Gained: A Journey into Phenomenology (Part 1). *British Journal of Midwifery*, 17(5), pp. 288–290. Worcester: Mark Allen Publishing Limited.

Tang, Y.H., Pang, S.M.C., Chan, M.F., Yeung, G.S.P. and Yeung, V.T.F. (2008) Health Literacy, Complocation Awareness, and Diabetic Control in Patients with Type 2 DM mellitus. *Journal of Advanced Nursing*, 62(1), pp. 74–83.

Thomas, S.B., Fine, M.J. and Ibrahim, S.A. (2004) Health Disparities: The Importance of Culture and Health Communication. *American Journal of Public Health*, 94(12), pp. 2050.

Thorne, S. (2000) EBN Notebook: Data Analysis in Qualitative Research. *Evidence Based Nursing*, 3(3), pp. 68–70.

Tongco, M.D.C. (2007) Purposive Sampling as a Tool for Informant Selection. *Ethnobotany Research and Applications*, 5(12), pp. 147–158.

Vashist, P., Singh, S., Gupta, N. and Saxena, R. (2011) Role of Early Screening for DR in Patients with DM Mellitus: An Overview. *Indian Journal of Community Medicine*, 36(4), pp. 247–252.

Ward, V., House, A. and Hamer, S. (2009) Developing a Framework for Transferring Knowledge into Action: A Thematic Analysis of the Literature. *Journal of Health Services Research and Policy*, 14(3), pp. 156–164.

Whitehead, D. (2001) Health Education, Behavioural Change and Social Psychology: Nursing's Contribution to Health Promotion. *Journal of Advanced Nursing*, 34(6), pp. 822–832.

Wilhot (2009) Bias and Values in Scientific Research. *Studies in History and Philosophy Part A*, 40(1), pp. 92–101.

Williams, R., Herman, W., Kinmonth, A.L. and Wareham, N.J. eds (2002) *The Evidence Base for DM Care*. Chichester: John Wiley and Sons Limited.

Willig, C. and Stainton-Rogers, W. eds (2008) *The Sage Handbook of Qualitative Research in Psychology*. London: Sage Publications Ltd.

WHO Universal Eye Health: A Global Action Plan 2014–2019. World Health Organization, Geneva (2013). http://www.who.int/blindness/actionplan/en/

Yau, J.W., Rogers, S.L., Kawasaki, R., Lamoureux, E.L., Kowalski, J.W., Bek, J., Chen, S.J., Dekker, J.M., Fletcher, A., Grauslund, J., Haffner, S., Hamman, R.F., Ikram, M.K., Kayama, T., Klein, B.E.K., Klein, R., Krishnaiah, S., Mayurasakorn, K. and O'Hare, J.P. (2012) Global Prevalence and Major Risk Factors of DR. *DM Care*, 35(3), pp. 558–584.

Zheng, Y., He, M. and Congdon, N. (2012) The Worldwide Epidemic of DR. *Indian Journal of Ophthalmology*, 60(5), pp. 428–431.

16

CHILDREN ON THE STREET

Chinyere Ihejieto

Introduction

This chapter offers insight into child labour within the context of street-working children, specifically children 'on' the streets of Benin City, Nigeria. In order to fully appreciate and understand the voices of children, it is important to set the scene and contextualise the narrative. Therefore, this chapter also discusses the methodological and theoretical framework adopted to tell the stories of working children in Benin City, in terms of what working means and how it affects their lives.

According to ILO (2018), child labour can be defined based on four premises, and they include work that deprives children of their childhood; work that deprives children of their potential and dignity; work that interferes with their schooling; and work that is physically, mentally, socially or morally harmful to the child. The practice is negatively portrayed in several works of literature, and rightfully so, due to numerous bodies of work documenting its physical, psychological and social impact on children. The focus on street work as a form of child labour is of particular interest not only because of the well documented impact on the well-being and education of children, emphasising the need for the phenomenon to be addressed, but also that this topic is of particular interest because the researcher was a street-working child. To learn about the lives of street-working children in Nigeria, the lived experiences of the researcher should not be considered a potential bias but rather a legitimate basis for making certain arguments regarding the context and the topic of interest.

DOI: 10.4324/9781003467601-19

Scope of Study

Within the context of Benin City, Nigeria, this study confines its attention to issues such as the role of poverty in child labour, the child labour-child education relationship and the sociocultural aspects of child work. There are many other significant aspects of child labour that are essential, especially around issues involving "unconditional worst forms of child labour". There are various forms of hazardous work, such as children working in mines, agriculture, manufacturing and so on. Discussions on hazardous child labour will centre only on street-working children, detailing the types of activities children perform on the streets and the characteristics and division of children who work on the street. This is because hazardous work and child street work are the most predominant and visible forms of child work in Nigeria (Edewor, 2014; Ekpiken-Ekanem, Ayuk and Adadu, 2014).

Defining Child Labour

Child labour continues to be a topic of academic concern and policy-making in Africa (Kazeem, 2013). For decades, the practice has been argued to be beneficial to children (Young Lives, 2016; Okyere, 2013, 2012; Katz, 2004; Robson, 2004), as well as detrimental to their well-being (Abubakar-Abdullateef, Adedokun and Omigbodun, 2017; Kazeem, 2013). There is still no academic consensus in child labour discourse in the region, as there is a divide in arguments on the phenomenon relating to its impact on children and its causes.

Global Trend

Child labour is a global concern, and many works of literature are calling for an end to the practice in all its forms. The latest joint publication by UNICEF/ILO (2021) suggests a global estimate of 160 million children in child labour—an increase of 8.4 million children in the last four years. This document is the most current and comprehensive publication on child labour, and as such, its findings significantly underpin several arguments presented in this study. At the beginning of the year 2020, 97 million boys and 63 million girls were child labourers, constituting almost 1 in every 10 children globally (UNICEF/ILO, 2021). Unlike the ILO (2017b) 2012–2016 Global Estimate report on the trend of child labour, which concluded that there had been a global reduction in child labour between years 2012 and 2016, this report cautions that for the first time in 20 years, the global progress to end child labour has stalled, recording a rise in cases of hazardous work among children aged 5–17 years by 6.5 million (to 79 million) since 2016. Extreme poverty, population growth and inadequate social protection measures have been blamed for the additional 16.9 million child labourers in Sub-Saharan Africa. A global prediction and warning of an additional 9 million children are at risk of being forced into child labour by the end of 2022 due to the COVID-19 pandemic (UNICEF/ILO, 2021).

Children on the Street V Children of the Street

The street-working child is not often represented as a diverse group, as it is mostly the case where they are seen and discussed as one group, ignoring their different and unique situations. For example, although the groups of street-working children are differentiated, Adewale and Afolabi (2013) propose that the phenomenon of "street children" is a "menace" and an "eye sore" among major cities that occurs as a result of poor welfare, neglect and faulty upbringing of certain groups of children. This statement epitomises how the street-working child is generally put across regardless of the form of labour they engage in, the level of support the child receives and the individual situation of street-working children.

In Nigeria, street-working children are geographically and culturally diverse (Abubakar-Abdullateef, Adedokun and Omigbodun, 2017). Street-working children in the southern part of Nigeria are typically referred to as "area boys", "street urchins" or the general term "street children", and they operate in motor parks or markets, either doing legitimate work (hawking, doing menial jobs) and/schooling, or conducting illicit activities (pickpocketing) alone.

There are two kinds of children that work on the street in Nigeria: *children of the street* and *children on the street* (Omiyinka, 2009). The former refers to children who typically earn a living and dwell on the streets with little or no adult supervision. These children run away from home, drop out of school or become orphaned, thus ending up in this situation. In contrast, *children on the street* refer to children who carry out activities on the street either on full- or part-time bases, under the supervision of their parents/guardian and return to their homes each day rather than residing/dwelling on the street.

The Child *of* the Street

Children of the street are boys and girls less than 18 years, who earn a living and reside on the street with inadequate protection and supervision. They have received enormous attention from both international, NGO's and individual researchers because of the severe impact such lifestyles have on a child's education, physical, psychological and moral well-being (Omiyinka, 2009). In Nigeria, these children sleep in unsecured places, such as in market stalls and under bridges. Circumstances like high striking poverty and the loss of their parents most times force children to be on the street (Okonkwo and Alhaji, 2014). They roam the streets, car parks and markets as their source of livelihood, and in some cases, they employ anti-social survival strategies to sustain themselves.

According to Bhukuth and Ballet (2015), they also face several difficulties, as they are marginalised and considered pariahs by their societies, and in some cases, businesses are threatened by their presence. As such, businessmen hire police to get rid of them from business vicinities. As a result of all these characteristics, they are particularly regarded as a vulnerable population.

These groups of children are commonly referred to in the literature as "street children". Other terms used to refer to them are "children without shelter" and "children in especially difficult circumstances". Their living situations expose them to more risk of sexual and physical assault, infections and diseases and mental health issues (anxiety, depression and insomnia), which is mainly because they are not under the consistent protection and supervision of their parents/guardians.

Consequently, in some cases, *children of the street* are sometimes catered for by street guardians—other grown-up, unemployed individuals who also grew up on the street (Emordi and Osiki, 2008). In Nigeria, these individuals are sometimes referred to as "Area Boys" or "Agberos", and they earn their living on the streets doing both illicit and legal activities (Uyieh, 2018). *Agberos* groom them on ways to make money on the streets via several means—illegal and, in some cases, violent means (such as pocket picking, gambling, begging and extortion), as well as legitimate street work (street hawking, trading, and running errands).

The Child *on* the Street

Children on the street refer to children under 18 years who carry out income-generating activities on the street either on full- or part-time basis. Unlike children *of* the street, they return to their homes each day, as they do not dwell on the street, and they often have parental/guardian supervision. They are a group of children who are classified as child labourers under the International Labour Organisation Conventions (ILO, 2017) either due to their age (Convention 138) or conditions under which they work (Convention 182).

Children on the street are the largest group of street-working children (Bhukuth and Ballet, 2015), as well as constitute the highest statistics of child workers in Nigeria. Ironically, they are less discussed than children *of* the street in Nigerian literature. Eliminating this group of child labour is not a priority for many international organisations, as the unconditional worst forms of child labour are the primary target of both action programmes and international research (ILO, 2017a).

Their profile varies as some of them either carry out street work on a full-time basis (apprenticeship) or combine it with school. From the literature and the researcher's experience of the street, *children on the street* are further categorised into two groups: children who combine work with school (Mosabo, 2017; Young Lives, 2016; Bourdillon, Crivello and Pankhurst, 2015) and children who work in informal sectors (Onodugo et al., 2016; Abbasi, 2013) as apprentices (Fajobi et al., 2017).

Working on the street is a combination of the child's external influence (family and peers) and the child's survival strategies to cope with existing circumstances (Terres Des Hommes, 2010). On the street, they do not all share similar backgrounds; they possess certain narratives that help them conduct business, form relations and make friends while working on the street. Such as working with family and education.

Child Labour in Benin City, Nigeria

Benin City is a commercial city with over 20 markets, with the major markets being Oba Market and New Benin Market. These markets are major locations for economic transactions; they are also located in significant transit areas with a substantial amount of human and motor traffic. Thus, these markets are common vending sites and are therefore used by adults and children to carry out trading activities regardless of the season. The city is located in a tropical equatorial zone characterised by wet seasons (April to October) and dry seasons (November to March) (Balogun and Orimoogunje, 2015). Furthermore, temperatures in Benin City are high throughout the year, with a mean average of 27°C, which permits for high demand and supply for cold sachet water, soft drinks and ice cream (Omofonmwan and Eseigbe, 2009).

The ancient kingdom of Benin, as it is popularly known, is in the South-South of Nigeria, a country located in Sub-Saharan Africa. Nigeria is commonly referred to as a key regional player in West Africa, with a population of approximately 184 million people (47% of West Africa's population) (The World Bank, 2018). Between 2006 and 2016, Nigeria experienced GDP growth at an average rate of 5.7% per year. With a population of 40 million children, such growth has seen some recent improvements in the situation of children. Although this economy has surpassed growth in previous years, according to the World Bank (2018), the volatility of the country's growth continuously imposes significant welfare costs on households. Also, Nigeria continues to experience significant developmental challenges such as insufficient infrastructure, unemployment, governance issues, diversifying the economy and addressing the living conditions of the population, among other issues (World Bank, 2008).

Child labour practice in Nigeria is prevalent and predominantly in the informal sector, as children often work on family enterprises, commercial farms and as domestic workers (Bureau of International Affairs, 2017). The practice cuts across economic, cultural, social and religious facets of the country (Federal Ministry of Labour and Productivity, 2017). ILO (2014) and UNICEF (2006) identified widespread poverty, a lack of enforcement of child protection instruments and rapid urbanisation as significant causes of child labour in Nigeria.

Street trading accounts for approximately 70% of urban employment in Nigeria, as many Nigerians generate income from entrepreneurial activities, and a significant amount of these activities occur on the street, often along the roadside amidst traffic (Emozozo, 2017). Several Nigerian studies conclude that poverty, low standard of living, low income, unemployment and culture result in child street activities (Oluwaleye, 2017; Johnson and Ihesie, 2015; Nduka and Duru, 2014; Dada, 2013; Clark and Yesufu, 2012; Ashimolowo, Aromolaran and Inegbedion, 2010; Umar, 2009).

The African Charter on the Rights and Welfare of the Child (ACRWC) is a declaration on the rights and welfare of the African child, and it was adopted in 1979 by the Heads of State and Government of the Organisation of African Unity (African Commission on Human and People's Rights, 2019). The ACRWC recognises that due to socioeconomic, traditional, cultural, armed conflict and natural disaster factors, most African children remain in critical situations. As a result, these children need special safeguarding and care with regards to their physical, mental, moral and social development (African Commission on Human and People, 2018). There are 48 articles contained in the ACRWC, which also cover the socioeconomic, cultural, family, education and health aspects of an African child's life.

It is interesting to note that the Nigerian government consistently makes attempts to clamp down on street activities, as street work falls into the country's category of what is and should be considered *hazardous* work in the country (Federal Ministry of Labour and Productivity, 2013). Although the list for hazardous work is not yet officially endorsed (IPEC, 2014), some states continue to implement measures to get street-working children off the street. For example, the Lagos State government banned street trading in 2016; street vendors are also similarly being intimidated and harassed on the street by government personnel in Benin City.

The actions of the Nigerian government, although needed to curb the worst forms of child labour, still fall short of promoting the overall well-being of children *on* the street for two reasons. Firstly, the government only just produced a document for categories of work activities classified as *hazardous work* for prohibition (as recommended by the ILO Convention 182) in 2013, and this document is yet to be officially endorsed as it functions only as a draft. Nevertheless, following Convention 182, interventions aimed at getting the working child off the street can be seen as going against the UN convention on the rights of the child, especially Article 3 (best interest of the child). This is because taking children off the street may further marginalise and deprive them of opportunities to survive and afford an education.

Secondly, imposing a ban and the use of intimidation on the street to clamp down on all street activities highlights the government's failure to differentiate between situations of street-working children and recognise that not every child on the street is necessarily in harm's way. Though the government has concerns about street activities causing overcrowding, disruption and congestion on main roadways (Emozozo, 2017) and concerns about higher incidences of road traffic accidents in areas with a higher concentration of street traders, child street work has not officially been classified as hazardous work in Nigeria, even in any of its forms. Also, hazardous work is yet to be clearly defined. It is confusing as to what legal and conventional backing interventions have for getting children *on the street* off the street.

Types of Street Work

The ILO (2018) agrees that not every work children indulge in should be classified as child labour to be targeted for elimination. This is because these types of work neither affect the child's personal development and health nor do they interfere with the child's schooling, as they are conducted outside school hours and during holidays. As such, they can generally be regarded as something positive. These activities include assisting parents with the family business and around the home or earning pocket money outside school hours. In contributing to their family's welfare, children develop skills and acquire experience that prepares them for adult life, which makes them grow up into productive members of society (ILO, 2018) (Figure 16.1).

In contrast, an open *street* space is one where there are fewer stalls/structures with no systematic arrangement and possesses a more extensive space available to pedestrians, motor cars and motorbikes. Open street spaces are sometimes scanty as they do not have structures (temporal or permanent) closely knitted. This may be the reason why it constitutes mostly of out-of-stall traders rather

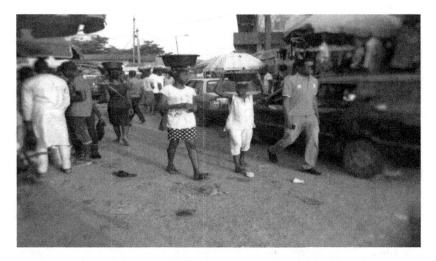

FIGURE 16.1 Oba Maret: child and adult street workers hawking and in temporary ST.

than stall traders, considering out-of-stall traders are mobile and can hawk goods or get patronised by individuals in cars, buses and motorbikes likewise pedestrians just passing through the street. The factors that decide whether the *street* is an open or clustered space are the presence of systematically arranged stalls and the space available and accessible to motor vehicles.

Nevertheless, whether clustered or open, the *street* is usually busy, overflowing with human and motor traffic. The human traffic constitutes of buyers, pedestrians, bus drivers and conductors, other drivers and sellers of goods and services. Therefore, there are a myriad of activities all happening at the same place, with different underlying intentions of the people present in that space at that time: buyers buying, sellers selling and pedestrians passing through or by the *street* without any economic reason.

Although both spaces are exposed to traffic (human and motor traffic in the open spaces and only human traffic in clustered spaces), they both have different exposure to the weather (rain, wind and sunshine) due to the presence/absence and arrangement of structures. For example, when it rains heavily, open 'street' spaces have limited trading, considering some traders do not hawk in the rain as water can destroy their commodities. Therefore, only traders with stalls can continue trading goods, regardless of the torrential downpour. Also, clustered street spaces usually have an opening and closing time. Traders in open-street spaces usually dictate their working hours with strategic customer routines. For example, markets in Benin City usually close by 6 pm; hawkers can, however, continue to trade along the roadside beyond this time. As a result, although they are locked out of the market space, out-of-stall traders continue to make sales to individuals who are returning from work, going out or even just passing through (Figure 16.2).

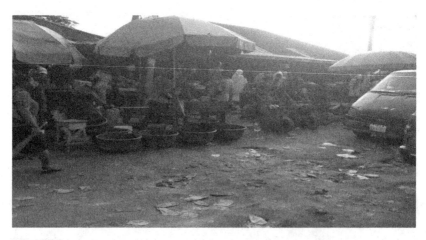

FIGURE 16.2   An open street space with out-of-stall vendors (teenage wheelbarrow pushers), stall traders (temporary structures) and motor traffic.

These characteristics make individuals aware of the best location to buy/sell goods and services at certain times and conditions. For example, from personal experience and observation, when thirsty during fieldwork, the researcher did not think of going inside the market to purchase *pure water*. The knowledge that *out-of-stall* traders operate on the street and usually hawk commodities resulted in the researcher's decision to remain seated in a public bus and wait to arrive at a busy area (heavy traffic) to buy *pure water* while seated on the bus rather than alighting to buy water from a supermarket or the market. Furthermore, sometimes traders that offer similar goods and services own stalls (permanent or temporary) in specific locations of the street, and as such, customers are attracted to certain parts of the street depending on what they want to buy.

Selected Groups of Children on the Street Included in This Study

The two main groups of street-working children identified in this study are children in apprenticeship and children who combine school and work.

Informal Apprentice

Informal apprenticeship is a form of education and training (Fajobi et al., 2017) that exists in different sectors whereby private business owners train apprentices (usually for a fee) in traditional skills over a period of three years or more. After the contracted period of apprenticeship, the apprentice is subsequently settled by the business owner (in the form of cash, equipment and similar endeavours). An example of such practice is in manufacturing, which produces skills in metal work, sewing and carpentry. Traditional apprenticeship in West Africa is a more important form of training than the vocational educational system (Adams, Johansson de Silva and Razmara, 2013). The role of apprenticeship training has been investigated to alleviate poverty (Igwe and Oragwu, 2014), supply occupational skills (Wallis, 2008) and promise youth employment.

Informal apprenticeship is quite popular in most urban cities in Nigeria, as it accounts for 85% of skill transfer and training across the country (Fajobi et al., 2017). Aside from being a significant source of livelihood, it is also a means of employment in an economically worthwhile venture. Nigeria is a country believed to have a significant amount of labour force that is not being adequately utilised; thus, the country has one of the highest rates of youth unemployment in the world. This is partly due to the lack of employment skills (which creates a wide skills gap) (Fajobi et al., 2017) and the failure of the government to initiate and provide adequate services and opportunities for its citizens both in the informal and formal sectors.

Apprenticeship is a universal practice that empowers youth and adolescents through skills acquisition and training in the ever-changing realities of globalisation (ILO, 2017a,b). This is no different in Nigeria, where apprenticeship is a significant driver for employment generation and poverty reduction at low investment costs (Fajobi et al., 2017). Thus, it improves not only the economy but also the well-being of citizens. As such, Fajobi et al. (2017) further suggest that the practice should be given reasonable consideration in the country as it affords young people the opportunity to contribute to several sectors of the economy, such as fashion and carpentry, among other related endeavours.

The set minimum age for an apprenticeship in Nigeria is 13 years (Nigerian Labour Act, Article 49), and the Federal Child's Right Act (2003) provides criminal sanctions for violation of this law. However, this law is only legally binding when adopted by an individual Nigerian state. So far, of the 36 Nigerian states, only eight states have adopted the law. Therefore, the potential of apprenticeship for growth and development in Nigeria is not duly exploited, and the pattern of decline in apprenticeship has increased through the socio-cultural process in Nigeria (Adekola, 2013; Ayadike, Emeh and Ukah, 2012). Young people in Nigeria have a negative attitude towards apprenticeship, as it is considered a low-class career path, one that is meant for people who cannot perform well in school or those whose parents cannot afford formal education (Adekola, 2013); likewise, it is a path that significantly offers lower prospects than academic training in higher education or the university (Fajobi et al., 2017). As such, young people in Nigeria do not consider or respect informal apprenticeship unless circumstance forces them to take it up.

Schooling Children

Today, skills of numeracy and literacy are essential and are empowering tools in the social, economic and political domains (Bourdillon, Crivello and Pankhurst, 2015). For this study, schooling children are a set of children on the street who combine work on the street and schooling. This situation is often seen in developing countries as large numbers of children engage in various forms of work alongside their schooling. Children work in difficult situations, and one common argument for child labour is that the practice hinders child education.

Though the study stated the need for the elimination of the worst forms of child labour, it further suggested that measures (such as strengthened social protection) should be provided to ensure flexibility so that children can better combine work and schooling. By so doing, the incidence of hazardous work could potentially decrease and maybe also reduce child labour statistics in these regions where the 'ideal' living situations are not always present. Considering children are sometimes trapped in difficult situations, likewise, parents are in compromising positions. Orkin (2010) strongly agrees, stating that when children work because of poverty or other family situations, schooling should be made flexible to facilitate compatibility with working.

Instead of "child labour" is often termed as the routine of child work and schooling 'children's work' because children mostly work within their households and communities, and such routine is considered an integral part of their everyday lives within a continuum of other activities. This places specific emphasis on why children are working at all.

It is also important to be aware that while schooling can enable a few children to break out of the circle of poverty, it cannot guarantee the same outcome for working children. On the contrary, work experience can help young people develop skills needed for life and work (Bourdillon, Crivello and Pankhurst, 2015). Besides, the effect of work on children's education depends on several factors, such as hours of work, nature of the job, relationship with the employer, flexibility of the schooling system, aptitude of the child and quality of schooling (Bourdillon et al., 2011).

Economic Determinants of Child Labour

A child may work to contribute to the basic survival of the family, most especially in situations of poverty where basic household human needs are unmet. This is a significant stance argued by Basu and Van (1998), a well-known classical work on luxury and substitute axioms. Although in their analysis of child labour, Basu and Van never precisely defined child labour or state activities that constitute the phenomenon, instead they stated that to meet household subsistence needs, children engage in some work activities. Their focus was on the multiple equilibria, which they claimed seemed to be an inherent characteristic of the child labour market: one in which wages are high and children do not work, or another in which wages are low and children work. This model gives primacy to household wealth as a determinant of child labour.

Luxury Axiom

In their definition, Basu and Van (1998) explained the luxury axiom as a situation when a family's income drops very low and they *only send their child to work* to increase the household income. Luxury axiom can also be described as a situation where non-child labour income is insufficient to meet the daily upkeep of the home; therefore, child labour is necessary to supplement the family's income for daily sustenance (ILO, 2007). Basu and Van argue that when children work, they are working to have a target income to complement overall household income. This target income would be the difference between the income needed for running the family and the income gotten without child labour.

The luxury axiom explains the supply of child labour by elucidating the decision-making process within the household. Consequently, grounds for declaring child labour practice illegal become significantly weaker, as child labour could be perceived as an act of desperation on the part of parents. If parents' employment prospects and wages were better, it seems reasonable not to expect parents to send their children to work.

Substitute Axiom

Substitute axiom is a situation where firms make child labour a substitute for adult labour. Under this assumption, if adult wages are higher than child wages in the market, firms will always prefer employing children instead of adults (Bhukuth and Ballet, 2006). Therefore, families would be left to solely rely on child labour as a significant source of the family's income, thus substituting adult labour for child labour. This hypothesis focuses on the demand side of labour.

Given the above assumption by Basu and Van (1998), it is possible that an increase in adult wages will result in parents not wanting to send their children to work. Basu and Van argue that child labour competes with adult labour in market-oriented activities. Nevertheless, Bhukuth and Ballet (2006) contradict this hypothesis, stating that labour substitution is not always feasible in every market-oriented situation.

Strategy for Inquiry

To illicit the opinions, experiences, beliefs and ideas of participants in Nigeria regarding child labour and child street work, grounded theory (GT)—a qualitative research methodology—was adopted. Qualitative research examines subjective human experiences utilising non-statistical methods (Ingham-Broomfield, 2015; Borbasi and Jackson, 2012). The use of GT principles (Fulton and Hayes, 2012) facilitated the researcher's ability to achieve theoretical sensitivity on the subject matter and subsequently investigate the study's research question. Besides, the process of constant comparison of participants' stories facilitated the development of concepts, and the theoretical sensitivity of the researcher promoted the understanding of these concepts.

The adopted methods of data collection for this study were observation, storytelling and semi-structured interviews with children and adult street workers. Five tools facilitated the data collection process: a comic leaflet, a participant information sheet, an emotion chart, market women facilitators and government participation. These methods provide a rich understanding of children's experiences and privilege children's voices, as well as help answer research questions that mainly focus on experiences, perspectives and meanings from the participant's standpoint (Hammarberg, Kirkman and Lacey, 2016).

Observation of participants on the street was carried out during every interaction with participants and even observation of the street/environment. This method complimented the use of semi-structured interview/storytelling.

Considering some children and adults might romanticise their street experiences, observation assisted the researcher not only in being aware of what participants said but also what they left out. Observations were also useful in gaining additional insight into the structure and process of working children, as the street was observed early in the mornings, during and after school hours and likewise during the close of the market at night. Aside from senses of sight and hearing, senses of smell and touch assisted the researcher in evaluating information about events and activities on the street, market structures and the distinct characteristics of each group of children on the street. Thus providing a holistic sense of the street. A field note (memo), voice recorder and camera were used to document observations.

Why Children on the Street of Benin City Work? The World of *Street* Children: Voices and Character

This section of this chapter presents the narratives of working children in Benin City, Edo State. These enduring stories capture aspects of a working child's activities while on the street. These stories also give insight into the child's life and facilitate understanding of the child's environment, culture and routines. Therefore, this understanding frames the subsequent interpretation of their stories within the right context in which children and families experience working. Through telling stories about themselves, their thoughts and their experiences, we are invited inside a participant's life (Denning, 2000). These are stories that children on the *street* shared repeatedly, and these stories are told alongside observations made by the researcher.

The findings are based partly on the stories of nine children. The starting point for the children's story was to explore the way the children regard and understand the practice of working. Children were interviewed in an empty market stall in *Oba* Market. Most of the children clearly articulated what they thought and felt, while others who do not attend school or have stopped attending school expressed themselves in *Pigin* English mixed with the English language.

Overall, within the context of this study, the incidence of child labour is greatly influenced by families, the government and the general perception and representation of the practice.

Ede: Experienced and Hardworking

Ede is a 16-year-old girl; she works in a stall with both her parents. The family sells snacks, drinks, cigarettes and other random household and bathroom items such as light bulbs and bathing sponges. The stall is located along New Benin Market Road and is surrounded by heavy human and motor traffic. In the stall is Mrs Asemota. Mrs Asemota runs the business with the help of her husband and daughter, Ede. In appearance, the family looked well-groomed and spoke good English. When starting her story, Ede made eye contact and appeared relaxed. At 16, she had finished secondary school and was attending lectures for the Joint Admissions and Matriculations Board (JAMB), which is a Nigerian entrance examination for tertiary-level institutions. These lectures are meant to assist students pass the JAMB entrance exams into universities.

Every morning, "*I say my prayers because we are Witnesses, we are Jehovah Witnesses*". Then, as early as 6:00 am in the morning, Ede leaves for the bakery to pick up fresh bread and then supply it to local stalls. She stated, "I get home by 10, 11:00 am" after the supply. Ede stated she repeatedly showers afterwards because of the sweet and dirt or muddy roads. She then proceeds to have her breakfast and rest. She said she would require rest because "*I have been trekking around town*". After resting, Ede has the day to herself, and she said, "if I have somewhere going to, I will go" and return by 4:00 pm. Ede uses that time to visit friends or attend lectures. She then sits at her mother's shop for the rest of the day, until it is closing hour. "*I don't cook regularly because I am always at the shop*", so when the shop closes, she eats and then retires to bed.

"*I am happy helping my parents at my young age*", and she believes that when she has children, they would also help her out, just like she has been helpful to her parents. Ede nonetheless stated, "*although I don't want my children to suffer the way I have suffered*". After stating this, Ede quickly adds, "*but am always happy helping my parents*". She said working in her mother's shop has "*a lot of benefits*"; Ede gets several incentives from family members and friends, as they always say to her, "*you are hard-working, so take this, take that*". Also, she said that because she is so helpful to her parents, they always pray for her, and these prayers "*guide me a lot*", Ede said. She also stated that she has the mentality that it is right to be hardworking: "*if you have this feeling that if you can work hard, I believe later on you're not going to suffer*". Ede reckons it is crucial for one to be hardworking, and working with her mother in the stall has helped her build that quality.

Ede said, "*to me child labour is…erm, I will use myself as an example*". She has been helping her parents manage the business for nine years, and she holds the opinion that children should help their parents provide for them, especially if they are not financially buoyant. Ede added that she interprets child labour as "*just to help your parents with things you can do*", "*like hawking if they* (parents) *ask you to hawk*". She continues by stating that some children work OST while others sit in stalls, but there is "*no significant difference*". The only difference she sees is that those who hawk only do so because they do not have shops/stalls, which may be because "*they may not have that money at that particular time to get a shop*".

Also, after Ede sells and makes a profit for her mother, she states that whenever she asks her parents for money, "*they will not hesitate*" to give her because they she has worked hard and made gains for the family. *"So I believe when I need anything I can go and ask them because I am also assisting them too"*, Ede said. When talking about children and their routines, Ede further said, *"every child should have their daily work"*, and this should start with prayers in the morning, doing morning and evening chores, attending school if they can, helping their parents out in the market, eating and sleeping.

Mekus: An Apprentice and a Hopeful Entrepreneur

On the 5th of October 2016, at 7:00 am, at the heart of the city centre of Benin City-Ring Road, the street was quiet, with few motor vehicles moving to various destinations. The temperature for that day was forecast to be about 25°C, and traders gradually made their way to *Oba Market*. The market opened at 8:00 am; therefore, when traders (and even buyers) got to the market, they had to wait for the gates to be opened. Children also accompanied their parent/guardian to the market to set up their various businesses. Some of the children were dressed in their school uniforms while assisting in setting up for the day.

At 9:00 am, the sun was out, the temperature was 29°C but felt like 35°C and trading activities had started. However, not every child had gone to school. Some children stayed and traded on the *street*, while others went to school.

Mekus is a 13-year-old boy who lives with his parents but works for a guardian in shoemaking/repair stall as an apprentice. He appeared pleased and excited to talk to the researcher. He gladly told the story of how the tortoise broke his shell (as an icebreaker to the storytelling session). Although his attempt to speak English was a mixture of *Pigin* English and correct grammar, he stated he was pleased to be working as an apprentice. According to Mekus, "some *Hausa* children beg for money on the *street*", and some families do have sufficient money to feed, clothe, or even cater to their children.

Mekus stated that when some parents cannot afford an education for their children due to a lack of money and the child gets work to self-sponsor their education, the parents would be very proud of that child:

> Their children come home daytime, started worrying their parents say, take me to education err… knowledge, they will say they don't have money. Their children will, their family will be crying say they did not have money. They will, their children, their brother will be working, they (the parents) will be clapping for you say you trying for the education.

Mekus made this statement not only about himself (being an apprentice) but also as a general statement affecting street-working children. Furthermore, he said he finished primary 5 and stopped schooling at that level, and he currently works in the stall to get the "best knowledge" he can understand in order to get "the good life" he wants. Fighting and running away from school, coupled with the fact that his parents did not have enough funds to continue paying for his schooling, Mekus said, this was the reason why his father decided to send him to apprentice handiwork. According to him, his father also believed that learning such work would *"help"* his life.

Findings from this study suggest that children on the street work mainly because of their desire for an education, formal or informal. Child labour has often been condemned for its role in stunting children's physical and educational growth, as well as maintaining low socio-class. Subsequently, continuing poverty and exploiting children (ILO, 2017a;)

Maya: Intelligent and Ambitious

Maya's house is located about 0.3 miles from New Benin Market; therefore, it is busy with both human and motor traffic. The house is a two-story building with several one-bedroom apartments on each floor. These houses are locally called "face-me-I-face-you" houses because each apartment entrance door faces each other along a walkway that leads to the main entrance of the building. At 2:00 pm, Maya and her siblings were not back from school. Several hawkers roamed the street, some carrying food items or goods on their heads, some pushing it in wheelbarrows, while others displayed items on their arms. These hawkers wear a waist pack around their waist, which serves the purpose of a cash register; sellers place money made from sales of items in them and likewise produce change for their customers from the waist pack.

Maya is a seven-year-old child who lives and hawks bitter kola for her mother, Mrs Ormon. She grew up without her father. Maya's father left before she was born, and Mrs Ormon has had to cater for Maya and her other older siblings. Although her father was unaware of her birth because of animosity between Mrs Ormon and her in-laws, when he later found out, he made promises to help take care of her. Although her father tries, Maya's mother stated that Maya still had to hawk to increase the family's income. After returning from school, Maya told her story. Every day, she prays during morning devotion with her mother and siblings, and then she has breakfast and walks about a mile to school.

Conclusion

It is problematic when researchers continuously present child labour arguments to either support or oppose the notion that children work for money. Each side of the argument does not sufficiently recognise the different narratives of these working families and the lives of children in different contexts, especially those that work on the street. With recognition and understanding, each side of the argument is valid and is right depending on the family's situation.

Furthermore, it helps reconcile the differences in opinions that, over time, have generated several arguments in child labour discourse. There may not be a no wrong on right answer to the justification of certain aspects of child labour, but rather an understanding of child work within different contexts. This approach provides consideration for work principles and the desires of working children and highlights the heterogeneity of child labour discussion and analysis.

Children *on* the street have a lifestyle and living circumstances different from popular perception. This makes them possess vital characteristics that influence the reasons for *street* work and its subsequent impact on the child. In comparison to children *of* the street, these characteristics produce nuances in their representation as child labourers. As such, these children should not be considered child labourers but rather assisted to work in ways that their education and well-being are not compromised in any foreseeable sense. Within the context of this study, children who work on the street stated that working offered them the opportunity to afford school, gain entrepreneurial and transferable skills and develop a sense of accomplishment and responsibility. For reasons of substitute axiom, children on the street obtained formal education either by working with parents or for/ with a guardian. In other cases, these children would get engaged with apprenticeship jobs and acquire knowledge through situated learning.

The acknowledgement and appreciation of knowing that street-working children are a heterogeneous group helps dismantle the assumption that every child found on the street is homeless, uneducated, suffering and needs saving. This assumption creates a stereotype that serves as the basis for discrimination and misrepresentation of street-working children both locally and in the international scene. The ubiquitous misconception that "children on the street" hold the same controversial meaning as "street of children" needs to be challenged, as the quality of life of *children on the street* is not fairly evaluated, much often overlooked and misrepresented or is not given as much attention to express their opinions. Involving children in research on issues affecting them is a contemporary way of thinking in research, and it is likely to be the future of social research.

Each form of street work ties in differently to the meaning of child labour as well as having a distinct impact on the child's education and well-being. As such, children that work on the street are a distinct subset of child labourers that, like other children, attend school and receive support from their parents/ guardians. This study's findings on child labour challenge the popular abolitionist approach, which supports the ban of all work children conduct. The abolitionist approach does not only ignore the circumstance/context of street work and appreciate the family's effort to support the child; a ban on their activities may also further marginalise them or deny them the opportunity for better futures. In extreme cases, it may force them into unconditional worst forms of child labour.

In viewing child labour as a coping strategy, interventions aimed at child labour should not only focus on eradicating the practice but also see the need to refine it in terms of redefining the meaning of child labour and promoting and protecting the child's overall health and well-being. Therefore, there is a need for a contextual definition of child labour beyond ILO Conventions 182 and 138, and in this case, one that recognises children's opinions and the context-specific nature of work. Regardless of whether children embark on work for economic or sociocultural reasons, the effect of working is the same and ranges on a spectrum from positives to negatives. Whether work is harmful or beneficial to a child is not determined merely by a straightforward answer.

References

Abbasi, A. (2013). *Societal Perception and Legal Interventions: Implications on the Well-being of Street Working Children in Pakistan*. Hungary: Central European University.

Abubakar-Abdullateef, A., Adedokun, B. and Omigbodun, O. (2017). 'A Comparative Study of the Prevalence and Correlates of Psychiatric Disorders in Almajiris and Public Primary School Pupils in Zaria, Northwest Nigeria', *Child and Adolescent Psychiatry and Mental Health*, 11(1), DOI:10.1186/s13034-017-0166-3.

Adams, A.V., Johanson de Silva, S. and Razmara, S. (2013). *Improving Skills Development in the Informal Sector: Strategies for Sub-Saharan Africa*. The World Bank, USA.

Adekola, G. (2013). 'Traditional Apprenticeship in the Old Africa and Its Relevance to Contemporary Work Practices in Modern Nigerian Communities', *British Journal of Education, Society & Behavioural Science*, 3(4), 397–406.

Adewale, A. and Afolabi, B. (2013). 'Street Children Phenomenon in Nigeria: The Challenges and Way Forward', *SSRN Electronic Journal*, DOI:10.2139/ssrn.2325114.

African Commission on Human and People's Rights (2018). *African Charter on the Rights and Welfare of the Child*. Available at: African Charter on the Rights and Welfare of the Child | African Commission on Human and Peoples' Rights (au.int). Accessed on: 20/07/2021.

African Commission on Human and People's Rights (2019). *African Charter on the Rights and Welfare of the Child/Legal Instruments/ACHPR*. Available at: https://www.acerwc.africa/acrwc-full-text/ Accessed on: 27/06/2024.

Ashimolowo, O.R., Aromolaran, A.K. and Inegbedion, S.O. (2010). 'Child Street - Trading Activities and Its Effect on the Educational Attainment of Its Victims in Epe Local Government Area of Lagos State', *Journal of Agricultural Science*, 2(4), 211, DOI:10.5539/jas.v2n4p211.

Ayadike, N., Emeh, I. and Ukah, O. (2012). 'Entrepreneurship Development and Employment Generation in Nigeria: Problems and Prospects', *Universal Journal of Education and General Studies*, 1, 88–102.

Balogun, O. and Orimoogunje, O. (2015). 'Geo-Spatial Mapping of Air Pollution in Benin City, Nigeria', *Journal of Geography, Environment and Earth Science International*, 3(3), 1–17.

Basu, K. and Van, P.H. (1998). 'The Economics of Child Labor', *The American Economic Review*, 88(3), 412–427.

Bhabha, H. (1994). *The Location of Culture*. London: Routledge.

Bhukuth, A. and Ballet, J. (2006). 'Is Child Labour a Substitute for Adult Labour?: A Case Study of Brick Kiln Workers in Tamil Nadu, India', *International Journal of Social Economics*, 33(8), DOI:10.1108/03068290610678734.

Bhukuth, A. and Ballet, J. (2015). 'Children of the Street: Why Are They in the Street? How Do They Live?', *Economics and Sociology*, 8(4), 134–148.

Borbasi, S. and Jackson, D. (2012). *Navigating the Maze of Research: Enhancing Nursing and Midwifery Practice*. Australia: Elsevier.

Bourdillon, M., Crivello, G. and Pankhurst, A. (2015). *In Children's Work and Labour in East Africa: Social Context and Implications for Policy*. Addis Ababa: OSSREA.

Bourdillon, M., Levison, D., Myers, W. and White, B. (2011). *Rights And Wrongs of Children's Work*. New Brunswick: Rutgers University Press.

Bureau of International Affairs (2017). *U.S Department of Labour's 2017 Findings on the Worst Forms of Child Labour: Required by the Trade and Development act 2000*. Available at: https://www.dol.gov/sites/default/files/documents/ilab/ChildLaborReport. pdf. Accessed on: 22/01/2019.

Clark, C. I. D., & Yesufu, S. (2012). Child street trading as an aspect of Child abuse and neglect: Oredo municipality of Edo State, Nigeria as a case study. *European Scientific Journal*, 8(5), 148–158.

Dada, O. (2013). 'A Sociological Investigation of the Determinant Factors and the Effects of Child Street Hawking in Nigeria: Agege, Lagos State, under Survey', *International Journal of Asian Social Science*, 3(1), 114–137.

Denning, S. (2000). *The Springboard: How Storytelling Ignites Action in Knowledge-Era Organizations*. Boston and London: Butterworth Heinemann.

Edewor, P. (2014). 'Homeless Children and Youths in Lagos, Nigeria: Their Characteristics, Street Life and Sexual Behaviour', *Mediterranean Journal of Social Sciences*, 5(1), DOI:10.5901/mjss.2014.v5n1p537.

Ekpiken-Ekanem, R., Ayuk, A. E., & Adadu, P. M. A. (2014). Causal effects of street children in Nigeria: Implications for counselling. *Journal of Education and Practice*, 5(8), 154-158.

Emordi, E.C. and Osiki, O.M. (2008). 'Lagos: The 'Villagized' City', *Information, Society and Justice*, 2(1), 95–109.

Emozozo, R. (2017). *Nigeria's Street Vendors Are Under Fire*. Foundation for Economic Education.

Fajobi, T., Olatujoye, O., Amusa, O. and Adedoyin, A. (2017). 'Challenges of Apprenticeship Development and Youths Unemployment in Nigeria', *Sociology and Criminology-Open Access*, 5(2), DOI:10.4172/2375–4435.1000172.

Federal Child Act (2003). *Child's Right Act*. Available at: Nigeria-Child-Rights-Act-2003. pdf (citizenshiprightsafrica.org). Accessed on: 22/01/2019.

Federal Ministry of Labour and Productivity (2017). *National Action Plan for the Elimination of Child Labour in Nigeria (2013–2017)*. Available at: https://www. ilo.org/wcmsp5/groups/public/---africa/---ro-addis_ababa/---ilo-abuja/documents/ publication/wcms_303410.pdf. Accessed on: 22/10/2019.

Fulton, J. and Hayes, C. (2012). 'Situational Analysis-Framing Approaches to Interpretive Inquiry in Healthcare Research'. *International Journal of Therapy & Rehabilitation*, 19(12), 662–669.

Hammarberg, K., Kirkman, M. and Lacey, S. (2016). 'Qualitative Research Methods: When to Use Them and How to Judge Them', *Human Reproduction*, 31(3), 498–501.

Igwe, L. and Oragwu, A. (2014). 'Techno-Vocational Skills Acquisition and Poverty Reduction Strategies in Vocational Institutions: A Case Study of Rivers State, Nigeria', *African Journal of Education and Technology*, 4(1), 47–58.

Ingham-Broomfield, R. (2015). 'A Nurses' Guide to Qualitative Research', *Australian Journal of Advanced Nursing*, 32(3), 34–40.

International Labour Organisation (2007). *Explaining the Demand and Supply of Child Labour: A Review of the Underlying Theories*. Available at: ICLS_rep_I_theories_ underlying_cl (1).pdf. Accessed on: 02/03/2017.

International Labour Organisation (2017a). *Hazardous Child Labour*. Available at: Hazardous child labour (IPEC) (ilo.org). Accessed on: 21/04/2017.

International Labour Organisation (2017b). *Report: Global Estimates of Child Labour: Results and Trends, 2012–2016*. Available at: wcms_575499.pdf (ilo.org). Accessed on: 02/05/17.

International Labour Organisation (2018). *What Is Child Labour*. Available at: What is child labour (IPEC) (ilo.org). Accessed on: 01/15/2019.

International Labour Organisation (2021). *ILO Convention on Child Labour*. Available at: ILO Conventions on child labour (IPEC). Accessed on: 20/07/21.

International Labour Organisation and United Nations Children Fund (2021). *Child Labour: Global Estimates 2020, Trends and the Road Forward*. Available at: wcms_797515.pdf (ilo.org). Accessed on: 04/09/21.

International Programme on the Elimination of Child labour (2014). *Compendium of Hazardous Child Labour List Nigeria: Country Overview*. Available at: CLP_ Compendium_of_HCL_List_Nigeria.pdf. Accessed on: 04/02/2019.

Johnson, O. and Ihesie, C. (2015). 'Social Implications and Factors Associated with Street Hawking Among Children in Uyo, Akwa Ibom State, Nigeria', *British Journal of Education, Society and Behavioural Sciences*, 11(2), 1–9.

Katz, C. (2004). *Growing Up Global: Economic Restructuring and Children's Everyday Lives*. Minneapolis: University of Minnesota Press.

Kazeem, A. (2013). 'Unpaid Work among Children Currently Attending School in Nigeria: With Focus on Gender, Ethnicity, Urban-Rural Residence and Poverty', *International Journal of Sociology and Social Policy*, 33(5/6), 328–346.

Mosabo, C.J. (2017). *Interface between Children's Work and Schooling in Rural Tanzania*. Norway: Norwegian University of Science and Technology.

Nduka, I. and Duru, C. (2014). 'The Menace of Street Hawking in Aba Metropolis, South-East Nigeria', *Journal of Medicine and Medical Sciences*, 5(6), 135–140.

Okonkwo, H.I. and Alhaji, I.M. (2014). 'Contemporary Issues in Nomadic, Minority and Almajiri Education, Problems and Prospects', *Journal of Education and Practice*, 5(24), 19–27.

Okyere, S. (2012). Re-examining the education-child labour Nexus: The case of child miners at Kenyasi, Ghana. *Childhoods Today*, 6(1), 1–20.

Okyere, S. (2013). 'Are Working Children's Rights and Child Labour Abolition Complementary or Opposing Realms?', *International Social Work*, 56(1), 80–91.

Oluwaleye, J.M. (2017). 'Child Labour among Nigerian Children: Implication for Development', *International Journal of Development and Sustainability*, 6(12), 2193–2215.

Omiyinka, F.O. (2009). 'Social Networks and Livelihood of Street Children in Ibadan, Nigeria', *International Journal of Sociology and Anthropology*, 1(15), 1–8.

Omofonmwan, S.I. and Eseigbe, J.O. (2009). 'Effects of Solid Waste on the Quality of Underground Water in Benin Metropolis, Nigeria', *Journal of Human Ecology*, 26(2), 99–105.

Onodugo, V.A., Ezeadichie, N.H., Onwuneme, C.A. and Anosike, A.E. (2016). 'The Dilemma of Managing the Challenges of Street Vending in Public Spaces: The Case of Enugu City, Nigeria', *Cities*, 59, 95–101, DOI:10.1016/j.cities.2016.06.001.

Orkin, K. (2010). 'In the Child's Best Interests? Legislation on Children's Work in Ethiopia', *Journal of International Development*, 22(8), 1102–1114.

Robson, E. (2004). 'Hidden Child Workers: Young Carers in Zimbabwe', *Antipode*, 36(2), 227–248.

Terres Des Hommes (2010). *Children in street situations*. Available at: TerreDesHommes. pdf (ohchr.org). Accessed on: 08/03/2018.

The World Bank in Nigeria (2018). *World Bank in Nigeria*. Available at: Nigeria Overview: Development news, research, data | World Bank. Accessed on: 22/01/2019.

Umar, F. (2009). 'Street Hawking: Oppressing the Girl Child or Family Economic Supplement? – ProQuest', *Journal of Instructional Psychology*, 36(2), 169–174.

Uyieh, J. (2018). 'Eko Gb'ole o Gbole': A Historical Study of Youth and Tout Culture in Shomolu Local Government Area, Lagos, 1976–2015', *Journal of African Cultural Studies*, 30(3), 323–338, DOI:10.1080/13696815.2018.1463844.

Wallis, P. (2008). 'Apprenticeship and Training in Premodern England', *Journal of Economic History*, 68, 832–681.

Young Lives (2016). *Children's Work*. Available at: https://www.younglives.org.uk/ content/childrens-work. Accessed on: 08/09/2018.

17

HEALTH-SEEKING BEHAVIOUR FOR CHILDHOOD DIARRHOEA

Benjamin Maduabuchi Aniugbo, Catherine Hayes and John Fulton

Introduction

> Diarrhea, 90 percent of which is caused by food and water contaminated by excrement, kills a child every fifteen seconds. That's more than AIDS, malaria, or measles, combined. Human feces are an impressive weapon of mass destruction.
>
> *Rose George (Journalist and Author)*

Introduction

Diarrhoea is the second leading cause of mortality in children under five years worldwide (WHO, 2013). Every year, an estimated 2.5 billion cases of diarrhoea are reported in children under five years of age, and these result in death and a huge economic burden worldwide. Walker et al. (2013) highlighted that 1.7 billion cases of diarrhoeal disease were reported, with 2% progressing to more severe cases. Of the 7.6 million deaths reported in children of less than five years in 2010, 10.5% were caused by diarrhoea (Liu et al., 2012).

Liu et al. (2012) highlighted that diarrhoeal mortality has reduced from 1.160 to 0.801 million, representing a 4% decrease per year from 2000 to 2010 in children aged under five years. Despite the decline recorded worldwide, probably due to the implementation of various child survival interventions, the situation in Africa remains an area of global concern. The average child in developing countries experiences three or more episodes of diarrhoeal disease each year, accounting for up to 4 billion cases annually (Black et al., 2010).

The incidence of diarrhoea in children varies substantially among different regions, with the highest rate found in low-income countries such as Nigeria

DOI: 10.4324/9781003467601-20

than high-income countries (Black et al., 2010). UNICEF (2009) reported that approximately 1.5 million deaths in children under five years occur each year because of diarrhoea, with 80% of these deaths occurring in Africa. The highest mortality rates occur in Sub-Saharan Africa, where 50% of total child mortality is caused by diarrhoea (Walker et al., 2013).

Owing to the evident impact of diarrhoeal illness in developing countries such as Nigeria, the Millennium Development Goals highlighted diarrhoea as a key public health challenge in developing countries, and organizations, such as UNICEF and WHO have both implemented strategic interventions to combat the effect of diarrhoea (UNICEF, 2012a,b). The Nigerian Ministry of Health has also adopted an array of procedures and policies to address the burden of diarrhoeal illness in children aged under five, which included the use of recommended zinc supplementation and oral rehydration therapy (Nigeria Zinc Study Team, 2008). Despite these interventions, Nigeria's National Demographic and Health Survey (National Population Commission, 2015) showed that despite increasing knowledge of the use of interventions such as oral rehydration therapy and zinc supplementation, the health-seeking behaviours of caregivers still remain poor, especially amongst caregivers in rural community settings. It also revealed that despite increased knowledge amongst rural dwellers in the South-Eastern region of Nigeria, with Enugu recording 86% awareness, health-seeking behaviour remained minimal (National Population Commission, 2015).

Aims of the Study

While research has been undertaken to examine factors influencing health-seeking behaviour in the treatment of childhood illness (Ezeoke et al., 2010), few have examined the factors relating specifically to diarrhoeal illness. There are thus a very limited number of studies that have examined the socio-demographic factors affecting access to healthcare for childhood diarrhoea in the rural communities of Enugu State. Those that are available engaged participants from urban areas and were conducted within tertiary healthcare facilities in urban cities (Ezeoke et al., 2010).

The aim of this study was to investigate the role of demographic and socio-economic characteristics in determining the health-seeking behaviours of those caring for children with diarrhoea and illness in rural communities in the Enugu state of Nigeria. The objectives of the study were focused on:

1 Establishing characteristic patterns of health-seeking behaviour for children with diarrhoeal illness in rural communities of Nkanu West LGA of Enugu State, Nigeria.
2 Investigating any relationship between evident social and demographic factors and the health-seeking behaviour of caregivers for children with diarrhoeal illness.

Testifiable Hypotheses for the Study

Null Hypothesis (HO): There is no association between socio-demographic factors and Health Seeking Behaviour of Caregivers for children with diarrhoeal illness aged under five years.

Alternative Hypothesis (H1): There is association between socio-demographic factors and Health Seeking Behaviour of Caregivers for children with hoeal illness aged under five years.

The Social Epidemiology of Diarrhoeal Illness

Diarrhoea is one of the leading causes of preventable death in children under five globally, especially in developing countries (WHO, 2013). Owing to the vulnerability of children under five years, diarrhoea grossly compromises their well-being, considerably creating a huge demand for health care services for the management (WHO, 2013). In 2011 alone, diarrhoea caused about 700,000 deaths in children under five years of age (Bhutta et al., 2013). Diarrhoea still represents the second leading cause of preventable deaths in children after pneumonia (Fischer-Walker et al., 2013; UNICEF, 2012b). Despite advancements in disease management, the prevalence has remained high, especially in developing countries (Liu et al., 2012). According to a report by UNICEF (2009), implementation of ORS, improved health care utilization and breast-feeding practices have led to a significant decline in mortality from 4.5 million in the 1980s to 1.3 million in 2008. Despite this decline, studies still suggest that diarrhoea remains a huge burden in developing countries (Black et al., 2010; Walker et al., 2012). In 2011, diarrhoea accounted for 9.9% of the over-all 6.9 million deaths among children under five (Fischer-Walker et al., 2013). According to the WHO (2013), there are 1.7 million incidences of diarrhoea every year.

Regional Distribution of Childhood b Illness

The burden of diarrhoea in children under five varies according to region. While it remains one of the major causes of mortality in children under five in America and Europe (Guarino et al., 2014), Africa still has the highest prevalence of diarrhoea in children (Black et al., 2010). Diarrhoea remains a significant cause of morbidity and mortality in children under five years in Sub-Saharan Africa (Aremu et al., 2011). In 2012, Sub-Saharan Africa and south Asia represented 82% of the global mortality in children under five, with diarrhoea accounting for 9% of the deaths (UNICEF, 2012a,b). A systematic analysis conducted by Liu et al. (2015) in 2013 reveals that half of the 578,000 deaths from diarrhoea occurred in Sub-Saharan Africa.

Variation in Epidemiology in a Global Context

The prevalence and mortality rates of diarrhoea in children under five years of age have shown variation across several countries (Bhutta et al., 2013). According to a report from UNICEF on childhood mortality, about half of the deaths occurring in children under five years globally are concentrated in developing countries like Nigeria, India, the Congo, China and Pakistan (UNICEF, 2012a). This suggests that diarrhoea remains a major public health challenge in developing countries like Nigeria. Evidence from a report published by the WHO on country-ranking mortality from diarrhoea in children under five suggests that there are 66.96 per 100,000 adjusted deaths (WHO, 2014).

A historical study conducted by Iyun and Oke (2000) in Nigeria estimated that about 25% of children in Nigeria die of diarrhoea before they celebrate their fifth birthday. Diarrhoea incidence varies with age, with the highest incidence occurring during the first two years of life (Boschi-Pinto et al., 2008). This reported vulnerability of children to diarrhoea is associated with biological predisposition (Khanal et al., 2015). During the second half of an infant's life, immunity is often weaker and diarrhoeal illness appears to have a higher incidence and prevalence rate at this age. This explains why some socio-demographic factors such as the age of the child, hygienic practices, worm infestation, contamination of weaning food, sanitary facilities and consumption of foods from street vendors play a significant role in the occurrence of diarrhoeal illness in children in developing countries such as Nigeria (Aziz et al., 2016; Cronin et al., 2016). Evidently, according to the WHO's (2013) report, globally, 780 million individuals lack access to improved drinking water and 2.5 billion lack improved sanitation. These factors appear to be why diarrhoeal illness appears to be more concentrated in developing countries.

While social and environmental factors have been attributed as predisposing risk factors in the development of diarrhoeal illness in children, research carried out in Nigeria to measure the effect of rotavirus in diarrhoea in children showed that rotavirus remains the commonest cause of severe diarrhoeal dehydration in children in Nigeria (Iyoha and Abiodun, 2015; Odimayo et al., 2008). This is estimated to cause approximately 111 million episodes of diarrhoeal illness, 2 million hospitalizations and 400,000 deaths in children under five years, annually with 82% of the deaths occurring in developing countries (Iyoha and Abiodun, 2015). However, in Sub-Saharan African countries such as Nigeria, it has been shown that factors such as child nutrition, dry season, age under 2, bottle feeding, low birth weight, male gender, maternal smoking, maternal age less than 20 and Human Immunodeficiency Virus (HIV) are associated with the incidence of rotavirus disease in children under five (Odimayo et al., 2008). The incidence of diarrhoea varies with the changing of the seasons in Nigeria (Boschi-pinto et al., 2008; Gyoh, 2011).

Dehydration and malnutrition due to the loss of fluid and nutrients are the major causes of death in diarrhoeal illness (UNICEF, 2012b). It is estimated that 88% of diarrhoea-associated deaths are directly attributable to unsafe water, inadequate sanitation and hygiene measures (Cronin et al., 2016). Most recently, rotavirus has played an important role in the aetiology of acute diarrhoea; it causes about 40% of diarrhoea in children under five especially in developing countries such as Nigeria (Liu et al., 2012; Tate et al., 2012). Evidence from research across developing countries demonstrates that poor sanitation practices, lack of access to clean water, poor hand washing hygiene and lack of proper feeding practices remain significant causes of diarrhoea in children (WHO, 2013).

Several studies have identified specific biological factors associated with the prevalence and incidence of diarrhoeal illness in children across the globe (Karambu et al., 2013). Some bacteria such as Enterotoxigenic E. coli, Salmonella Paratyphi, Shigella species and virus appear to be the most common infective agents; however, other environmental factors have been associated with the burden of diarrhoeal illness in children (Brown et al., 2015). Factors associated with the incidence of diarrhoea vary across regions and countries. In Sub-Saharan African countries like Nigeria, lack of access to clean water and effective sanitation remain a huge burden (Oloruntoba et al., 2014). According to WHO report in 2010, about 884 million people lack access to clean water, whereas 2.6 million people do not have access to effective sanitation facilities (WHO, 2010). Consequently, about 25% of people in developing countries defecate in open spaces and consequently this waste has the potential of being washed into major streams used as drinking water resources (Segecha, 2013; UNICEF, 2012b). Since children have developing immunity, which is still weak, they remain most vulnerable to diarrhoeal illnesses (Schilling, 2010). However, research by Finkbeiner et al. (2008) observed that about 40% of the cause of diarrhoea are of an unknown aetiology. Nigeria, in common with other developing countries in Sub-Saharan Africa and Asia lacks access to safe water and proper sanitation in the majority of rural communities (Oloruntoba et al., 2014). The majority of people in rural communities do not have access to appropriate sanitation facilities; hence, people defecate in open spaces which are effectively act as discharges of infectious disease to environments where children are most at risk of contracting infectious gastrointestinal disease.

Similarly, other factors such as fly infestation and the consumption of street foods have contributed to the increased incidence of diarrhoea in children (Oadi and Kuitunen, 2005). In addition to this, evidence reveals poor infant feeding practices contribute directly to the incidence of diarrhoea in children (WHO, 2012). Research has shown that lack of exclusive breastfeeding for up to six months, as well as introduction of complementary feeding at an early stage, increases the risk of development of diarrhoeal illness in children across Africa (Mohammed and Tamiru, 2014).

The Social Epidemiology of Health-Seeking Behaviour

Different models and theories have been proposed to explain the social epidemiology of health-seeking behaviour/healthcare utilization in individuals, alongside the wider determinants of health. They predict various factors that influence health-seeking behaviour in individuals. However, specific theories can be used to explain the relationship between health-seeking behaviour and social, economic and demographic factors. Health belief model (HBM) (Becker, Strecher and Rosenstock, 1988) highlighted that an individual's ability to seek care can be influenced by their perceived vulnerability and susceptibility to illness and health consequences. To support this view, evidence from studies also suggests that caregivers are more likely to adopt an appropriate health-seeking behaviour when they perceive the illness to be severe and threaten the lives of their children (Lamberti et al., 2015).

Bourdieu (1986) argued that the social capital (social and cultural network) affiliated with individuals plays a significant role in contributing to their ability to manage health and utilize health services. According to his idea, social capital can include the family, relatives and community. This proposition is in congruence with the Graham and White (2016) commentaries on the wider determinants of health, which included the social environment as one of the major influencers of health and health care utilization. Moreover, a study found that caregiver's choices for health seeking outside the home can be influenced by significant others (Gera et al., 2015).

Enabling factors are logistics necessary for healthcare utilization. These factors must be available even in the presence of predisposing factors. They are necessary to purchase healthcare services. They include income, the presence of health facilities in the community, accessibility to health facilities and the presence of health insurance. Finally, need factors, according to Andersen and Newman (2005), are perceived needs for health care, which include perceived severity, vulnerability, susceptibility and past experience. Caregivers need for health seeking outside the home may be influenced by these factors.

This study adopted a positivist approach to enquiry, which assumed that the existence of an observable reality could be uncovered via statistical analysis of collated information from tangible variables (Bruce et al., 2007). As the study sought to investigate the numerical relationship between caregiver utilization of healthcare services for children with diarrhoea and socio-demographic factors, quantitative methodology was deemed appropriate. However, the design adopted used aggregate data, which could only provide information about the sample chosen and not on the basis of the individual. This may suggest that any association found in the aggregate data may not necessarily mean the same on an individual level (Spicker, 2008). This design, therefore, could show correlation but not causality, hence the need to apply a qualitative approach in the context of individual attribution of its findings.

This study involved a quantitative research approach using a cross-sectional survey design to systematically collect information from purposively recruited participants with the aim of predicting a phenomenon in a population of interest (Rovai et al., 2013). Survey design deals with the recruitment of a sample that is representative of the population of interest in order to understand a phenomenon within the population (Levy and Lemeshow, 2013). Additionally, it uses statistics to measure outcomes of phenomena that can be generalized within the population of interest (Rovai et al., 2013). Another characteristic of cross-sectional survey design is its ability to estimate a degree of certainty from a sample that can be inferred for the entire population of interest. To achieve this, random sampling of intended communities from the entire population was adopted, thus giving every community a chance of being selected (Levy and Lemeshow, 2013). Usually, to ensure very reliable sampling, some defined techniques are adopted, such as the use of computers. However, this study adopted manual random sampling (this is discussed in detail in the sampling section).

Study Setting

This study was conducted in the Nkanu West Local Government Area of Enugu State, Nigeria. Enugu State is in the eastern part of Nigeria, West Africa. Nkanu West on itself is located within the eastern part of Enugu State under the Enugu East senatorial district. According to the 2006 census, it has a population of 147,385 (F = 74,679, M = 72,706) (National Population CommissionNigerian Data P 2006). It is constituted of nine communities/villages with 18 political wards. The local government secretariat/headquarters are at Agbani. The predominant ethnicity is Igbo, with majorly Christians and few traditional religious practices. Also, the predominant language is Igbo and rarely English. Basic amenities such as roads, market and schools are available; however, health facilities are majorly primary health care centres and traditional birth attendants (TBAs), which provide mainly preventive and promotive health services.

Target PopulationNi

The study population for this study was made up of caregivers of children under five years of age in the Nkanu West Local Government area of Enugu State, Nigeria. Research was conducted between June and July 2016.

Inclusion Criteria

This study included participants who were primary caregivers of children under five years of age who have had diarrhoeal illness in the last three months. The participants were residents of the Nkanu West local government area of Enugu

State for the last five years. Participants must have visited the primary health centres (PHCs) for any healthcare reasons.

Sampling

A multi-stage sampling technique was used to select communities, wards, health facilities (PHC) and participants for this study. This sampling method was used because of its ability to provide equal opportunity for each community/village, health nd except for participants, to be selected (Bryman, 2016). The procedures are as follows:

Step 1 (Selection of Communities): Six communities were randomly selected by simple random sampling using the lottery method. First, each community was written on separate paper and folded into a container. The container was shaken vigorously, and a research assistant was asked to pick the communities randomly until the desired number of wards was reached.

Step 2 (Selection of Wards and Primary Healthcare Centres): Some of the six selected communities had more than one PHC, which is allocated according to the political ward. Political wards are electoral subdivisions created for people who share more similar demographic features. Each ward had a political leader known as the councillor. Therefore, this study adopted the use of political wards to select PHC instead of communities. This is to give every PHC in each ward an opportunity to be selected. Moreover, this approach coincides with the Ward Health System (WHS) policy in Nigeria. To select the wards, simple random sampling using the lottery method as applied in stage one was adopted. A number was assigned to each of the 13 political wards. Any community that has more than 1 ward but only 1 PHC is classified as 1 ward, and vice versa. The selected communities were made up of 13 wards. Six PHCs were selected by simple random sampling using the lottery method (as in stage one).

Step 3 (selection of respondents): A total of 150 respondents (25 from each PHC) were sampled by purposive sampling. Purposive sampling was adjudged appropriate because the respondents had already been predetermined. Although it has been argued to lack strong reliability in randomizing respondents, the use of purposive sampling in this study was considered appropriate to select the required respondents. Additionally, purposive sampling was used because of its easy access to the participants, flexibility, time and high response rate (Uprichard, 2013). Eligible participants were given questionnaires to complete until the required number was reached. An initial sample size calculation was attempted through an online medium to determine the significant size of the sample at the confidence level (CI) of 95%. However, because sample size is unlikely to be significant for non-probability sampling, the calculation is therefore not used.

Pilot Study

A pilot study is the collection of data about the study before the main study. This process allows the researcher the opportunity to interview a few participants who share similar characteristics with the original participants required for the main study (Leon et al., 2011) so as to make amendments based on the responses from the piloted participants. According to Williams (2014), it is useful to ensure if the participants understand the use of terminologies in the questionnaire as well as a measure of the reliability and validity of the questionnaire.

The questionnaire was piloted on six conveniently selected participants from different PHCs who shared similar characteristics with the intended participant. Those were mothers of children who have had diarrhoea in the last three months. The reason for the piloting was to test the reliability and validity of the questionnaire and restructure the questionnaire to match the backgrounds of the participants in the Nkanu West Local Government area of Enugu State. The result of the piloting resulted in a few modifications to the question. This new modification therefore included the actions of mothers should their children had diarrhoea that lasted longer than 14 days. This was part of a behaviour risk assessment that is of great significance to health promotion strategies in the region.

Data Collection

A structured, self-administered questionnaire was used for data collection. A self-administered questionnaire was considered appropriate to allow respondents to complete the questionnaire themselves with minimal influence from the researcher. The validity of the questionnaire was determined through the pilot study. Six caregivers who have children under five years who have had diarrhoea were given the questionnaire to complete. The analysis of the completed questionnaire aligns with the intent of the researcher. This therefore shows that the actual respondents who have the same characteristics as those used for the pilot can be able to complete the question.

The study chose three months as the maximum period a child will have had diarrhoea for the caregiver to participate in the study. The validity of these indicators is influenced by the caregiver's perception of diarrhoea as a disease and her capacity to recall any event of diarrhoea in the child. In addition, this time covered the period when diarrhoea usually occurs in children due to variations in the weather (raining season). The researcher acknowledged the challenge of recall bias; however, where needed, the researchers used the names of market days to elicit the recall of any event of diarrhoea.

However, because the predominant language of the respondents was Igbo language, the researcher therefore utilized and trained four student nurses to assist in administering and interpreting the questionnaires where necessary. According to Phellas et al. (2011), the interviewer can guide the participant to complete a questionnaire. This is different from an interviewer-administered questionnaire. However, the use of interpreters and assistants may have offered potential limitations to the study due to the risk of social desirability and bias (Krumpal, 2013). Questions translated may have led to mistranslation, and the researcher may have filtered the answers provided verbally. Despite these potential limitations, the questionnaires provided a basic view of the proportion of caregivers who have used different PHCs.

The questionnaire consists of 23 questions divided into three sections: A, B and C. Section A comprises the caregiver's bio-demographic data and is meant to help the researcher determine any correlation between the caregiver's and healthcare-seeking behaviour. Section B is comprised of the child's bio-demographic data and information about significant orders, such as the father. This information will help to examine any correlation between child-factors such as sex and age and caregiver's health-seeking behaviour. Finally, Section C explores caregiver's health-seeking behaviour for DIC. The questionnaires were distributed to the respondents, completed and returned to the researchers on the same day. The returned questionnaires were kept in a secured bag.

Data Analysis

Data analysis is a significant component of quantitative research because it provides insight and meaning to the data collected from participants. It comprises all test tools and processes employed for transforming raw data from respondents into useful information (Treiman, 2014). In this research, both descriptive and inferential statistical analyses will be done. The analyses were done using the statistical package for social science version 21.

In data analysis, descriptive statistics are generally useful in generating and organizing original data from respondents into a meaningful pattern of information. According to Romero and Ventura (2013), descriptive statistics usually calculate the frequency and percentage of each response from respondents. Therefore, this explains reason why it is usually the first statistical analysis in quantitative research, as recommended by Romero and Ventura (2013). Contrary to descriptive statistics, inferential statistics are used to make predictions about the population from a sample randomly selected for the study (Jackson, 2015). According to Pallant (2013), inferential statistics are used to estimate that the relationship observed in a sample is depended or not on observed variables. In this study, descriptive analysis was conducted on the entire 23 questions and responses. As with traditional descriptive statistics, responses will be displayed in frequency tables and graphs.

Furthermore, because inferential statistics are used to estimate relationships between variables that are observable in a group, special statistical test packages are specially used for the analysis of responses. Therefore, it is used to test hypotheses. However, the choice of package used depends on the type of data, such as whether it is ordinal, nominal or categorical (Pallant, 2013). In this study, chi square was used as the preferred inferential data analysis tool. This was used because both the independent and dependent variables are nominal in nature. This is in congruence with the recommendatiy Duke et al. (2020) who recommends the use of chi square as an ideal when both the independent and dependent variables are nominal data. The level of significance set out in which to either accept or reject the null hypothesis was a = 5% = 0.05. This means that a p value less than 0.05 accepts the null hypothesis, and vice versa. The results will be presented in tables and graphs.

Results

For the purpose of this study, the results have been presented in two different forms namely, descriptive and inferential analyses.

A descriptive analysis has been used to describe the frequencies and percentages of the results. Additionally, to ensure accessibility of the data, it has been presented in frequency tables and graphs. Inferential statistics have been used to address the specific objectives of the research. The Chi-square testing was used to analyse the data.

Response Rate

150 questionnaires were administered to consenting participants who visited PHCs in the six randomly selected wards in the Nkanu West local government area of Enugu State, Nigeria. Of the 150 administered questionnaires, 140 were completed and returned:

$$Response\ Rate\ = \frac{No.\ of\ completed\ survey\ questionnaires\ returned}{No.\ of\ survey\ questionnaires\ administered} \times 100\%$$

$$= \frac{140 \times 100\%}{150} = 93.3\%$$

This response rate is similar to the 92.8% recorded in a similar study conducted in rural Ghana by Daniels, Ahenkan and Poku (2013) to examine factors affecting maternal health service utilization. Although response rate is not a significant determinant of the validity of a result in purposive sampling, a response rate of 93.3% has been considered as significant rate (Abiodun et al., 2013).

Descriptive Statistics of Independent Variables

Participant Gender

Participants in this study represent primary caregivers of children under five years. 100% (140) of the participants were female.

Caregivers Age

Of the total participants, 42.1 (59) are within the age range of 26–30 years, 22.9% (32) are within 31–35 years, 20.7% (29) are within 36–40 years and only 14.3% (20) are within 20–25 years (Table 17.1; Figure 17.1).

TABLE 17.1 Tabulation of Caregiver Age

Variable	Frequency (n = 140)	Valid Percent (%)
20–25	20	14.3
26–30	59	42.1
31–35	32	22.9
35–40	29	20.7
Total	140	100

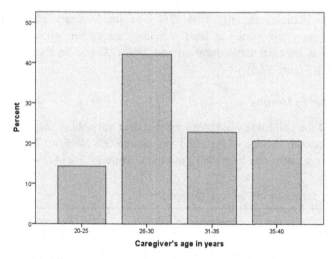

FIGURE 17.1 "Caregivers' Occupation", is a bar chart with the bottom axes entitle Caregivers' Occupation, the occupations are listed as housewife, farmer, artisan, employee, unemployed, student and trader. The side axes are the percentages of each occupation. The percentages are illustrated as follows: housewife just under 10%, farmer just under 20%, artisan just under the housewife figure, employee as 20%, unemployed as 10%, student as the mid-point between 0 and 10% and trader as 30%.

Religion/Faith

100% (140) of the participants reported belonging to the Christian faith.

Ethnicity

100% of the participants are from the Igbo ethnic group in the eastern part of Nigeria, where the study was conducted.

Caregiver Occupation

Occupation was used as an indicator for the wealth quantile of the participants. () was adopted to describe the occupation. Those within the socio-economic status of the middle class are employees, self-employed traders and artisans. Housewives, farmers, students and the unemployed are classified as lower-class. However, the wealth described for each occupation may not be a true representative of the socio-economic status of the participants. 30.0% (42) of the participants are traders, while 19.3% (27) are employees, 17.9% (25) are farmers, 9.3% (13) are unemployed, 8.6% (12) are housewives, 7.9% (11) are artisans and 7.1% (10) are students (Table 17.2; Figure 17.2).

Caregivers Educational Status

Out of the participants, only 15% (21) completed tertiary education. 35% (49) participants completed at least secondary education, whereas 30% (42) completed at least primary education and 20% (28) had no formal education (Table 17.3; Figure 17.3).

Age of Child in Months

The age of the child was used as an independent variable to measure the relationship between the age of the child and caregiver's HSB. 40.7% (57) of the children were under one year (0–12 months), while 29.3% (41) are within two

TABLE 17.2 Tabulation of Caregiver Occupation

Variables	Frequency (n = 140)	Valid Percent (%)
Housewife	12	8.6
Farmer	25	17.9
Artisan	11	7.9
Employee	27	19.3
Unemployed	13	9.3
Student	10	7.1
Trader	42	30.0
Total	140	100

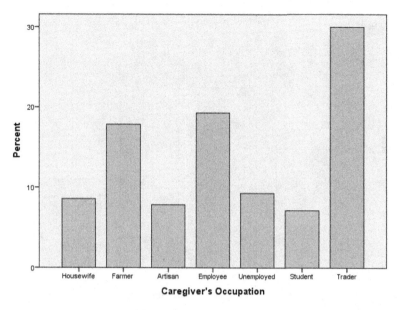

FIGURE 17.2   Tabulation of Caregiver Occupation

TABLE 17.3 Tabulation of Caregiver Educational Status

Variables	Frequency (n = 140)	Valid Percent (%)
No formal education	28	20.0
Primary education	42	30.0
Secondary education	49	35.0
Tertiary education	21	15.0
Total	140	100

years (13–24 months), 16.4% (23) are under three years (25–36 months) and 13.6% (19) are under five years (37–48 months) (Table 17.4).

Child Gender

Gender is an independent variable used to measure the relationship between a child's age and caregiver's HSB. Around 52.1% (73) are males, and 47.9% (67) are females (Table 17.5).

Father's Occupation

Caregivers were asked about the father's occupation. 25.7% (36) were artisan, 24.3% (34) were traders, 21.4% (30) were employees, 14.3% (20) were

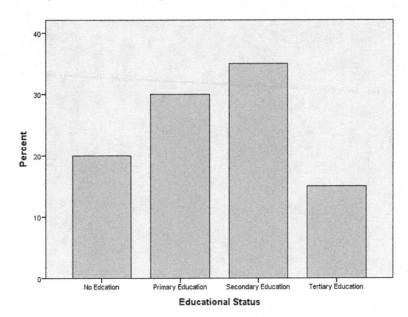

FIGURE 17.3 "Educational Status" has a bottom axis showing four types of education levels: No Education, Primary Education, Secondary Education, Tertiary Education. The side axes are the percentage of each education level. No Education is showing as 20%, Primary Education is showing as just under 30%, Secondary Education is showing as mid-way between 30% and 40% and Tertiary Education is showing as just over 10%.

TABLE 17.4 Tabulation of Child Age in Months

Variables	Frequency (n = 140)	Valid Percent (%)
0–12	57	40.7
13–24	41	29.3
25–36	23	16.4
37–48	19	13.6
Total	140	100

TABLE 17.5 Tabulation of Child Gender

Variables	Frequency (n = 140)	Valid Percent (%)
Male	73	52.1
Female	67	47.9
Total	140	100

commercial bus drivers, 9.3% (13) were farmers and 5.0% (7) were clergy. This dependent variable was used to measure the relationship between a father's occupation (wealth) and appropriate health-seeking behaviour (Table 17.6).

Descriptive Statistics of Dependent Variables

Frequency of Diarrhoea

Frequency was used to examine the severity of diarrhoea. Respondents were asked whether the diarrhoea lasted for 14 days or longer. Out of 140 respondents, only 10 (7.1%) reported the child's diarrhoea lasting up to 14 days (Table 17.7).

Seeking Health Care Outside of the Home

Respondents were asked in the questionnaire if they sought any kind of health services outside of the home. Around 74.3% (104) answered yes. Only 25.7% (36) did not seek health services outside of the home (Table 17.8).

TABLE 17.6 Tabulation of Father's Occupation

Variables	Frequency (n = 140)	Valid Percent (%)
Farmer	13	9.3
Artisan	36	25.7
Employee	30	21.4
Commercial bus driver	20	14.3
Clergy	7	5.0
Trader	34	24.3
Total	140	100

TABLE 17.7 Tabulation of Frequency of Diarrhoea

Variable	Frequency (n = 140)	Valid Percent (%)
Yes	10	7.1
No	130	92.9
Total	140	100

TABLE 17.8 Tabulation of Seeking Health Care Outside of the Home

Variable	Frequency (n = 140)	Valid Percent (%)
Yes	104	74.3
No	36	25.7
Total	140	100

Place of Visit

Those who sought health services outside of the home were asked to choose from the list where they visited. 38 (27.1%) reported visiting a PHC, 25 (17.9%) visited a TBA, 17 (12.1%) visited chemists, 15 (10.7%) visited hospital and 10 (7.1%) sought help from a traditional healer (Table 17.9).

Factors Influencing Health Choice of Place Visited

Respondents who sought health care outside the home were asked the specific reason for their choice. The majority reported accessibility, 37.1% (39). Other reasons include affordability, 24.8% (26), recommendation from relatives/friends, 20.0% (21), to receive specialist care, 10.5% (11) and for better service, 7.6% (8) (Table 17.10).

Barriers to Health Seeking Outside Home

Respondents who did not seek for care outside the home were asked their reasons. Barriers reported by respondents include perceived severity (not serious), 45.7% (16), cost of treatment, 31.4% (11) and health care facility being far from home, 22.9% (8). Therefore, this suggests that perceived severity of illness played a major role in not seeking care outside the home (Table 17.11).

TABLE 17.9 Tabulation of Place of Visit

Variables	Frequency (n = 140)	Valid Percent (%)
Traditional Birth Attendant	25	23.8
Primary Health Centre	37	36.2
Chemist	17	16.2
Hospital	15	14.3
Traditional healer	10	9.5
Total	104	100
Total	140	

TABLE 17.10 Tabulation of Factors Influencing Health Choice of the Places Visited

Variables	Frequency (n = 140)	Valid Percent (%)
Affordability	26	24.8
Accessibility	38	37.1
Recommended by relatives/friends	21	20.0
Specialist care	11	10.5
Better service	8	7.6
Total	104	100

Use of Oral Rehydration Therapy

As part of the recommended regimen for diarrhoea in children, oral rehydration therapy use was included as health-seeking behaviour/ health care utilization. Respondents were therefore asked to give their children oral rehydration solutions during the episode of diarrhoea. 86.4% (121) answered yes, while only 13.6% (19) answered no (Table 17.12).

Those who answered no were further asked why they did not (table 14). 68.4% (13) answered lack of knowledge of the use, whereas 31.6% (6) answered lack of access to oral rehydration solution (Table 17.13).

Inferential Statistics of the Relationship between Socio-Demographic Characteristics and Health-Seeking Behaviour

The Chi square test was used to develop the inferential statistics, which explained the relationship between measured variables such as socio-demographic factors and health-seeking behaviour. Null and alternative hypotheses were tested to either accept or reject the null hypothesis. The level of significance adopted for the measurement was a p value of 0.05.

TABLE 17.11 Tabulation of Barriers to Health Seeking Behaviours Outside of the Home

Variables	Frequency (n = 140)	Valid Percent (%)
Distance	9	22.9
Cost of treatment	11	31.4
Not serious (perceived severity)	16	45.7
Total	36	100

TABLE 17.12 Tabulation of Use of Oral Hydration Therapy

Variables	Frequency (n = 140)	Valid Percent (%)
Yes	121	86.4
No	19	13.6
Total	140	100

TABLE 17.13 Factors Affecting Non Use of Oral Rehydration Therapy

Variable	Frequency (n = 140)	Valid Percent (%)
Knowledge	13	68.4
Lack of access to recipe/ORS	6	31.6
Total	19	100

Hypothesis One: There Is No Significant Relationship between Socio-Demographic Characteristics and Caregivers' Health-Seeking Behaviour

Education versus Health Seeking Outside Home

A Chi-square test showed that a significant relationship exists between the education of caregivers and health care seeking outside for children under five years who have diarrhoea ($p = 0.000$). However, the result also shows that parents with secondary education are more likely to take their children for health care outside the home (Table 17.14).

Education Versus Place Visited

The Chi-square test result showed a significant relationship between education and place of visit. This therefore provides evidence to reject the null hypothesis that there is no relationship between caregivers' education and health service utilization (Table 17.15).

TABLE 17.14 Result of Chi Square Test on the Relationship between Caregiver's Education and Health Seeking Outside Home

Variables	Visit to Health Care Facility		Total
	Yes	No	
No formal education	16	12	28
Primary education	23	19	42
Secondary education	46	3	49
Tertiary education	19	2	21
Total	104	36	140

Chi square = 25.417; df = 3; Asymp. Sig. (2-sided) = 0.000, Phi = 0.426
Significant = $p < 0.05$; Non-significant = $p > 0.05$

TABLE 17.15 Result of Chi Square Test on the Relationship between Caregiver's Education and Place Visited

Variables	TBA	PHC	Chemist	Hospital	Traditional Healer	Total
No formal education	6	2	5	0	4	17
Primary	6	5	6	2	4	23
Secondary	9	21	4	10	2	45
Tertiary	4	10	2	3	0	19
Total	25	38	17	15	10	104

Chi square = 26.137; df = 12; Asymptotic Sig. = 0.010, Phi = 0.499
Significant = $p < 0.05$; Non-significant = $p > 0.05$

Education versus the Use of Oral Rehydration Therapies

Chi square test analysis indicated a significant relationship between caregiver's education and ORT use. P value = 0.001. Therefore, this result presented no sufficient evidence to accept the null hypothesis that age does not influence HSB. P value = 0.001 (Table 17.16).

In summary, a statistically significant relationship was observed between caregiver's educational status and seeking care outside of home (df = 3; $p < 0.000$), choice of place visited (df = 12; $p < 0.010$) and use of ORT (df = 3; $p < 0.001$). This result therefore provided sufficient evidence to reject the null hypothesis, which proposed that caregiver's education is completely independent of seeking care outside of home, the place visited and the use of ORT.

Occupation

The Chi-square test above showed that no significant relationship between caregiver's occupation and health seeking outside the home existed. This suggests sufficient evidence to accept the null hypothesis that caregiver's occupation does not influence health-seeking behaviour outside of the home (Tables 17.17–17.19)

TABLE 17.16 Result of Chi Square Test on the Relationship between Caregiver's Education and Use of ORT

Variables	Yes	No	Total
No formal education	18	10	28
Primary education	36	6	42
Secondary education	48	1	49
Tertiary education	19	2	21
Total	121	19	140

Chi square = 17.570; df = 3; Asymptotic Sig. = 0.001, Phi = 0.354
Significant = $p < 0.05$; Non-significant = $p > 0.05$

TABLE 17.17 Result of Chi Square Test on Relationship between Caregiver's Occupation and Health Seeking Outside Home

Variables	Yes	No	Total
Housewife	9	3	12
Farmer	16	9	25
Artisan	8	3	11
Employee	24	3	27
Unemployed	7	6	13
Student	10	0	10
Trader	30	12	42
Total	104	36	140

TABLE 17.18 Tabulation of Occupation

	Value	df	Asymptotic Significance (2-sided)
Pearson chi-square	10.900	6	0.092
Likelihood ratio	13.519	6	0.035
Linear-by-linear association	0.130	1	0.719
N of valid cases	140		

4 cells (28.6%) have expected count less than 5. The minimum expected count is 2.57, Phi = 0.279
Significant = p < 0.05; Non-significant = p > 0.05

TABLE 17.19 Result of Chi Square Test on Association between Caregiver's Occupation and Place of Visit

	Value	df	Asymptotic Significance (2-sided)
Pearson chi-square	48.958	24	0.002
Likelihood ratio	55.063	24	0.000
Linear-by-linear association	1.351	1	0.245
Phi	0.683		
N of valid cases	104		

Significant = p < 0.05; Non-significant = p > 0.05

Evidence from the result of the Chi-square test showed a significant association between caregiver's occupation and health care seeking. This therefore provides sufficient evidence to reject the null hypothesis (p < 0.002) (Table 17.20).

Although the statistical results showed no significant relationship between health seeking outside the home and caregivers occupation (df = 6; p > 0.092), appropriate health seeking, described as visiting either a hospital, PHC or TBAs, was measured using the Chi-square test. Results showed a significant relationship between caregiver's occupation and appropriate health seeking. Therefore, this suggests sufficient evidence to reject the null hypothesis that caregiver's occupations do not influence appropriate health seeking.

Caregivers Age

The results from Chi Square show no association between caregivers' ages and health seeking outside the home. Therefore, this provides sufficient evidence to reject the null hypothesis with a p value > 0.444 (Table 17.21).

Caregivers Age versus Place Visited

The result from Chi-square test shows no association between caregivers age and place of visit. Therefore, this provides sufficient evidence to accept the null

TABLE 17.20 Result Of Chi Square Test on Relationship between Caregiver's Occupation and Appropriate Health-Seeking Behaviour

	Value	df	Asymptotic Significance (2-sided)
Pearson chi-square	25.046	12	0.015
Likelihood ratio	32.417	12	0.001
Linear-by-linear association	0.129	1	0.720
Number of valid cases	78		

Significant = p < 0.05; Non-significant = p > 0.05

TABLE 17.21 Result of Chi Square Test on the Relationship between Caregiver's Age and Health-Seeking Behaviour Outside of the Home

Variables	Yes	No	Total
20–25	17	3	20
26–30	43	16	59
31–35	24	7	32
36–40	19	10	29
Total	104	36	140

Chi-square = 2.677; df = 3; p > 0.0444; Phi = 0.138
Significant = p < 0.05; Non-significant = p > 0.05

TABLE 17.22 Result of Chi Square Test on Relationship between Caregiver's Age and Place Visited

Variables	TBA	PHC	Chemist	Hospital	Traditional Healer	Total
20–25	6	3	3	1	4	17
26–30	10	18	7	7	1	23
31–35	7	7	4	6	1	45
36–40	2	10	3	1	4	19
Total	25	38	17	15	10	104

Chi square = 19.054; df = 12; asymptotic Sig. = 0.087; Phi = 0.426
Significant = p < 0.05; Non-significant = p > 0.05

hypothesis, which suggests that caregiver's age is totally independent of the place of visit (p value > 0.444) (Table 17.22).

Caregiver's Age versus Use of Ort

The Chi-square test result estimates no statistically significant relationship between the use of ORT and caregiver's age. This therefore provides sufficient evidence to accept the null hypothesis, which predicted that caregiver's age is independent of the use of the ORT (p value = 0.960) (Table 17.23).

Child Gender

The result of the Chi-square test to determine whether there was a statistically significant relationship between a child's gender and seeking care outside the home yielded a p value = 0.765. This value indicates no relationship between the two variables. Therefore, this suggests evidence to accept the null hypothesis that a child's gender does not affect care seeking outside the home. However, in order to estimate the level of significance between the gender of the child and the place visited during the episode of diarrhoea, the Chi-square test indicated no significant evidence to suggest any positive relationship (p value = 0.845). This therefore proves the null hypothesis (Tables 17.24 and 17.25).

TABLE 17.23 Result of Chi Square Test on the Relationship between the Caregiver's Age and Oral Rehydration Therapy Use

	Value	df	Asymptotic Significance (2-sided)
Pearson chi-square	0.298	3	0.960
Likelihood ratio	0.298	3	0.960
Linear-by-linear association	0.016	1	0.900
Phi	0.046		
Number of valid cases	140		

3 cells (37.5%) have expected count less than 5. The minimum expected count is 2.71
Significant = p < 0.05; Non-significant = p > 0.05

TABLE 17.24 Result Of Chi Square Test on Relationship between Child's Gender and Health Seeking Outside Home

	Value	df	Asymptotic Significance (2-sided)	Exact Significance (2-sided)	Exact Significance (1-sided)
Pearson chi-square	0.089	1	0.765		
Continuity correction	0.011	1	0.916		
Likelihood ratio	0.089	1	0.765		
Fisher's exact test				0.847	0.458
Phi	0.025				
Linear-by-linear association	0.089	1	0.766		
Number of valid cases	140				

0 cells (0.0%) have expected count less than 5. The minimum expected count is 17.23
Significant = p < 0.05; Non-significant = p > 0.05

Child's Age

The chi square test to measure the level of significance between a child's age and care seeking outside the home revealed no statistically significant relationship between the age of a child and seeking health care outside the home (df = 3; p > 0.686). similarly, no statistically significant relationship was also observed between a child's age and the place visited (df = 12; p > 0.514) (Table 17.26 and 17.27).

In summary, there was no statistically significant relationship between a child's age and seeking care outside the home (df = 3; p > 0.686) or place visited during a diarrhoea episode (df = 12; p > 0.514). This finding therefore provides sufficient evidence to accept the null hypothesis, which proposed no relationship between both variables.

Hypothesis two: affordability (cost of treatment), accessibility (distance from home) and significant others) are independent of the choice of place visited.

TABLE 17.25 Result Of Chi Square Test on Relationship between Child's Gender and Place Visited

	Value	*df*	*Asymptotic Significance (2-sided)*
Pearson chi-square	1.396	4	0.845
Likelihood ratio	1.402	4	0.844
Phi	0.115		
Linear-by-linear association	0.001	1	0.971
Number of valid cases	104		

1 cells (10.0%) have expected count less than 5. The minimum expected count is 4.76
Significant = p < 0.05; Non-significant = p > 0.05

TABLE 17.26 Result of Chi Square Test on Relationship between Child's Age and Health Care Seeking Outside Home

Variables	*Yes*	*No*	*Total*
0–12	44	13	57
13–24	30	11	41
25–36	15	8	23
37–48	15	4	19
Total	104	36	140

Chi square = 1.485; df = 3; asymptotic Sig. = 0.686; Phi = 0.103
Significant = p < 0.05; Non-significant = p > 0.05

TABLE 17.27 Result of Chi Square Test on Relationship between Child's Age and Place of Visit

	Value	df	Asymptotic Significance (2-sided)
Pearson chi-square	11.174	12	0.514
Likelihood ratio	13.601	12	0.327
Linear-by-linear association	0.822	1	0.365
Phi	0.326		
Number of valid cases	104		

11 cells (55.0%) have expected count less than 5. The minimum expected count is 1.43
Significant = p < 0.05; Non-significant = p > 0.05

TABLE 17.28 Result of Chi Square Test on Relationship between Cost of Treatment and Place of Visit

	Value	df	Asymptotic Significance (2-sided)
Pearson chi-square	14.900	4	0.005
Likelihood ratio	17.251	4	0.002
Linear-by-linear association	0.144	1	0.704
Phi	0.377		
Number of valid cases	104		

Significant = p < 0.05; Non-significant = p > 0.05

The Chi-square analysis shows a relationship between the cost of treatment and the place visited. Although this association appeared to be weak (Phi = 0.377), it suggests that cost is a determinant of HSB (Table 17.28).

Accessibility vs Place of Visit

The result above shows a statistically significant relationship between accessibility and the choice of place visited. This therefore suggests that accessibility is a determinant of HSB (Table 17.29).

Significant Others versus Place of Visit

Summary of relationship between accessibility, affordability (cost of treatment), family influence (significant others) and health utilization (place visited) (Table 17.30).

The table above shows a statistically significant relationship between place visited and accessibility (df = 4; p < 0.005), affordability (df = 4; p < 0.002) and family influence (significant others) (df = 4; p < 0.005). Therefore, this provided strong evidence to reject the null hypothesis (Table 17.31).

TABLE 17.29 Result of Chi Square Test on Relationship between Accessibility and Place of Visit

	Value	df	Asymptotic Significance (2-sided)
Pearson chi-square	16.884	4	0.002
Likelihood ratio	22.449	4	0.000
Linear-by-linear association	13.871	1	0.00
Phi	0.401		
Number of valid cases	104		

1 cells (10.0%) have expected count less than 5. The minimum expected count is 3.71
Significant = p < 0.05; Non-significant = p > 0.05

TABLE 17.30 Result of Chi Square Test on Relationship between Significant Others (Family and Friends) and Place of Visit

	Value	df	Asymptotic Significance (2-sided)
Pearson chi-square	14.857	4	0.005
Likelihood ratio	12.765	4	0.012
Phi	0.376		
Linear-by-linear association	11.534	1	0.001
Number of valid cases	104		

Significant = p < 0.05; Non-significant = p > 0.05

TABLE 17.31 Tabulation of Significant Others versus Place of Visit

Variables	Chi-square	df	P value
Affordability (cost of treatment)	14.900	4	0.005
Accessibility (distance of health facility from home)	16.884	4	0.002
Family influence (significant others)	14.857	4	0.005

Significant = p < 0.05; Non-significant = p > 0.05

Discussion

Diarrhoea in children has remained the major cause of child mortality worldwide, especially in Sub-Saharan African counties, like Nigeria (Aremu et al., 2011). While factors such as poor sanitation, viral infection, worm infestations and unhygienic infant feeding practices have been majorly linked with the cause of diarrhoea in children, evidence still suggests that these causes are preventable (Oloruntoba et al., 2014). Policies and programmes have focused on preventive and promotive activities. However, appropriate health-seeking behaviour remains a significant approach to reducing the disease burden of diarrhoea in children under five years of age as well as mortality (Ogunlesi and Olanrewaju,

2010). Evidence from studies has shown that appropriate health seeking reduces the complication of diarrhoea in children (Tagbo et al., 2014). However, reports have shown that the health-seeking behaviour of caregivers, especially in rural communities in developing countries like Nigeria, is still poor. Several factors, such as social, economic and demographic factors, have been documented to affect the health-seeking behaviour.

Therefore, the aim of this study was to examine the health-seeking behaviour and socio-demographic factors that influence caregiver's health-seeking behaviour for diarrhoea in children in rural communities in Nkanu West LGA of Enugu State, Nigeria. The study employed the use of statistical tools to determine the pattern of socio-demographic characteristics and the relationship between them and health-seeking behaviour.

Health-Seeking Behaviour

Unexpectedly, the result of this study showed that the majority of caregivers sought care outside the home during the episode of diarrhoea [104 (74.3)]. However, perceived severity was majorly reported as the reason by caregivers who did seek care outside (36, 25.7%). However, this finding may not be conclusive evidence on the role of perceived severity and health-seeking behaviour. This is because no question was asked to ascertain the duration between the notice of symptoms of diarrhoea and health seeking and the reason for any gap that could have been observed. However, a study showed that caregivers are more likely to seek care outside the home when they perceive the diarrhoea to be severe and often accompanied by dehydration (Salami and Adesanwo, 2015). Therefore, understanding how caregivers perceive illness hinders health seeking outside the home explains the importance of perceived severity on HSB and thus suggests the need to focus education on timely health seeking.

Moreover, the majority (37, 36.2%) sought care in primary centres compared to other facilities. This result may have been influenced by the fact that data were collected in PHC, thus introducing bias in reporting health care utilization. However, this result is consistent with findings from other studies (Kahabuka et al., 2011).

Relationship between Socio-demographic Characteristics and Health-Seeking Behaviour

This study found that health-seeking is generally high in the area. This is concurrent with other studies that examined HSB for childhood illnesses, including diarrhoea, in rural communities (Awoke, 2013). This interpretation may not be the actual representation of the HSB of the target population, apparently because of the sample size and setting where data were collected. However, knowledge of the pattern of these behaviours among the people interviewed gives insight into the pattern of health-seeking behaviour.

Caregiver's Education: As discussed in the literature review, education has a strong association with health seeking and health acre utilization. This study found that education has a strong relationship with health seeking for diarrhoea in children in Nkanu West LGA. This finding is consistent with other studies (Kanté et al., 2015). The reason for this relationship may be explained by the proposition that women who have more education are empowered, which thus improves their decision-making ability. This rejects the assumption of Mukiira (2015), which suggests that women with higher education are less likely to seek care because they assumed that women with higher education tend to have better knowledge of treatment for diarrhoea and, thus, find it not useful to seek care.

Caregiver's Occupation: Evidence from a literature review reveals that the relationship between occupation and health seeking has been controversial. This study found no significant relationship between occupation and the likelihood of seeking healthcare outside of the home. However, a sufficient relationship was observed between caregiver's occupation and the choice of health service visited, as well as the use of ORT. This is consistent with other studies in Nigeria (Aremu et al., 2011). In Nigeria, this association can be explained by the report that the burden of diarrhoea in children under five is associated with income (Aremu et al., 2011). Thus, due to the high burden of diarrhoea among lower income people, health-seeking tends to be higher among them.

Child's Gender: Due to cultural and religious beliefs and practices in Sub-Saharan Africa, gender discrepancy exists when it comes to the distribution and use of basic amenities at home and in the community, where males are more inclined to be taken for appropriate healthcare services. However, no significant relationship was observed between the gender of the child and health seeking.

Child's Age: Child's age has been a significant predicator of health care seeking, especially in Africa (Chandwani and Pandor, 2015). Although no statistically significant association was found between a child's age and health-seeking behaviour, the results of this study showed that caregivers were more likely to seek care for younger children (0–12 months) compared to older children between 37 and 48 months. This finding is consistent with other studies in Kenya, Tanzania and Nigeria (Kanté et al., 2015). Conversely, this does not agree with the results of a similar study by Mukiira (2015). However, the variation between the findings of this study and Mukiira (2015) could be due to the fact that my study focused on whether the caregivers sought care or not, as opposed to whether they sought appropriate care. This therefore argues that the caregiver sought care for younger children, but the care was not appropriate. This study therefore provides an alternative answer.

Accessibility: Physical access to healthcare services and facilities has played a major role in health seeking and healthcare utilization. According to Mukiira

(2015), accessibility plays a major role, especially in rural communities where basic health and social amenities are limited. Congruently, this study observed a statistically significant relationship between accessibility (distance to a health facility) and health-seeking behaviour. Caregivers reported visiting health facilities due to easy access. This finding is consistent with findings from other studies conducted in Nigeria (Kahabuka et al., 2011) and other countries. This finding could be due to the lack of a proper road transport network in rural communities. Contrary to Uzochukwu et al. (2008), who observed that individuals in rural areas are likely to visit traditional healers when physical access to higher (PHC and hospitals) health facilities is not possible, this study found this to be the case with visiting TBA. Despite the association between accessibility and HS, the results still showed that accessibility was not a barrier when caregivers considered the quality of service provided in a health facility (government hospital). This is in congruence with findings from other studies. Perceived service quality plays an important role in healthcare service utilizations (Kahabuka et al., 2011). However, the finding finds reflection in Andersen and Newman's (2005) model of health care utilization, which suggests access to health facilities as a significant determinant of health care utilization.

Family Influence/Significant Orders: The study found an association between significant others and HSB. Studies that examined the influence of significant others on caregiver's health-seeking behaviour for childhood illnesses are limited. However, some theories have explained this relationship. Foucault (1980) explained the role of power and hegemony in health service usage. His opinion centred on the role of the family figure head in every decision-making process, including health service utilization. However, this may not be the case in this study, as the study did not ask whether the influence was from family health or friends and relatives. Meanwhile, this finding can be explained using Andersen and Newman's (2005) model of health care utilization, which explained the importance of social interaction in health seeking and service utilization.

Conclusion

This study sought to examine caregivers HSB and socio-demographic determinants of caregivers HSB for children with diarrhoea in the Nkanu West LGA area of Enugu State Nigeria. An extensive literature review reveals the magnitude of the burden of diarrhoea in children in developing countries (Aremu et al., 2011; Liu et al., 2015; Walker et al., 2013; WHO, 2013). However, the literature also suggests that the morbidity and mortality resulting from diarrhoea in children can be minimized through the adoption of appropriate health-seeking behaviour by caregivers (Awoke, 2013; Ogunlesi and Olanrewaju, 2010). An extensive review of literature on caregivers HSB showed variations in the pattern of HSB across Sub-Saharan African countries, especially Nigeria. Various studies showed that caregivers visited both hospitals, PHCs, traditional healers, chemists or adopted Self-management with and without the use of ORT (Kanté et al., 2015). However, the choice of HSB adopted is influenced by factors such as educational status, socio-economic status, child's age and gender, place of residence, accessibility, cost of treatment, significance orders, perceived severity of illness, etc. (Gera et al., 2015; Kanté et al., 2015; Omotoso, 2010).

The result of this study showed a significant level of HSB among the caregivers in the geographical area. Unexpectedly, contrary to many studies that examine HSB in rural areas, cultural and religious factors were not found to influence the HSB of the caregivers for diarrhoea in children. Instead, social, economic and demographic factors such as cost of treatment, education, occupation, accessibility (distance from a health facility) and significant others were found to be the major determinants of HSB. Moreover, these findings could therefore suggest a positive effect of health promotion and a shift in the religious-cultural definition of illness and practices to appropriate health care utilization and practices. However, the perceived severity of the illness was the major determinant of not seeking care outside the home. These findings can be explained by the application of theories such as Andersen and Newman's (2005) health utilization model, which suggests that factors such as socio-economic, demographic, perceived vulnerability, susceptibility and severity influence health-seeking behaviour.

Evidence from the findings of this study suggests that policies targeted at improving and promoting appropriate HSB and healthcare utilization among caregivers in rural communities in Nigeria for diarrhoea in children under five years of age should include strategies that will improve child health through:

- Improving awareness of health promotion and appropriate HSB.
- The development of focused intervention programmes to meet the needs of rural dwellers, with the aim of improving child health that could lead to a reduction in child morbidity and mortality, was the aim of the MDGs and the SDGs.
- Inclusion policy through the implementation and reinforcement of Rural Communities Social Health Insurance Programme (RSHIP), which will improve access to affordable basic child healthcare services in rural communities in Nigeria.
- Training of TBAs by the Ministry of Health through the National Primary Health Care Development Agency (NPHCDA) to assist in managing childhood illnesses in the communities.
- Implementation of the WHS through the construction of PHCs in each rural community to improve access to basic child health services.
- Inclusion of others in health education regarding a child's health
- A multi-sectoral approach to health promotion and education
- However, the design adopted uses aggregate data, which can only provide information about the sample chosen and not the individual's sample unit. This may suggest that any association found in the aggregate data may not

necessarily mean the same on an individual level (Spicker, 2008). Therefore, this design can show only statistical correlation; hence, the need to apply a qualitative approach to examine the how and why.

• Furthermore, the study only asked question on general health seeking and not specific ones. It is important for other studies looking at HSB to examine whether or not the care sought is in an appropriate facility in order to measure whether the care is appropriate. This is because if the care sought is inappropriate, it could worsen the child's health, leading to increased child mortality.

Nursing practices involve different roles both in the inter-disciplinary approach and independent functions at various facets of individual care, such as counselling for behaviour change and strategies to improve access. Nursing roles have increased, including health promotion and improvement both at the primary and secondary intervention levels. Therefore, understanding an individual's health-seeking behaviour is crucial to nursing practice both in the clinical and community settings (Ogunlesi and Olanrewaju, 2010). Generally, nursing interventions at the community and clinical levels help improve health. Understanding the health-seeking behaviour of caregivers for children with diarrhoea in rural communities will necessitate nursing interventions to strengthen efforts to make every contact with caregivers count. This is because nurses, when compared to other healthcare professionals, have more and longer contact and interaction with individuals in healthcare facilities. Knowledge of the caregiver's health-seeking behaviours for children with diarrhoea will help develop strategies for developing community-based nursing interventions and health promotion plans that will help caregivers adopt positive and recommended health behaviours. Promoting positive health behaviours among caregivers will help to minimise child mortality and morbidity from diarrhoea and improve the health outcomes of children under five in rural communities, which is one of the major goals of the sustainable development goal (United Nations Development Programme, 2000).

References

Abiodun, A. A., Adebayo, S. B., Oyejola, B. A., and Anyanti, J. (2013). A Spatial Analysis of Age at Sexual Initiation Among Nigerian Youth as a Tool for HIV Prevention: A Bayesian Approach. In Advanced Techniques for Modelling Maternal and Child Health in Africa (pp. 279–302). Dordrecht: Springer Netherlands.

Andersen, R., and Newman, J. F. (2005). Societal and Individual Determinants of Medical Care Utilization in the United States. *The Milbank Quarterly*, 83(4), 1–28.

Aremu, O., Lawoko, S., Moradi, T., and Dalal, K. (2011). Socio-Economic Determinants in Selecting Childhood Diarrhoea Treatment Options in Sub-Saharan Africa: A Multilevel Model. *Italian Journal of Pediatrics*, 37(2), 13.

Aziz, F., Rubio, J. P., Ouazzani, N., Dary, M., Manyani, H., Morgado, B. R., and Mandi, L. (2016). Sanitary Impact Evaluation of Drinking Water in Storage Reservoirs in Moroccan Rural Area. *Saudi Journal of Biological Sciences*, 7(3), 57–59.

Becker, M., Haefner, D., and Maiman, L. (1977). The Health Belief Model in the Prediction of Dietary Compliance: A Field Experiment. *Journal of Health and Social Behaviour*, 18(1), 348–366.

Bhutta, Z. A., Das, J. K., Rizvi, A., Gaffey, M. F., Walker, N., Horton, S., and Maternal and Child Nutrition Study Group. (2013). Evidence-based Interventions for Improvement of Maternal and Child Nutrition: What Can Be Done and at What Cost? *The Lancet*, 382(9890), 452–477.

Black, R. E., Cousens, M., Johnson, H. L., Lawn, J. E., Rudan, I., Bassani, D. G., et al. (2010). Global, Regional, and National Causes of Child Mortality in 2008: A Systematic Analysis. *Lancet*, 375(9730), 1969–1987.

Boschi-Pinto, C., Velebit, L., and Shibuya, K. (2008). Estimating Child Mortality due to Diarrhoea in Developing Countries. *Bulletin of the World Health Organization*, 86(9), 710–717.

Bourdieu, P. (1986). *The Forms of Capital; Cultural Theory: An Anthology.* Available at: https://books.google.co.uk/books?hl=en&lr=&id=tK_KhHOkurYC&oi=fnd&pg=PA 81&dq=bourdieu+social+capital&ots=NVFsdZuUSI&sig=KaSsjASNAT2hTNIql8z chlJPlqQ#v=onepage&q=bourdieu%20social%20capital. Accessed: 20/08/23.

Brown, J., Cumming, O., Bartram, J., Cairncross, S., Ensink, J., Holcomb, D., et al. (2015). A Controlled, before-and-after Trial of an Urban Sanitation Intervention to Reduce Enteric Infections in Children: Research Protocol for the Maputo Sanitation (MapSan) Study, Mozambique. *BMJ Open*, 5(6), e008215.

Bruce, C. D. (2007). Questions arising about emergence, data collection, and its interaction with analysis in a grounded theory study. *International Journal of Qualitative Methods*, 6(1), Article 4. Available from http://www.ualberta.ca/~iiqm/backissues/6_1/bruce.htm accessed 01/07/2024

Bryman, A., 2016. *Social research methods.* Oxford university press.

Chandwani, H., and Pandor, J. (2015). Healthcare-Seeking Behaviors of Mothers Regarding their Children in a Tribal Community of Gujarat, India. *Electronic Physician*, 7(1), 990.

Cronin, A. A., Sebayang, S. K., Torlesse, H., and Nandy, R. (2016). Association of Safe Disposal of Child Feces and Reported Diarrhea in Indonesia: Need for Stronger Focus on a Neglected Risk. *International Journal of Environmental Research and Public Health*, 13(3), 310.

Daniels, A. A., Ahenkan, A., and Poku, K. A. (2013). Factors Influencing the Utilisation of Maternal Health Services: The Perspective of Rural Women in Ghana. *Journal of Public Administration and Governance*, 3(2), 121–141.

Duke, C., Park, K. and Ewing, R., 2020. Chi-square. In *Basic quantitative research methods for urban planners* (pp. 133–149). Routledge.

Ezeoke, U. E., Nwobi, E. A., Ekwueme, O. C., Tagbo, B., Aronu, E., and Uwaezuoke, S. (2010). Pattern of Health Seeking Behaviour of Mothers for Common Childhood Illnesses in Enugu Metropolis South East Zone Nigeria. *Nigerian Journal of Clinical Practice*, 13(1), 37–40.

Finkbeiner, S.R., Kirkwood, C.D. and Wang, D., 2008. Complete genome sequence of a highly divergent astrovirus isolated from a child with acute diarrhea. *Virology journal*, 5, pp.1-7.

Fischer-Walker, C. L., Rudan, I., Liu, L., Nair, H., Theodoratou, E., Bhutta, Z. A., et al. (2013). Global Burden of Childhood Pneumonia and Diarrhea. *Lancet*, 381(9875), 1405–1416.

Foucault, M. (1980). Language, Counter-memory, Practice: Selected Essays and Interviews. Ithaca, NY: Cornell University Press.

Gera, A., Ramachandran, S., Gera, R., and Singh, A. P. (2015). Comparison of Health Care Seeking Behavior in Rural versus Urban Women in Uttarakhand. *Indian Journal of Child Health*, 2(3), 122–125.

Graham, H., and White, P. C. L. (2016). Social Determinants and Lifestyles: Integrating Environmental and Public Health Perspectives. *Public Health*.141;270-278

Guarino, A., Ashkenazi, A., Gendrel, D., Vecchio, A. L., Shamir, R., and Szajewska, H. (2014). European Society for Pediatric Gastroenterology, Hepatology, and Nutrition/ European Society for Pediatric Infectious Diseases Evidence-Based Guidelines for the Management of Acute Gastroenteritis in Children in Europe. *Journal of Pediatric Gastroenterology and Nutrition*, 59(1), 132–152.

Gyoh, S. (2011). An Epidemic of Faecal Fistulae. *Africa Health*, 23, 4–8.

Iyoha, O., and Abiodun, P. O. (2015). Human Rotavirus Genotypes Causing Acute Watery Diarrhea among under-Five Children in Benin City, Nigeria. *Nigerian Journal of Clinical Practice*, 18(1), 48–51.

Jackson, M.R., 2015. Resistance to qual/quant parity: Why the "paradigm" discussion can't be avoided. Qualitative Psychology, 2(2), p.181.

Iyun, B. F., and Oke, E. A. (2000). Ecological and Cultural Barriers to Treatment of Childhood Diarrhoea in Riverine Areas of Ondo State, Nigeria. *Social Science and Medicine*, 50(1), 953–964.

Kahabuka, C. (2013). *Care Seeking and Management of Common Childhood Illnesses in Tanzania: Questioning the Quality of Primary Care Services*. The University of Bergen, Bergen.

Kahabuka, C., Kvåle, G., Moland, K.M. and Hinderaker, S.G., 2011. Why caretakers bypass Primary Health Care facilities for child care-a case from rural Tanzania. BMC health services research, 11, pp.1-10.

Kanté, A. M., Gutierrez, H. R., Larsen, A. M., Jackson, E. F., Helleringer, S., Exavery, A., et al. (2015). Childhood Illness Prevalence and Health Seeking Behavior Patterns in Rural Tanzania. *BMC Public Health*, 15(1), 1.

Karambu S, Matiru V, Kiptoo M, Oundo J. Characterization and factors associated with diarrhoeal diseases caused by enteric bacterial pathogens among children aged five years and below attending Igembe District Hospital, Kenya. Pan Afr Med J. 2013 Oct 4;16:37. doi: 10.11604/pamj.2013.16.37.2947. PMID: 24570797; PMCID: PMC3932116.

Kahabuka, C., Kvåle, G., Moland, K.M. and Hinderaker, S.G., 2011. Why caretakers bypass Primary Health Care facilities for child care-a case from rural Tanzania. BMC health services research, 11, pp.1-10.

Khanal, V., Bhandari, R., and Karkee, R. (2015). Non-medical Interventions for Childhood Diarrhoea Control: Way Forward in Nepal. *Kathmandu University Medical Journal*, 11(3), 2256-261

Krumpal, I., 2013. Determinants of social desirability bias in sensitive surveys: a literature review. *Quality & quantity*, *47*(4), pp.2025-2047

Lamberti, L. M., Fischer-Walker, C. L., Taneja, S., Mazumder, S., and Black, R. E. (2015). The Influence of Episode Severity on Caregiver Recall, Care-seeking, and Treatment of Diarrhoea among Children 2–59 Months of Age in Bihar, Gujarat, and Uttar Pradesh, India. *American Journal of Tropical Medicine and Hygiene*, 93(2), 250–256.

Leon, A.C., Davis, L.L. and Kraemer, H.C., 2011. The role and interpretation of pilot studies in clinical research. Journal of psychiatric research, 45(5), pp.626-629.

Levy, P.S. and Lemeshow, S., 2013. *Sampling of populations: methods and applications*. Toronto: John Wiley & Sons.

Liu, L., Johnson, H. L., Cousens, S., Perin, J., Scott, S., Lawn, J. E., et al. (2012). Child Health Epidemiology Reference Group of WHO and UNICEF. Global, Regional, and

National Causes of Child Mortality: An Updated Systematic Analysis for 2010 with Time Trends since 2000. *Lancet*, 379(9832), 2151–2161.

Liu, L., Oza, S., Hogan, D., Perin, J., Rudan, I., and Lawn, J. E. (2015). Global, Regional, and National Causes of Child Mortality in 2000–13, with Projections to Inform Post-2015 Priorities: An Updated Systematic Analysis. *Lancet*, 385, 430–440.

Mohammed, S., and Tamiru, D. (2014). The Burden of Diarrheal Diseases among Children under Five Years of Age in` Arba Minch District, Southern Ethiopia, and Associated Risk Factors: A Cross-Sectional Study. *International Scholarly Research Notices 24 (1), 654901*

Mukiira, C. K. (2015). *Healthcare-seeking Practices of Caregivers of under-Five Children with Diarrheal Diseases in Two Informal Settlements in Nairobi, Kenya* (Doctoral dissertation, University Of Witwatersrand, Johannesburg).

Nigerian Data Portal (2006) available at https://nigeria.opendataforafrica.org/ifpbxbd/state-population-2006 accessed 01/07/2024

Nigeria Zinc Study Team (2008). *Report of the Operational Research on Inclusion of Zinc in the Household Management of Childhood Diarrhea in Nigeria.* Study Report Submitted to UNICEF, Abuja, Nigeria.

Oadi, K., and Kuitunen, M. (2005). Childhood Diarrheal Morbidity in the Accra Metropolitan Area, Ghana: Socio-economic, Environmental and Behavioral Risk Determinants. *Journal of Health and Population in Developing Countries*, 17646, 33–46.

Odimayo, M. S., Olanrewaju, W. I., Omilabu, S. A., and Adegboro, B. (2008). Prevalence of Rotavirus-induced Diarrhoea among Children under 5 Years in Ilorin, Nigeria. *Journal of Tropical Paediatrics*, 54(5), 343–346.

Ogunlesi, T. A., and Olanrewaju, D. M. (2010). Socio-demographic Factors and Appropriate Health Care-Seeking Behavior for Childhood Illnesses. *Journal of Tropical Pediatrics*, 56(6), 379–385.

Oloruntoba, E. O., Folarin, T. B., and Ayede, A. I. (2014). Hygiene and Sanitation Risk Factors of Diarrhoeal Disease among under-Five Children in Ibadan, Nigeria. *African Health Sciences*, 14(4), 1001–1011.

Omotoso, D. (2010). Health Seeking Behaviour among the Rural Dwellers in Ekiti State, Nigeria. African Research Review, 4(2). }, url={https://api.semanticscholar.org/CorpusID:1439513

Pallant, J. S. (2013). *A Step by Step guide to data analysis using IBM SPSS.* (5th edition). Milton Keynes: Open University Press.

Phellas, C.N., Bloch, A. and Seale, C., 2011. Structured methods: interviews, questionnaires and observation. Researching society and culture, 3(1), pp.23–32.

Romero, C. and Ventura, S., 2013. Data mining in education. Wiley Interdisciplinary Reviews: Data mining and knowledge discovery, 3(1), pp.12-27

Rosenstock, I.M., Strecher, V.J. and Becker, M.H., 1994. The health belief model and HIV risk behavior change. In *Preventing AIDS: Theories and methods of behavioral interventions* (pp. 5-24). Boston, MA: Springer US.

Rovai, A.P., Baker, J.D. and Ponton, M.K., 2013. *Social science research design and statistics: A practitioner's guide to research methods and IBM SPSS.* Chesapeake: VA Watertree Press LLC.

Salami, K. K., and Adesanwo, O. J. (2015). The Practice of Self-medication for Treatment of Illnesses for under-Five Children by Mothers in Ibadan, Nigeria. *Research Journal of Drug Abuse*, 2(1), 2.

Schilling, K. A. (2010). Characteristics and Etiology of Moderate-to-Severe Diarrhea of Acute, Prolonged Acute, and Persistent Duration among Children Less than 5 Years Old in Rural Western Kenya, 2008–2010.

Segecha, S. (2013). *Etiology of Diarrhea in Children under 5 Yrs in Mbagathi District Hospital, Nairobi Province* (Doctoral dissertation).

Spicker, P. (2008). *Social Policy: Themes and Approaches*. Bristol : Policy Press.

Tagbo, B. N., Mwenda, J. M., Armah, G., Obidike, E. O., Okafor, U. H., Oguonu, T., Ozumba, U. C., Eke, C. B., Chukwubuike, C., Edelu, B. O. and Ezeonwu, B. U. (2014). Epidemiology of Rotavirus Diarrhea among Children Younger than 5 years in Enugu, South East, Nigeria. *The Pediatric Infectious Disease Journal*, 33, pp.S19–S22.

Tate, J. E., Burton, A. H., Boschi-Pinto, C., Steele, A. D., Duque, J., and Parashar, U. D. (2012). 2008 Estimate of Worldwide Rotavirus-Associated Mortality in Children Younger than 5 Years before the Introduction of Universal Rotavirus Vaccination Programmes: A Systematic Review and Meta-analysis. *Lancet*, 12(1), 136–141.

Treiman, D.J., 2014. Quantitative data analysis: Doing social research to test ideas. Toronto: John Wiley & Sons.

UNICEF (2012a). *Levels and Trends in Child Mortality: Report 2012*. Available at: http://www.childmortality.org/files_v9/download/Levels and Trends in Child Mortality Report 2012.pdf. Accessed: 20/08/23.

UNICEF (2012b). *Pneumonia and Diarrhea: Tackling the Deadliest Diseases in the World*. New York: UNICEF.

UNICEF/WHO (2009). *Diarrhea: Why Children Are Still Dying and What Can Be Done*. New York: UNICEF.

United Nations Development Programme (2000). *Millennium Development Goals*. Available at: http://www.un.org/millenniumgoals/childhealth.shtml. Accessed: 10/12/2016.

Uprichard, E. (2013). Focus: Big Data, Little Questions? *Discover Society*, (1). Available at https://archive.discoversociety.org/2013/10/01/focus-big-data-little-questions accessed 02/07/2024

Uzochukwu, B. S., Onwujekwe, E. O., Onoka, C. A., and Ughasoro, M. D. (2008). Rural-urban Differences in Maternal Responses to Childhood Fever in South East Nigeria. *PLoS One*, 3(3), e1788.

Walker, C. L., Aryee, M. J., Boschi-Pinto, C., and Black, R. E. (2012). Estimating Diarrhea Mortality among Young Children in Low and Middle Income Countries. *PLoS One*, 7(1), 151–156.

Walker, C. L. F., Rudan, I., Liu, L., Nair, H., Theodoratou, E., Bhutta, Z. A. and Black, R. E. (2013). Global Burden of Childhood Pneumonia and Diarrhoea. *The Lancet*, 381(9875), 1405–1416.

Williams, N., 2014. The AUDIT questionnaire. Occupational Medicine, 64(4), pp.308-308.

World Health Organisation. (2010). *Integrated Management of Childhood Illness (IMCI)*. Available at: https://www.who.int/teams/maternal-newborn-child-adolescent-health-and-ageing/child-health/integrated-management-of-childhood-illness/

World Health Organisation (2012). World Health Statistics, available at https://www.who.int/docs/default-source/gho-documents/world-health-statistic-reports/world-health-statistics-2012.pdf accessed 01/12/2021

World Health Organisation (2013). *Diarrhoeal Disease, Fact Sheet N°330 2013*. Available at: http://www.who.int/mediacentre/factsheets/fs330/en/. Accessed: 20/08/23.

World Health Organisation (2014). *Diarrhoeal Diseases Death Rate Per 100,000 Standardized*. http://www.worldlifeexpectancy.com/cause-of-death/diarrhoeal-diseases/by-country/. Accessed: 20/08/23.

INDEX

Note: **Bold** page numbers refer to tables and *italic* page numbers refer to figures.

Printed in the United States
by Baker & Taylor Publisher Services